CANCER IN FEMALE ADOLESCENTS

Cancer in Female Adolescents

Margarite T. Moorland
Editor

Nova Science Publishers, Inc.
New York

For permission to use material from this book please contact us:
Telephone 631-231-7269; Fax 631-231-8175
Web Site: http://www.novapublishers.com

Library of Congress Cataloging-in-Publication Data

Cancer in female adolescents / Margarite T. Moorland (editor).
P. : cm.
Includes bibliographical references and index.
ISBN 978-1-60456-421-1 (hardcover)
1. Cancer in women. 2. Teenage girls—Diseases. I. Moorland, Margarite T.
[DNLM: 1. Neoplasma. 2. Adolescent. 3. Womenr's Health. QZ 275 C2148 2008]
RC281.W65.C352 2008
616.99'40082—dc22 2008005112

Published by Nova Science Publishers, Inc. ✦ New York

Contents

Preface

This new book is devoted to research on cancer in female adolescents which one would logically assume to be a decreasing amount but the numbers indicate just the opposite is true.

Chapter I - Adolescence is the developmental period between childhood and adulthood, a period during which rapid biological as well as psychological maturation occurs. Although opinion regarding the adolescent age group varies, in most of the recent reports, cancer in adolescents concerned individuals between 15-19 years of age. Since adolescent girls' health plays an important role in determining the health of the future generation, adolescence in girls has been recognized as a special period in their life cycle that requires specific and special attention. However, factors such as poor nutritional status and early consummation of marriage in the developing world and the behaviors or conditions that begin or occur during adolescence in the developed countries–for example tobacco and alcohol use, poor eating habits, sexual abuse, and risky sex, contributes significantly to disease burden including precancer and cancer, and premature deaths among adults. In children aged less than 15 years, common malignancies are leukemias, CNS tumors, and childhood embryonal tumors. After the age of 10 years, embryonic tumors almost disappear, whereas other cancers become more frequent, notably lymphomas, carcinomas, germ-cell tumors, and bone tumors. The highest incidence rates for cancers among adolescents (15-19 years) include those for lymphomas, followed by carcinomas, CNS tumors, germ-cell tumors, and leukemias. In the west, lymphomas are the most common malignancy in adolescent females, followed by carcinomas, leukemias, CNS tumors, bone tumors, melanomas, soft tissue sarcomas, and germ-cell tumors. In a developing country like India lymphomas and leukemias are also most common cancer in adolescent females, followed by malignancies of bone and soft tissue, urogenital system, CNS, head and neck, thyroid, gastrointestinal system, and breast. Because of the relatively low cancer incidence, the adolescent and young adult population has not been the focus of attention in cancer control and prevention strategy in the past. However, there is clear evidence of an increase in cancer incidence in children, adolescents and young adults during the past decades. Therefore, over the past 10 years, ever-increasing attention has been paid to the needs of adolescents with cancer world-wide.

Methods of diagnosis of cancer include clinical, imaging, microscopic examination, and others. The main microscopic studies include histology, hematology (blood film and bone marrow), and cytology including exfoliative and fine needle aspiration (FNA) cytology.

Exfoliative cytology in the form of Pap test and ancillary tests on this sample helps in early detection of squamous intraepithelial (precancerous) lesions and human papillomavirus infections in adolescent females, so that necessary intervention is offered to prevent the development of invasive cancer during adulthood. Review of literature shows that the most common site of FNA in children and adolescents is lymph node (41.2%), followed by bone and soft tissue (17.1%), head and neck lesions excluding thyroid (9.4%), abdominal and pelvic masses (9.0%), breast (8.4%), thyroid (7.4%), thorax (5.8%), and central nervous system (1.7%). The averages of benign, suspicious, malignant, and inadequate cytology reports in a review of seven studies in children and adolescents were 55.2%, 0.9%, 41.0%, and 3.0%, respectively indicating that malignancy is very common in the FNA material in this age group. The diagnostic efficacy of this tool is also very high. The sensitivity, specificity, and diagnostic accuracy of FNA in children and adolescents, based on 6 studies, were 91.8 ± 8.29%, 97.4 ± 3.08%, and 95.2 ± 4.37%, respectively. The averages of frequency of malignancy for various sites in FNA cytology reports in the literature were as follows: head and neck excluding thyroid (14.6%), thyroid (13.6%), lymph nodes (5.6%), thorax and abdomen (46.3%), and bone and soft tissue (58.0%).

FNA is useful in the management of cases with mass lesions in the body by offering a quick diagnosis and by reducing additional and costly procedures. The efficacy of FNA as a diagnostic tool for various sites is generally high. In literature, the sensitivity and specificity for diagnosis of malignancies in various anatomic sites were as follows: head and neck (97.2 ± 3.96% and 95.1 ± 2.90%, respectively), thyroid (90.3 ± 15.71% and 80.4 ± 12.91%, respectively), lymph nodes (92.8 ± 5.74% and 94.5 ± 3.11%, respectively), abdomen and pelvis (93.4 ± 2.80% and 100.0%, respectively), and bone and soft tissue (90.2 ± 16.91% and 94.8 ± 5.97%, respectively). Information on diagnostic accuracy, available for limited sites, were as follows: thyroid (84.6 ± 4.95%), abdominal visceras (95.7 ± 1.72%), and bone and soft tissue (96.0 ± 1.05%). Further, exfoliative cytology in the form of examination of serous cavity fluids following ascitic or pleural tap and FNA cytology on samples from the space occupying lesions in various organs of the body cavities, which are difficult to be accessed by surgical procedures, especially in very sick adolescents, make enormous contribution to the management of patients. However, in certain situations the cytopathologists face diagnostic difficulties, which are largely solved with the help of ancillary studies like cytochemistry, immunocytochemistry, flow cytometry, cytogenetics, ultrastrucure, and molecular biologic techniques.

Chapter II - Persistent anogenital infection with oncogenic human papillomaviruses (HPVs) is a prerequisite for HPV related squamous and adenocarcinoma anogenital malignancies of the cervix, vulva, vagina and anus of the female anogenital tract. Integration of the E6 and E7 HPV genes of the oncogenic HPVs into the host genome in the presence of co-carcinogens may result in cellular proliferation, and malignant transformation. Ano-genital HPV infection is primarily sexually transmitted and very common after sexual debut, yet anogenital malignancies are very rare in adolescents. This is largely due to high clearance rates of initial HPV infection, plus the fact that development of neoplasias from the precancerous lesions of high-grade dysplasia (such as cervical intraepithelial neoplasia grade 2 or 3 [CIN2/3]) takes around 15-20 years. In adolescents, apart from genital warts (caused largely by low risk genotypes 6/11) HPV infection is asymptomatic. Both high and low risk genotype infection may cause cell abnormality, otherwise recognized on cytology as low-grade dysplasia, although these really just represent manifestations of cellular infection. They are highly prevalent within a couple of years of initial HPV infection, but generally have a high chance of regression, not requiring treatment. Furthermore there is good evidence that excisional biopsy is associated with future adverse obstetric outcome, such as preterm labour. Therefore national organisations in the UK and USA have recently revised their protocols for young women, recommending cervical screening to commence at a later age, with more conservative management of early stage dysplasias. However while overall rates of cervical cancer have significantly declined with the introduction of well-organized nationalized Pap screening programmes, a trend of increasing rates in young women has been seen in some countries, with cervix cancer being second in incidence in genital tract cancers for the age group 20-24 years.

Whilst various risk factors predisposing to anogenital carcinomas are recognized, it is unclear if those cancers occurring in adolescents represent infection with more virulent types of HPV (a particular variant) or if they are due to other risk factors in childhood, such as immunosuppression or a result of earlier acquisition of HPV due to sexual abuse.

American Pap screening guidelines have suggested that earlier screening may be required in those who have been sexually abused or are immunosuppressed, although other national organizations have not made these recommendations. There have been significant recent advances in the treatment of early stage cervical carcinomas in young women, meaning that fertility sparing surgery may be offered to a larger number of young women with invasive cervical cancer without compromising survival. The introduction of prophylactic HPV vaccines has been a monumental step in the fight against anogenital carcinomas, with the distinct possibility that these cancers can be largely prevented in the future with wide coverage of such vaccines. However as immunity is largely type specific, a successful vaccine programme at best will be 70% preventative for cervical cancer. Australia is the first country that has introduced the quadrivalent HPV vaccine as part of a widespread federally funded school-based public health initiative, with a current uptake of around 80% in the target age, compared to a other countries using family physician based reimbursable schemes where uptake is more in the order of 30%. Moreover with the extremely high cost of the current vaccines HPV infection and anogenital cancer, particularly cervical cancer will continue to be a problem worldwide for decades to come, with maximal burden of disease occurring in developing nations. Vertical transmission from the maternal genital tract of low risk HPV genotypes 6/11 is also known to play an aetiological role in the rare, but recalcitrant to treatment, juvenile onset recurrent respiratory papillomatosis (JORRP). JORRP usually presents within the first 5 years of life and runs a protracted course, with malignant transformation occurring rarely. This review will therefore also discuss the implications for adolescents who have this rare but debilitating condition.

Chapter III - With the improvements in anticancer treatment, the survival rate of adolescent cancer victims is increasing. As a consequence of this therapy, many female adolescents suffer from ovarian failure and premature ovarian failure. The level of infertility varies by patient age (the younger the patient, the lesser the likehood of severe ovarian failure) as well as by drug dose, treatment duration, type of treatment (alkylating agents cause severe ovarian damage), and number of agents used. The highest risk is associated with high-dose chemotherapy combined with total body irradiation before bone marrow transplantation. Ovarian damage caused by irradiation is also correlated to the anatomical location of the ovaries in relation to the radiation field in the abdomen. Unfortunately, cancer patients have limited options for fertility preservation. Most survivors require oocyte donation. However, there is a shortage of donated oocytes in Western countries on the one hand, and most women prefer fertility restoration with self-oocytes on the other. Of the feasible possibilities for fertility preservation from self-oocytes, embryo cryopreservation after in vitro fertilization (IVF) as well as cryopreservation of mature human oocytes are in most cases unsuitable for minors. Therefore, cryopreservation of ovarian tissue containing small immature ovarian follicles remains almost the only practical option. So far, the autologous transplantation of cryopreserved-thawed ovarian tissue in women has resulted in four pregnancies, including two live births. Attempts to establish an in vitro maturation system are still in their infancy. This technology followed by routine IVF would eliminate the risks of reseeding malignant cells by ovarian grafts, and could possibly be offered in the future to infertile survivors of adolescent cancer, particularly of hematological malignancies. Obtaining ovarian tissue for cryopreservation requires a surgical procedure, usually laparoscopy, under general anesthesia, which may harbor risks that need to be discussed with the patient and her guardians. Other issues, such as the optimal surgical technique and the amount of tissue that needs to be removed for successful cryopreservation, have yet to be resolved. Although fertility-restoration techniques are still in the experimental stage, ovarian tissue removed from prepubertal and adolescent cancer patients is being frozen-stored in some medical centers worldwide. Sustaining the option of parenthood for young female patients may convey a message of hope, with a positive psychological effect.

Chapter IV - Currently thousands of teen and adult women are submitted to cancer treatment every year and estimates point to the existence of one survivor of malignant disease during childhood for each group of 250 adults. Improvements in medical care became absolutely necessary, demanding the development of new strategies to diminish the toxic consequences of chemotherapy and improve quality of life of treated patients. Ovarian failure is a frequent complication following cancer treatment, due to the cytotoxic effect of radio and chemotherapy. Temporary or permanent absence of endocrine and reproductive ovarian functions depends, mainly, on patients' age at the moment the gonadotoxic treatment was performed and also on the administered doses. The ovarian failure and consequently the installed hypogonadism culminate with several complications as the augmented incidence of cardiovascular diseases, reduced bone mass density and osteoporosis, precocious climacteric symptoms and infertility. Scientific advances progressively increase the knowledge on ovarian follicular and hypothalamic-pituitary axis dynamics. Furthermore cryobiology development has permitted physicians to plan and offer distinct strategies intending to maintain gonadal function for patients submitted to malignant neoplasm treatment. This chapter aims to discuss the available options in fertility preservation, especially focusing hormonal/pharmacological methods and cryobiology techniques (oocytes, embryos and ovarian cortical tissue cryopreservation).

Chapter V - Solid-pseudopapillary tumor (SPT) of the pancreas is an uncommon malignant tumor that predominantly affects young females. In this study, the clinical and histological features of pancreatic SPT are reviewed.

Over 19 years, 5 patients with SPT were seen in the authors' practice. They were all females, ranging in age from 21 - 66 years. Three tumors were located in the head of the pancreas, and two were located in the body and tail of the pancreas. Clinically, pancreatic SPT patients usually have vague abdominal symptoms, including discomfort, abdominal pain, increased abdominal girth, and the presence of a palpable mass. Three patients had pancreaticoduodenectomy, and two patients had distal pancreatectomy. No patients had metastasis to other sites. All patients are currently alive without recurrent disease. The histological findings were similar in all patients, and included: fairly uniform, round or oval eosinophilic cells concomitant with numerous thin-walled blood vessels in the solid component; red blood cells in the spaces between the pseudopapillary structures; and rare mitoses. The following immunohistochemical findings were confirmed: no reaction was evident with anti-chromogranin A, amylase, lipase or pancreatic polypeptide antibodies. The most useful markers for making a conclusive diagnosis were alpha-1-antitrypsin, neuron-specific enolase (NSE), and vimentin. Alpha-1-antitrypsin- and NSE-positive cells were present in all cases. All tumor cells were progesterone receptor-positive and estrogen receptor-negative. These findings show a close relationship between the tumor and sex hormones.

Pancreatic SPT occurs most frequently in young females and has low-grade malignant potential; it is associated with distinctive pathological and immunohistochemical features. Surgical resection should be considered even if metastases or local invasion is present, since it offers the patients an excellent prognosis.

Chapter VI - Breast cancer etiology researchers and those examining puberty regulation may think they have little in common, yet the conclusion that, "...breast feeding and late age at menarche protect against both ER^+PR^+ and ER^-PR^- breast cancer" (estrogen/progesterone receptor status) from the 2006 publication of Ma et al. a meta-analysis of reproductive factors and breast cancer risk [1] would argue otherwise. In a number of studies, early menarche has been identified as an important risk factor for breast cancer which has been explained by increased hormonal exposure. But among monozygotic twins, this risk becomes much stronger, implicating genetic factors as well [2]. The focus of recent female cancer epidemiological study designs has shifted from adult cohort studies to the ontogeny of female reproductive organs [2–5], presenting potential causal data either leading to or resulting from precocious puberty, late versus early breast development, parity, and age at first birth.

In a recent microarray gene expression study the authors found a group of related genes known to regulate the cell cycle and suppression of tumor growth (termed tumor related genes or TRGs) to be one of the most prominent groups of genes to increase hypothalamic expression throughout female puberty [6]. When the above factors are considered within the context of the newly unveiled hypothalamic polygenic TRG network, compelling research questions demanding multi-dimensional approaches emerge to investigate possible links. They also cast new hope for understanding and managing cancer predispositions as we expand the dimensions and details regarding this genetic network operating within the neuroendocrine brain.

Chapter VII - Ovarian masses in children and adolescents are a heterogeneous group of lesions that are predominantly neoplastic. Ovarian malignancies are uncommon, accounting for 1% of all malignant pediatric neoplasms. The pathology of ovarian neoplasms differs significantly from those occurring in adults. The majority of ovarian neoplasms in the pediatric and adolescent age group are of germ cell origin, as opposed to the predominance of surface epithelial-derived neoplasms in adults. Metastatic tumors to the ovary such as rhabdomyosarcoma are rare and are often bilateral.

Ovarian tumors usually present as abdominal or pelvic masses and may secrete hormones and other tumor markers that help in preoperative diagnosis and monitoring. However, preoperative evaluation alone is insufficient in the evaluation of these neoplasms. Pathology of the resected ovarian tissue remains an important tool for accurate diagnosis and staging. Histology with the aid of immunohistochemistry, as well as chromosomal karyotyping in some cases is an important tool in making accurate diagnosis and predicting a patient's prognosis.

In: Cancer in Female Adolescents
Editor: Margarite T. Moorland

ISBN: 978-1-60456-421-1

Expert Commentary

Future Directions and Challenges for HPV Education and Adolescent Immunization: Prevention of Cervical Cancer and Beyond

Luisa L. Villa[1] and Heather L. Sings[2]
[1] Ludwig Institute for Cancer Research,
Hospital Alemão Oswaldo Cruz, R. João Julião 245,
01323-930 São Paulo, SP, Brazil
[2] Merck Research Laboratories, PO Box 1000, UG3C-06,
North Wales, PA 19454-1099

On June 8, 2006, the United States Food and Drug Administration approved the first quadrivalent HPV vaccine. It has been designed for the prevention cervical cancer and genital warts, as well as vulvar and vaginal cancers (Gardasil, Merck and Co., Inc. Whitehouse Station, NJ, USA). The vaccine has been approved in 98 countries. In this commentary, we present a summary of the current data for the quadrivalent HPV vaccine in the prevention of female cancers, as well as future directions and challenges for HPV education and adolescent immunization in both developed and developing countries. Further areas of research such as efficacy in men and mid-adult women, the potential impact of the vaccine in head and neck cancers and recurrent respiratory papillomatosis (RRP), are also highlighted.

The multinational phase II/III trials of the quadrivalent vaccine enrolled over 20,000 women, the majority aged 16 to 23, from the Americas, Europe and Asia Pacific. Data on the efficacy of the vaccine was published among four articles which appeared in the *New England Journal of Medicine*[1, 2] and the *Lancet*[3, 4] in May and June of 2007. In summary, prophylactic administration of the quadrivalent vaccine was up to 100% effective in preventing development of HPV 16/18-related cervical, vulvar, and vaginal cancer (via surrogate markers); HPV 6/11/16/18-related low grade cervical dysplasia; and HPV 6/11/16/18-related genital warts. In 2006, a study published in the journal *Pediatrics[5]* showed that vaccination of 9- to 15-year-old boys and girls induced antibody levels that were higher than those seen in young adult women. On the basis of this immunogenicity bridging, the efficacy of the quadrivlanet vaccine in 9- to 15-year-old girls was inferred. An extension of a Phase II study showed the vaccine is highly effective through at least 5 years post-vaccination[6] and induces a robust anamnestic response, a hallmark of vaccines which provide long-term protection.[7] In these adolescent and adult studies, vaccination has been well-tolerated. Extensive safety information has been published as supporting information for the *New England Journal of Medicine* articles.[1,2] This includes data on pregnancy outcomes, as well as all serious adverse events, and systemic adverse events, categorized by organ system. The U.S. Food and Drug Administration has classified the HPV vaccine as a pregnancy Category B medication. Pregnancy Category B is given to medicines that have not been studied in pregnant humans, but do not appear to cause harm to the fetus in animal studies. Although this is the first vaccine designated as pregnancy category B, vaccination is not recommended during pregnancy.

In the literature published to date, there has been no evidence of protection from disease caused by vaccine-HPV-types for which subjects were positive at vaccination onset.[1,2] On the other hand, women who are infected with 1-3 of the HPV types included in the quadrivalent vaccine derive significant protection from the remaining HPV type(s) to which they are naïve.[8] Vaccination of women with HPV-6, 11, 16 or 18 DNA or antibodies pre-vaccination has been well-tolerated.[8]

The minimum antibody titer which will confer protection from HPV is not known. Because HPV is a global disease and vaccines will be offered to diverse ethnic/racial groups, it was important to evaluate the impact of demographic and behavioral parameters on the immunogenicity of the quadrivalent vaccine. An article which describes the effect of baseline subject characteristics on vaccine-induced immune responses was published in October 2007.[9] Covariates of interest included day 1 HPV serostatus, age, race, region of residence, lactation status, hormonal contraceptive usage, smoking status, Pap test diagnosis, immunosuppressant/anti-inflammatory agent use, and number of sexual partners. The study showed that younger age at vaccination and seropositivity to a particular HPV type pre-vaccination (indicating previous exposure) resulted in more robust antibody responses. Antibody responses were comparable among the remaining demographic subgroups.

The current data indicate that the vaccine will be highly effective in preventing female anogenital cancers, and the vaccine is most effective if administered to women who are naïve to the respective HPV type pre-vaccination. It is well known that the 5 years following sexual debut represent the period of highest risk for acquisition of HPV infection and in most countries, the median/mean age of sexual debut is between 15 and 16 years of age. Therefore the major targets of HPV vaccination campaigns are pre- and early adolescents. On June 29, 2006, the Advisory Committee on Immunization Practices (ACIP) of the Centers for Disease Control and Prevention recommended that the quadrivalent HPV vaccine be administered routinely to all females 11 to 12 years of age as well as 13–26-year-olds who have not previously received the vaccine. Females 9–10 years of age may be vaccinated at the discretion of the provider. This position is endorsed by the Society of Adolescent Medicine.[10] In Europe, several countries have publicized HPV vaccination recommendations including the UK, Austria, Belgium, France, Germany, Italy, Luxembourg, Norway and Switzerland. In developing countries, there is great interest in facilitating the implementation of a vaccine capable of preventing 70% of cervical cancers; however, recommendations are still under discussion. The major problem for developing countries is vaccine cost. Efforts to bring the vaccine to the lowest of income nations are being made by the vaccine's manufacturer. On September 27, 2007, Merck and Co., Inc committed to donating 3 million doses for use in demonstration projects in lowest income nations throughout the world

A vaccination program aimed at adolescents presents several unique challenges for both developed and developing countries. Barriers to adolescent vaccination have been grouped into four categories: parent/adolescent, health care provider, governmental and economic.[11] These barriers are relevant to implementation to most vaccines, however, for a vaccine that prevents a sexually transmitted infection, there may be unique barriers to acceptance.[12] Some recent reviews have been published on acceptability of HPV vaccines. However, most studies were performed pre-licensure, thus the data may be limited by the hypothetical nature of the topic.[13] Given that an HPV vaccine is now commercially available, post-licensure data are needed to reassess HPV knowledge and vaccine acceptance among parents, adolescents, and health care providers. In most studies to date from interviews conducted pre-licensure, young women had positive attitudes about HPV vaccination. Correlates of acceptance included parent's attitudes, efficacy, physician recommendation, and low cost. Knowledge of HPV sequele appears to be one of the most important factors for acceptability among parents. A study of 575 American parents/guardians published in 2004 found that about 23% of parents would not accept an HPV vaccine and an equal number of parents were undecided. After reading a one-page information sheet about HPV infection, transmission, and cancer risk, 20% of those who initially rejected the vaccine and 65% of those who were initially undecided changed their minds. The study highlights the importance of education on the impact of vaccine acceptability.

Some studies on vaccine acceptance by parents have been published post-licensure; however, even most studies published in 2007 report data from questionnaires that were administered before the vaccine was approved. In one of the first statewide studies reported (parents of daughters in California; questionnaire administered in spring and summer of 2006), 75% of the parents surveyed said they would be likely to vaccinate a daughter before 13 years of age.[14] Similar results were obtained in a study conducted in England (questionnaires administered between February and June 2006).[15] In the US study, Hispanic parents were more likely to accept vaccination than were non-Hispanic parents, whereas African-American and Asian-American parents were less likely. In the UK study white mothers were more in favor of earlier vaccination than non-white mothers. Further studies which examine the source of these apparent subgroup disparities are particularly important, as cervical cancer mortally rates are twice as high in African-Americans compared with white women.

Cervical cancer rates are highest in developing countries, however, there is little information regarding acceptance of an HPV vaccine in these areas. Most research studies have come out the United States and other English-speaking countries.[16] A study of mothers of adolescent girls in Mexico found them highly in favor of a theoretical vaccine against cervical cancer.[17] In Vietnam, cervical cancer is the most commen cancer among women and the leading cause of cancer-related death. A study published in 2007 (questionnaire administered to 194 mothers in Vietnam in June 2005), found 11% of the women surveyed had heard of an HPV vaccine and 94% agreed that such a vaccine would be effective in protecting their daughter from cervical cancer; however, 37% of mothers who believed vaccines are important to protect public health reported never having a child immunized.[18] A clinic based survey of young Brazilian women indicated overall a fairly poor knowledge of HPV infections and cervical cancer. However, being sexually active and perception of high risk of cervical cancer were predictors of participation in HPV vaccine trials.[19] In contrast, a recent study conducted in Australia indicated that most women aged 18-30 years had heard about HPV and HPV vaccines. Interestingly, those who did not know of a vaccine stated they would likely ask their general practitioner for information.[20]

Given the target age range for HPV vaccination, pediatricians will have an important role in promoting HPV vaccination. A survey conducted between September and October 2006 among 175 primary care pediatricians, 160 hospital pediatricians and 65 pediatric residents in Italy found a lack of knowledge concerning HPV disease and its prevention.[21] The findings highlight the need to improve pediatrician knowledge of HPV to ensure the optimal implementation of HPV vaccination. A review published in 2005 reported that the majority of research studies indicate that health care providers are less comfortable vaccinating younger versus older adolescents and that endorsement of an HPV vaccine by professional organizations is of great importance.[22] Several studies have established that adult as well as adolescent women have limited understanding of HPV,[22] and health care providers are identified as important sources of education. The authors of the review acknowledge that pediatricians and other health care providers will need to develop the knowledge base and skills necessary to effectively communicate the advantages of vaccination to adolescents and their parents, and suggest strategies by which providers of adolescent health care can discuss and recommend HPV vaccine with parents and their children. An additional barrier to vaccination of adolescents is that few adolescents see physicians regularly and physicians are concerned that it will be difficult to administer a 3-dose regimen to this population. Studies designed to simplify the use of quadrivalent HPV vaccine in adolescents by demonstrating that it is appropriate to co-administer the vaccine with other adolescent vaccines may allay these concerns. It has been demonstrated that co-administration of quadrivalent HPV vaccine and hepatitis B vaccine (Recombivax, Merck and Co., Inc) resulted in robust antibody responses and near 100% seroconversion rates for the quadrivalent vaccine, and >96% of subjects achieved a protective anti-HBs seroprotection level (≥10 mIU/ml). Co-administration of the vaccines was generally well-tolerated.[23]

There are additional practical challenges to implementation of HPV vaccination programs in adolescents: (1) visits to the pediatrician are infrequent, because few preventative medicine interventions are routinely administered; (2) some pediatricians are uncomfortable in managing the health of adolescent girls, and the transition from their practices to adolescent medicine specialists or gynecologists may result in long gaps in physician visits; (3) parents may have difficulty in compelling their adolescent children to undergo 3 separate vaccinations, and even among those who receive the 3-dose regimen, compliance with the 0, 2, 6 visit windows may be challenging; and (4) vaccination may not occur prior to sexual debut. While these provide a compelling argument for vaccination of infants, the duration of efficacy is not known, the infant vaccination schedule is already crowded, and the vaccine has not been tested in infants.

It is clear that the introduction of an HPV vaccine into national health care systems will raise difference questions for individual countries. Vaccination must take in account the country's disease burden, health care infrastructure, and its capacity for initiating and sustaining an immunization program for adolescents.[24] In January 2007, a working group of The World Health Organization's United Nations Population Fund identified several potential delivery strategies such as national immunization programs, school-based vaccination, and sexual and reproductive health services for adolescents.[25] The working group rightly states the challenge for policy-makers and opinion leaders is to ensure cervical cancer prevention has a high priory on the global public health agenda. In should also be noted that immunosuppression (HIV, use of immunosuppressive medications, malnutrition) results in severe exacerbation of HPV-related disease, thus developing world implementation strategies must include evaluations of the vaccine in immuno-compromised populations. Implementation would require the use of the vaccine in non-refrigerated settings, posing an additional challenge for the vaccine's manufacturer for delivery of the vaccine to developing nations. In countries with the fewest resources, direct assistance and public-private partnerships can help deliver needed medicines to the population at or below development costs. PATH, Harvard University, the International Agency for Research on Cancer, and the WHO, with funding from the Bill and Melinda Gates Foundation, are undertaking activities for making HPV vaccine available, acceptable, and affordable.[26] The vaccine's manufacturer is also pursuing arrangements to make the vaccine available to those in need.

Future directions for the prevention of female cancers will include studies in mid-adult women.[27] The ongoing clinical program for the quadrivalent vaccine is designed to further expand the indication to 27- to 45-year-old women for the prevention of cervical, vulvar, and vaginal cancers and precancers, and genital warts, as women in this age range remain at risk for HPV-related disease.

Men are a primary vector for HPV transmission to women and are also affected by HPV-related cancers. In men, HPV is a cause of genital warts, anal and penile cancers.[28] Men are also at substantial risk for development of HPV-related oropharyngeal cancer. Compared to women, less is known about the natural history of HPV infection in men, however more knowledge on the incidence, duration, and host response to HPV infections in men is being obtained. A recent study has shown that genital HPV infection is common and multifocal in young men, its incidence is higher than that previously reported, and detection of HPV DNA under the fingernail tips is common.[29] The authors of this new study conclude that the high rates of HPV infection in men should be considered when strategies for the prevention of HPV infection in female adolescent and young women are being developed. However, the efficacy of the vaccine in men has not been established; studies are ongoing.[27] In a study of male and female college students, there were no significant differences in acceptance by gender and both were more likely to accept an HPV vaccine if it was recommended for universal coverage.[30] In Australia and Canada, a limited use of the vaccine in boys has been accepted.

HPV causes other life-threatening diseases. HPV types 6 and 11 cause most recurrent respiratory papillomatosis (RRP). RRP is characterized by rapidly growing, histologically benign laryngeal tumors. The disease causes choking and recurrent super-infections. Patients must undergo frequent laser excision; some cases progress to death. Thus, HPV 6/11 cause a disease that may be considered as bad as cancer, impacting vulnerable populations (infants). Otolaryngologists and the RRP lay community are highly interested in investigating the impact of the vaccine on the burden of RRP. Their interest stems from the dismal state of available therapeutic options. Though a randomized controlled clinical trial which demonstrates prevention of RRP may not be feasible, in theory prevention of RRP can be demonstrated if RRP rates are lower in children of vaccinated women, compared with children of unvaccinated women. Such data can only be gathered once there is sufficient uptake of the vaccine in the general population.

In summary, a vaccine which prevents female cancers is now available. Further areas of research include efficacy in men, mid-adult women, the potential impact of the vaccine in head and neck cancers and recurrent respiratory papillomatosis (RRP). There are many practical challenges to implementation of HPV vaccination programs in adolescents. Historically, there has been significant delay in the introduction of new vaccines in developing countries. These challenges may be easier to overcome if cervical cancer prevention and education has a high priory on the global public health agenda, as well as if there is a full understanding of the burden of HPV diseases.

References

[1] Garland SM, Hernandez-Avila M, Wheeler CM et al. Quadrivalent vaccine against human papillomavirus to prevent anogenital diseases. *N. Engl. J. Med.* 2007; 356:1928-1943.

[2] The FUTURE II Study Group. Quadrivalent vaccine against human papillomavirus to prevent high-grade cervical lesions. *N. Engl. J. Med.* 2007; 356:1915-1927.

[3] Joura EA, Leodolter S, Hernandez-Avila M et al. Efficacy of a quadrivalent prophylactic human papillomavirus (types 6, 11, 16 and 18) L1 virus-like-particle vaccine against high-grade vulval and vaginal lesions: a combined analysis of three clinical trials. *Lancet.* 2007; 369:1693-1702.

[4] The FUTURE II Study Group. Effect of prophylactic human papillomavirus L1 virus-like-particle vaccine on risk of cervical intraepithelial neoplasia grade 2, grade 3 and adenocarcinoma in situ: a combined analysis of four randomised clinical trials. *Lancet.* 2007; 369:1861-1868.

[5] Block SL, Nolan T, Sattler C et al. Comparison of the immunogenicity and reactogenicity of a prophylactic quadrivalent human papillomavirus (types 6, 11, 16, and 18) L1 virus-like particle vaccine in male and female adolescents and young adult women. *Pediatrics.* 2006; 118:2135-2145.

[6] Villa LL, Costa RLR, Petta CA et al. High sustained efficacy of a prophylactic quadrivalent human papillomavirus types 6/11/16/18 L1 virus-like particle vaccine through 5 years of follow-up. *Br. J. Cancer.* 2006; 95:1459-1466.

[7] Olsson S-E, Villa LL, Costa R et al. Induction of immune memory following administration of a prophylactic quadrivalent human papillomavirus (HPV) types 6/11/16/18 L1 virus-like-particle vaccine. *Vaccine.* 2007; 25:4931-4939.

[8] The FUTURE II Study Group. Prophylactic efficacy of a quadrivalent HPV vaccine in women with virologic evidence of HPV infection. *Journal of Infectious Diseases.* 2007; 196:1438-1446.

[9] Giuliano A, Lazcano-Ponce E, Villa L et al. Impact of baseline covariates on the immunogenicity of a quadrivalent (types 6, 11, 16, and 18) human papillomavirus virus-like-particle vaccine. *J. Infect. Dis.* 2007; 196: 1153-1162..

[10] Friedman LS, Kahn J, Middleman AB, Rosenthal SL, Zimet GD. Human papillomavirus (HPV) vaccine: a position statement of the Society for Adolescent Medicine. *J. Adolesc. Health.* 2006; 39:620.

[11] Schaffner W, Brooks DA, Jenson HB, Juszczak L, Word BM. Adolescent Vaccination: Bridging from a Strong Childhood Foundation to a Healthy Adulthood. Bethesda, MD: National Foundation for Infectious Diseases. Available at http://www.nfid.org/pdf/ publications/adolescentvacc.pdf. Accessed September 24, 2007.

[12] Kahn JA. Maximizing the potential public health impact of HPV vaccines: a focus on parents. *J. Adolesc. Health.* 2007; 40:101-103.

[13] Liddon N, Zimet G, Stanberry LR. STI Vaccines: Status of Development, Potential Impact, and Important Factors for Implementation. In: Aral SO, Douglas JM, editors. *Behavioral Interventions for Prevention and Control of Sexually Transmitted Diseases.* New York: Springer Science+ Business Media, LLC; 2007 p. 248-273.

[14] Constantine NA, Jerman P. Acceptance of human papillomavirus vaccination among Californian parents of daughters: a representative statewide analysis. *J. Adolesc. Health.* 2007; 40:108-115.

[15] Marlow LA, Waller J, Wardle J. Parental attitudes to pre-pubertal HPV vaccination. *Vaccine.* 2007; 25:1945-1952.

[16] Zimet GD, Liddon N, Rosenthal SL, Lazcano-Ponce E, Allen B. Chapter 24: Psychosocial aspects of vaccine acceptability. *Vaccine.* 2006; 24 Suppl 3:S201-S209.

[17] Lazcano-Ponce E, Rivera L, Arillo-Santillán E, Salmerón J, Hernández-Avila M, Muñoz N. Acceptability of a human papillomavirus (HPV) trial vaccine among mothers of adolescents in Cuernavaca, Mexico. *Arch. Med. Res.* 2001; 32:243-247.

[18] Dinh TA, Rosenthal SL, Doan ED et al. Attitudes of mothers in Da Nang, Vietnam toward a human papillomavirus vaccine. *J. Adolesc. Health.* 2007; 40:559-563.

[19] Moreira ED, Jr., de Oliveira BG, Neves RC, Costa S, Karic G, Filho JO. Assessment of knowledge and attitudes of young uninsured women toward human papillomavirus vaccination and clinical trials. *J. Pediatr. Adolesc. Gynecol.* 2006; 19:81-87.

[20] Giles M, Garland S. A study of women's knowledge regarding human papillomavirus infection, cervical cancer and human papillomavirus vaccines. *Aust. N. Z. J. Obstet. Gynaecol.* 2006; 46:311-315.

[21] Esposito S, Bosis S, Pelucchi C et al. Pediatrician knowledge and attitudes regarding human papillomavirus disease and its prevention. *Vaccine.* 2007; 25:6437-6446.

[22] Zimet GD. Improving adolescent health: focus on HPV vaccine acceptance. *J. Adolesc. Health.* 2005; 37:S17-S23.

[23] Wheeler CM, Bautista OM, Tomassini JE, Nelson M, Sattler CA, Barr E. Safety and immunogenicity of co-administered quadrivalent human papillomavirus (HPV)-6/11/16/18 L1 virus-like particle (VLP) and hepatitis B (HBV) vaccines. *Vaccine* 2008; 26:686-696.

[24] Agosti JM, Goldie SJ. Introducing HPV vaccine in developing countries--key challenges and issues. *N. Engl. J. Med.* 2007; 356:1908-1910.

[25] Pollack AE, Balkin M, Edouard L, Cutts F, Broutet N. Ensuring access to HPV vaccines through integrated services: a reproductive health perspective. *Bull. World Health Organ.* 2007; 85:57-63.

[26] Herdman C, Demspey, M. Introducing HPV vaccines in developing countries: Overcoming the challenges. Available at. http://www.path.org/publications/ pub.php?id=1121.Accessed Sept 24, 2007 .

[27] Barr E, Tamms G. Quadrivalent human papillomavirus vaccine. *Clin. Infect. Dis.* 2007; 45:609-7.

[28] Partridge JM, Koutsky LA. Genital human papillomavirus infection in men. *Lancet Infect. Dis.* 2006; 6:21-31.

[29] Partridge JM, Hughes JP, Feng Q et al. Genital human papillomavirus infection in men: Incidence and risk factors in a cohort of university students. *J. Infect. Dis.* 2007; 196:1128-1136.

[30] Boehner CW, Howe SR, Bernstein DI, Rosenthal SL. Viral sexually transmitted disease vaccine acceptability among college students. *Sex. Transm. Dis.* 2003; 30:774-778.

In: Cancer in Female Adolescents
Editor: Margarite T. Moorland

ISBN: 978-1-60456-421-1

Chapter I

Role of Cytology in Diagnosis and Management

Dilip K. Das*

Department of Pathology, Faculty of Medicine, Kuwait University

Abstract

Adolescence is the developmental period between the childhood and adulthood, a period during which rapid biological as well as psychological maturation occurs. Although opinion regarding the adolescent age group varies, in most of the recent reports, cancer in the adolescence concerned individuals between 15-19 years of age. Since adolescent girls' health plays an important role in determining the health of future generation, adolescence in girls has been recognized as a special period in their life cycle that requires specific and special attention. However, factors such as poor nutritional status and early consummation of marriage in the developing world and the behaviors or conditions that begin or occur during adolescence in the developed countries–for example tobacco and alcohol use, poor eating habits, sexual abuse, and risky sex, contributes significantly to disease burden including precancer and cancer, and premature deaths among adults. In children aged less than 15 years, common malignancies are leukemias, CNS tumors, and childhood embryonal tumors. After the age of 10 years, embryonic tumors almost disappear, whereas other cancers become more frequent, notably lymphomas, carcinomas, germ-cell tumors, and bone tumors. The highest incidence rates for cancers among adolescents (15-19 years) include those for lymphomas, followed by carcinomas, CNS tumors, germ-cell tumors, and leukemias. In the west, lymphomas are the most common malignancy in adolescent females, followed by carcinomas, leukemias, CNS tumors, bone tumors, melanomas, soft tissue sarcomas, and germ-cell tumors. In a developing country like India lymphomas and leukemias are also most common cancer in adolescent females, followed by malignancies of bone and soft tissue, urogenital system, CNS, head and neck, thyroid, gastrointestinal system, and

* Address for Coresspondence: Dr. Dilip K. Das, MBBS, MD, PhD, DSc, FRCPath. Associate Professor; Department of Pathology, Faculty of Medicine, Kuwait University, P.O. Box: 24923; Safat 13110, Kuwait. Tel: 00965-5319456 Fax: 00965-5338905; E-mail: dilip76@hotmail.com, dilip@hsc.kuniv.edu.kw

breast. Because of the relatively low cancer incidence, the adolescent and young adult population has not been the focus of attention in cancer control and prevention strategy in the past. However, there is clear evidence of an increase in cancer incidence in children, adolescents and young adults during the past decades. Therefore, over the past 10 years, ever-increasing attention has been paid to the needs of adolescents with cancer worldwide.

Methods of diagnosis of cancer include clinical, imaging, microscopic examination, and others. The main microscopic studies include histology, hematology (blood film and bone marrow), and cytology including exfoliative and fine needle aspiration (FNA) cytology. Exfoliative cytology in the form of Pap test and ancillary tests on this sample helps in early detection of squamous intraepithelial (precancerous) lesions and human papillomavirus infections in adolescent females, so that necessary intervention is offered to prevent the development of invasive cancer during adulthood. Review of literature shows that the most common site of FNA in children and adolescents is lymph node (41.2%), followed by bone and soft tissue (17.1%), head and neck lesions excluding thyroid (9.4%), abdominal and pelvic masses (9.0%), breast (8.4%), thyroid (7.4%), thorax (5.8%), and central nervous system (1.7%). The averages of benign, suspicioius, malignant, and inadequate cytology reports in a review of seven studies in children and adolescents were 55.2%, 0.9%, 41.0%, and 3.0%, respectively indicating that malignancy is very common in the FNA material in this age group. The diagnostic efficacy of this tool is also very high. The sensitivity, specificity, and diagnostic accuracy of FNA in children and adolescents, based on 6 studies, were 91.8 ± 8.29%, 97.4 ± 3.08%, and 95.2 ± 4.37%, respectively. The averages of requency of malignancy for various sites in FNA cytology reports in the literature were as follows: head and neck excluding thyroid (14.6%), thyroid (13.6%), lymph nodes (5.6%), thorax and abdomen (46.3%), and bone and soft tissue (58.0%).

FNA is useful in the management of cases with mass lesions in the body by offering a quick diagnosis and by reducing additional and costly procedures. The efficacy of FNA as a diagnostic tool for various sites is generally high. In literature, the sensitivity and specificity for diagnosis of malignancies in various anatomic sites were as follows: head and neck (97.2 ± 3.96% and 95.1 ± 2.90%, respectively), thyroid (90.3 ± 15.71% and 80.4 ± 12.91%, respectively), lymph nodes (92.8 ± 5.74% and 94.5 ± 3.11%, respectively), abdomen and pelvis (93.4 ± 2.80% and 100.0%, respectively), and bone and soft tissue (90.2 ± 16.91% and 94.8 ± 5.97%, respectively). Information on diagnostic accuracy, available for limited sites, were as follows: thyroid (84.6 ± 4.95%), abdominal visceras (95.7 ± 1.72%), and bone and soft tissue (96.0 ± 1.05%). Further, exfoliative cytology in the form of examination of serous cavity fluids following ascitic or pleural tap and FNA cytology on samples from the space occupying lesions in various organs of the body cavities, which are difficult to be accessed by surgical procedures, especially in very sick adolescents, make enormous contribution to the management of patients. However, in certain situations the cytopatholoists face diagnostic difficulties, which are largely solved with the help of ancillary studies like cytochemistry, immunocytochemistry, flow cytometry, cytogenetics, ultrastrucure, and molecular biologic techniques.

Introduction

Adolescence is the developmental period between the childhood and adulthood, and a unique stage of life during which rapid physical (biological), cognitive, intellectual (psychological), and emotional maturation occurs.[1, 2] World Health Organization (WHO) defines three time periods from 10 to 25 years of age: the preadolescence (10-14 years), the adolescence (15-19 years), and the post-adolescence (20-25 years).[1] There are 1.2 billion adolescents worldwide and one in every five people in the world is an adolescent.[3] Although, in most of the recent reports from USA and European countries, cancer in the adolescence concerned individuals between 15-19 years of age,[1, 4-9] there are many other studies in which the age group for adolescence has been considered as of 12-18 years,[10] 13-19 years,[11] 14-21 years,[12, 13] 15-20 years,[14] and 12-21 years.[15] A report on adolescent females,[16] defines adolescence as the time for growth spurts and puberty, during which the adolescent female not only experiences initiation of changes in physical, mental and social parameters earlier in life than the male counter part, but also endowed with additional changes. This may justify the use of separate age ranges for adolescent boys (15-19 years) and adolescent girls (10-19 years) by Singh et al [17] while describing some uncommon tumors of childhood and adolescence.

Because of the relatively low cancer incidence, the adolescent and young adult population has not been the focus of attention in cancer control and prevention programs, [9] however, everybody is not free from concerns in this age group. There are adolescents who carry with them a the memory of childhood cancer, while remaining in a state of remission or apparent cure; those whose immediate relatives suffer from cancers, especially familial types; and finally those who are drawn into an mileau of carcinogens by virtue of their owns acts or others' contribution. Childhood cancers, which were regarded as ominous signs leading to sure death once upon a time, are viewed as some of the most treatable and curable cancers (in more than 70% cases) due to the cooperative efforts of pediatric hematologists/oncologists, pediatric surgeons, radiation therapists, and pathologists.[18, 19] Acute lymphoblastic leukemia (ALL) is the most common cancer in children and is among the most curable of the pediatric malignancies.[20] The other curable neoplasms are common and uncommon primitive and embryonic neoplasms of childhood.[18, 21-23] Malignant ovarian germ cell tumors [24] and rhabdomyosarcoma of the genital tract [25] are also some of the example of curable cancers in adolescent females. As their intellectual development takes shape, the adolescents (in a state of remission or cure of childhood cancer) begin to realize that there is a chance of recurrence of their past illness, even if it is slim, and this haunts the young mind. Considering the high survival rates of childhood cancers, physical and psychological long term effects (LF) as well as the estimation of Quality of Life (QoL) are now becoming a new focus of clinical research.[26]

Studies on perceptions of children (<18 years of age) of their mother's breast cancer reveal that awareness of cancer as a life threatening illness existed even among most of the youngest children.[27] These children experience multiple worries concerning their mother, and their families, and themselves. They attempt to make sense of their mothers' illness for themselves and imagine how it may affect their own lives in future.[28] Further, children growing up in hereditary breast and ovarian cancer families may experience diminished psychological well-being because of the efforts to cope with having a cancer-affected parent and the thought on their own health risk in light of the shared genetic information.[29] It is also observed that undergoing genetic testing and learning one's BRCA1/2 status, may affect family relationships.[30]

Adolescence in girls, being recognized as a special period in their life cycle, requires specific and special attention, because adolescent girls' health plays an important role in determining the health of future population. However, in large part of the world, they have a lesser access to food, and a lesser share in household distribution of health care facility, goods, and services as compared to men and boys, which leads to a poor nutritional status and a state of ill health for most of the adolescent girls.[31] Despite international agreements and national laws, marriage of girls <18 years of age is common worldwide and affects millions. Further child marriage is driven by poverty and has many effects on girls' health including increased risk of sexually transmitted diseases, cervical cancer, malaria, death during child birth, and obstetrics fistula.[32] Early consummation of marriages, multiple pregnancies, and lack of proper sanitation leading to genital infections, are some of the factors linked to precancer and cancer of uterine cervix, the commonest cancer in the females of the developing world. Although adolescents appear to be a relatively healthy group in developed countries like U.S.A., the behaviors or conditions that begin or occur during adolescence –for example tobacco and alcohol use, poor eating habits, sexual abuse, and risky sex, contributes to 33% of the disease burden and about 60% of premature deaths among adults.[33] Case-control studies from Europe [34, 35] and USA [36] have identified smoking as an important risk factor for lung cancer in young adults. A study from Norway reveals that the lung cancer incidence rate in young Norwegian women now equals that of men and lung cancer incidence rates at age 40-44 were highly correlated with smoking prevalence at age 15-19 in males and females within the same birth cohort.[37] A 1991 report on the current trends of premarital sexual experience among adolescent women (15-19 years of age) in the United States revealed that there was at least 55% increase during 1970-1988 and an accelerated increase occurred from 1986 to 1988.[38] The incidence and prevalence of sexually transmitted diseases (STDs) including chlamydia, HSV-2, tricomonas, and HBV, was found to be extremely high among female adolescents in a study of sexually active females aged 14-19 years.[39] According to WHO estimates, 50% of all new HIV infections are among young people (about 7,000 young people become infected everyday), and that 30% of the 40 million people living with HIV/AIDS are in the 15-24 year age group.[40] In a study conducted at Indiana University School of Medicine, it was observed that four out of five sexually active adolescent females were infected with human papillomavirus, a common sexually transmitted infection, responsible for genital warts, precancer and cancer of the uterine cervix.[41] Cervical abnormalities were also found to be higher among HIV infected adolescents than among non-HIV-infected counterparts.[42]

Adolescent Cancers: Magnitude of the Problem

International patterns of childhood cancers are well documented but equivalent information relating to adolescence is scarce. Total incidence of cancer in the adolescents ranges from 95 to 255 per million person years and the highest rates are recorded in Australia and among Jews in Israel and the lowest in India and Japan.[43] The overall rate of adolescent (15-19 year age group) cancer was 144 per million (14.4 per 100,000) in England.[7] As compared to the annual incidence rate per million in England, those in Netherlands (193.3) and U.S.A. (202.2) were higher.[6] Cancer incidence varies not only between adolescents of developed and developing countries but also between various regions of these countries and according to socioeconomic status.[44] There is clear evidence of an increase in cancer incidence in children, adolescents and young adults during the past decades on both sides of the Atlantic.[8,45] The incidence of cancer in the young patients aged 15-30 years is higher (220- 250 cases per million youths) and rising faster than children. As per United States SEER program data during 1975-1995, the incidence of cancer in adolescents increased by 30%, while that in childhood rose by only 10%.[4] Subsequent statistical review of data from the SEER program and the UK cancer registry indicate that cancer in 15-19 year old adolescents is 50% higher than in younger persons.[45] In Europe, the age specific cancer rates in adolescents per millions were 147 in 1970s, 165 in 1980s, and 193 in 1990s, on the basis of 15460 cases.[8] Therefore, over the past 10 years, ever-increasing attention has been paid to the needs of adolescents with cancer world-wide.

Change of Cancer Pattern from Childhood to Adolescence

In English children aged less than 15 years, the most common malignancy is leukemia (33% of all malignancies), followed by CNS tumors (25%), childhood embryonal tumors (16%), lymphomas (9%), and bone and soft tissue sarcomas (9%). Less than 2% of childhood cancers are carcinomas.[46,47] In Europe, the most common tumor types in children were also leukemias (age-standardized incidence rates or ASR 44.8), CNS tumors (29.8), and lymphomas (15.5).[8] Although it is often stated that 15-19-year-old adolescents more commonly suffer from pediatric tumors, a closer look at epidemiological and incidence data does not support this observation. Hodgkin's disease and germ cell tumors, the two commonest adolescent malignancies, occur at an incidence 3-6 times higher than the pediatric one. Epithelial carcinomas, thyroid cancer and melanomas are seldom, if ever, encountered in children, while ALL, NHL, CNS tumors, and osteosarcoma/Ewing family tumors (EFT) are almost as common in adolescence as in childhood.[45] After the age of 10 years, embryonic tumors such as retinoblastoma, nephroblastoma (most renal tumors), and hepatoblastoma (most hepatic tumors) almost disappear in European children, whereas other cancers become more frequent, notably lymphomas, carcinomas, germ-cell tumors, and bone tumors.[8] A report on international pattern of cancer by Stiller,[43] reveals that osteosarcoma, ovarian germ cell tumors and, in some populations, nasopharyngeal carcinoma have their highest incidence at age 15-19 years. The highest incidence rate for cancers among adolescents (15-

19 years) in Europe includes lymphomas (age-specific rate 47.4 per million), followed by carcinomas (38.1), CNS tumors (24.6), germ-cell tumors (24.5), and leukemias (23.4).[8] According to National Cancer Institute's Surveillance Epidemiology and End Results (SEER) program cancer statistics review (1973-1998), the most common tumors among 15-19-year-old adolescents are Hodgkin's disease (16%) and germ cell tumors (15%) by far, followed by central nervous system tumors (10%), non-Hodgkin's lymphoma (8%), thyroid cancer (7%), malignant melanoma (7%), and acute lymphoblastic leukemia (6%).[45] The striking increase in incidence of cancers in adolescence as compared to childhood during 1975-1995 was mainly due to malignant germ cell tumors and lymphoid neoplasm.[4]

Cancers in Adolescent Females Versus Adolescent Males

In France, the overall incidence of cancers in adolescent females (15-19 year age group) was 159.5 per million individuals and among them lymphoma and leukemias were the most common (49.3 per million), followed by carcinomas and other epithelial tumors (41.8), malignant bone and soft tissue tumors (24.7), CNS and miscellaneous intracranial and spinal tumors (17.1), and germ cell, trophoblastic and other gonadal tumors (16.6).[1] Lymphomas were also the most common malignancy in adolescent females (27.33 per million) in England too, followed by carcinomas (largely contributed by thyroid carcinomas, 15.72), leukemias (13.52), CNS tumors (11.14), bone tumors (8.57), melanomas (8.17), soft tissue sarcomas (6.07), and germ-cell tumors (4.51).[7] In population-based cancer registries of India, 900 cancers were recorded in adolescent females (15-19 year age group) during 1990-1996. Lymphomas and leukemias were most common cancer (29.7%), followed by malignancies of bone and soft tissue (16.7%), urogenital system (15.8%), brain and CNS (11.3%), head and neck (6.4%), thyroid (4.9%), gastrointestinal system (4.8%), and breast (4.1%).[48] In USA, the overall incidence of cancer is 19.9 per 100,000 for adolescent white females and 13.7 in black adolescent females. The top five common cancers among white adolescent females were Hodgkin's lymphoma (4.0 per 100,000), thyroid cancers (3.0), leukemias (1.9), melanomas (1.9), and brain and CNS tumor (1.6). In their black counter parts, the top five malignancies were Hodgkin's lymphoma (1.8), soft-tissue sarcoma (1.8), leukemias (1.3), brain and CNS tumors (1.2), and nonHodgkin's lymphomas (0.9).[9]

A study on international pattern of cancer in adolescence shows that the total cancer incidence is higher in adolescent males than females, but there is often a female excess in melanoma and thyroid carcinoma; Hodgkin lymphoma is atleast as frequent among females as males in several countries with relatively high incidence.[43] As per SEER data from U.S.A., the male: female ratio in most cancers, viz., acute lymphoblastic leukemia, nonHodgkin lymphoma, Ewing's sarcoma, osteogenic sarcoma, germ cell tumors, CNS tumors, and soft tissue sarcoma ranged from 1.2 to 2.2 in adolescents. However, in Hodgkin's lymphoma, malignant melanoma, and thyroid carcinoma, there was a female predominance with male to female ratio ranging from 0.1 to 0.8.[4] In England, four of the top five cancers, i.e., lymphomas, leukemias, CNS tumors and bone tumors were common between adolescent males and females; the only difference was germ cell tumors in males and carcinomas in females, which found places among the top five.[7] Top five cancers in French adolescents males and females were the same neoplasms, if lymphomas and leukemias were combined into one group.[1] In USA, comparing adolescents of opposite sexes (white males and females, black males and females) revealed testicular cancer and NHL were among five top cancers in white males but NHL was not found among top five cancers in their female counterparts. On the other hand thyroid cancers and melanomas were among the top five in white females and not in males. There was no difference between black males and females, except in the order among top five cancers.[9] Data from Indian cancer registries shows that the higher rate of thyroid, breast, urogenital and CNS cancers were observed in female adolescents (15-19 years age group) than adolescent males; on the other hand lymphoma/leukemias, and bone and soft tissue malignancies were higher in male adolescents when the top five caners were compared.[48]

Methods of Cancer Diagnosis: Impact of Age

Methods of diagnosis of cancer include clinical, imaging, microscopic examination, and others. The common microscopic studies include histology, cytology, and hematology (blood film and bone marrow). The main cytologic parameters are exfoliative and fine needle aspiration (FNA) cytology, which will be the subject of this chapter. FNA from children and adolescents appear to form a small part of the procedure performed in all age groups. Of the 7487 fine-needle aspirations (FNAs) reported by Eisenhut et al,[49] 288 (3.8%) were observed in the pediatric age group (≤19years). Among 7000 procedures, Cohen and associates[50] reported 92 FNA biopsies (1.3%) form 84 patients younger than 16 years of age. Although one of the greatest merits of cytologic techniques is the scope for quick diagnosis, it has been found that older adolescents and young adults with cancer in the United States are likely to have a delay in the diagnosis because of inadequate health insurance and consequently present with a more advanced stage of disease.[51] On the other hand, children and adolescents treated for cancer in pediatric units of Canada experience short waiting times to key diagnostic and treatment events, once they enter the healthcare system.[52]

Cytodiagnosis Cancers with Special Reference to Adolescent Females

Exclusive reports on FNA diagnosis of cancers in adolescents are few and most of them are isolated case reports.[53-56] Publications on FNA cytology diagnosis of cancers in adolescent patients are either an integral part of reports on cancers in broad pediatric age group or combined reports on children and adolescents. As per five studies (table 1), the most common site for FNA in children and adolescents was lymph nodes (41.2% cases), followed by bone and soft tissue masses (17.1%), head and neck lesions (9.4%), abdomen and pelvic masses (9.0%), breast (8.4%), thyroid (7.4%), thorax (5.8%), and central nervous system (1.7%).[49, 50, 57-59]

Table 1. Sites of Fine Needle Aspiration (FNA) in Children and Adolescents

Authors and Year	Total no of cases	Sites of FNA: No of cases (%)							
		Head & neck	Thyroid	Lymph node	Breast	Thorax	Abdomen	Bone & soft tissue	CNS
Tailor & Nunez (1984)[57]	64	5	0	9	3	16	20	9	2
Wakely et al (1988)[58]	112	5	12	44	2	8	5	34	2
Cohen et al (1989)[50]	92	33	1	23	0	6	11	18	0
Silverman et al (1991)[59]	135	7	16	41	24	10	26	3	8
Eisenhut et al (1996)[49]	288	15	22	168	29	0	0	54	0
Total	691	65 (9.4)	51 (7.4)	285 (41.2)	58 (8.4)	40 (5.8)	62 (9.0)	118 (17.1)	12 (1.7)

CNS= central nervous system.

Table 2. Fine Needle Aspiration (FNA) in Children and Adolescents: Cytodiagnosis of Lesions

Author (s) and year	Age range (mean/median)	No of patients (No of FNAs)	Male: female	FNA cytodiagnosis: No of cases (%)			
				Benign	Suspicious	Malignant	Inadequate
Taylor and Nunez (1984)[57]	Newborn to 18 yrs	58 (64)	33:25	38 (59.4)	0 (0.0)	19 (29.7)	7 (10.9)
Wakely et al (1988)[58]	Newborn to 16 years	107 (112)	52:55	70 (62.5)	2 (1.8)	39 (34.8)	1 (0.9)
Cohen et al (1989)[50]	9 m-16 yrs (5.8yrs)	84 (92)	43:41	51 (55.4)	2 (2.2)	33 (35.9)	6 (6.5)
Almeida et al (1991)[60]	11m-16yrs	46	34:12	4 (8.7)	2 (4.3)	28 (60.9)	12 (26.1)
Silverman et al (1991)[59]	1 d-18 yrs (10.5 yrs)	123 (135)	1:1.4	93 (68.9)	8 (5.9)	28 (20.7)	6 (4.4)
Eisenhut et al (1996)[49]	1 d-19 yrs	276 (288)	142:134	275 (95.5)	0 (0.0)	13 (4.5)	0 (0.0)
Drut et al (2005)[61]	<18 years*	829 (899)	-	372 (41.4)	0 (0.0)	510 (56.7)	17 (1.9)
Total	Newborn-19yrs	1523 (1636)	-	903 (55.2)	14 (0.9)	670(41.0)	49 (3.0)

*except one who was 24 yrs, d= day, m= month, yrs= years.

Table 3. Efficacy of Fine-Needle Aspiration (FNA) Cytology in Children and Adolescents

Authors and year	Age range in yrs	No of patients (FNAs)	Male: female	Diagnostic efficacy in percentages		
				Sensitivity	Specificity	Accuracy
Taylor and Nunez (1984)[57]	Newborn-18 yrs	58 (64)	33:25	76	100	89
Wakely et al (1988)[58]	Newborn-16 yrs	107 (112)	52:55	97	97	-
Cohen et al (1989)[50]	9 m-16 yrs	84	43:41	97	95	-
Silverman et al (1991)[59]	1 d-18 yr	125 (135)	52:73	90.6	100	96.5
Eisenhut et al (1996)[49]	1m-19 yrs	276 (288)	142:134	92.3	99.6	99.3
Drut et al (2005)[61]	<18 yrs*	829 (899)	-	98	92.6	95.8
Total	Newborn-19yrs	1479 (1582)	-	91.8±8.29	97.4±3.08	95.2±4.37

*Except one who was 24 yrs-old, d= day, m= month, yrs= years.

Malignancy rate varies widely in FNA cytology studies in children and adolescents. A review of 7 studies [49, 50, 57-61] on FNA cytodiagnosis of lesions in children and adolescents (table 2) revealed benign, suspicious, malignant, and inadequate aspirates in 54.2%, 0.9%, 41.4%, and 3.6%, respectively. Rate of malignancy was as low as 4.5% [49] but exceeded 50% in two of the seven studies.[60,61]

The sensitivity, specificity, and diagnostic accuracy of FNA cytology in mass lesions of children and adolescents as observed in seven studies are very high (table 3). The average sensitivity, specificity, and diagnostic accuracy were 91.8%, 97.4%, and 95.2%, respectively in these studies. [49, 50, 57-59, 61] Unlike FNA, there are limited number of studies on imprint cytology [62] and exfoliative cytology [15, 63, 64] in the diagnosis of precancerous lesions and malignancies in children and adolescents.

Head and Neck Cancers (Excluding Thyroid)

Pediatric head and neck malignancies comprise 4 to 5% of all childhood cancers.[65,66] These neoplasms consist of a mixed bag and differ from the adult head and neck tumors in many aspects.[67] Whereas about 80% of adult neck malignancies are epidermoid, ~90% of pediatric malignancies are mesenchymal.[68] Dave et al [69] in a study of pediatric head and neck tumors in children, observed that hemolymphoid malignancies were the predominant tumor, followed by other small round-cell tumors of childhood. Most reports on FNA cytodiagnosis of pediatric head and neck tumors include children up to the age of 18 years (table 4).[68, 70-72] Liu et al [68] reported a bimodal age distribution, with most patients either between ages 0 and 6, or 13 and 18; thus, the second peak did correspond to adolescent age group.

FNA is an extremely useful tool in the management of head and neck masses in children.[71] According to Liu et al [68] FNA reduces the need for more invasive and costly procedures and is a valuable diagnostic tool in the management of children (including adolescents) with the clinical presentation of head and neck masses. The frequency of malignancies among pediatric FNA cytology of head and neck masses (table 4) ranges from 6% to 21.3%, with an average of 14.6% [68, 70-72] and the common malignancies encountered in children are non-Hodgkin lymphoma, Hodgkin's lymphoma, Langerhans cell histiocytosis, nasopharyngeal carcinoma, papillary thyroid carcinoma, metastatic neuroblastoma and medulloblastoma, and osteogenic sarcoma. The nasopharyngeal carcinoma (NPC) frequently presents as lymph node metastasis in cervical lymph nodes and its detection by FNA (figure 1), points towards the primary, which is often occult and difficult to detect clinically.[73] FNA cytology has also been utilized for cytodiagnosis of rhabdomyosarcoma of oral cavity [74] and parotid gland of children.[75] Mathew and Ali [76] also correctly diagnosed an embryonal rhabdomyosarcoma in a 2 year-old male child and a mucoepidermoid carcinoma in a 15-year old female by FNA cytology of the parotid gland. However, a lymphoma diagnosed by them [76] turned out to be Ewing's sarcoma and a pleomorphic/monomorphic adenoma revealed an acinic cell carcinoma in histology.

Table 4. Fine-Needle Aspiration (FNA) Cytology Diagnosis of Pediatric Head and Neck Masses

Author (s) and year (Sites of FNA)	Age range (mean/median)	No of patients (FNAs)	Male: female	FNA cytodiagnosis: No (%)			
				Benign	Suspicious	Malignant	Inadequate
Mobley et al (1991)[70] (Head and neck)	≤16yrs	89	44:45	68 (76.4)	1 (1.1)	19 (21.3)	1 (1.1)
Ramadan et al (1997)[71] (Head and neck)	1d-17yrs (8.9yrs)	26 (29)	16:10	25 (86.2)	0 (0.0)	2 (6.9)	2 (6.9)
Liu et al (2001)[68] (Head and neck)	3m-18yrs (8.9yrs)	40 (50)	-	38 (76.0)	0 (0.0)	3 (6.0)	9 (18.0)
Rapkiewicz et al (2007)[72] (Head and neck)	4m-18yrs (9yrs)	85	59:26	71 (83.5)	1 (1.2)	13 (15.3)	0 (0.0)
Raab et al (1995) [84] (Thyroid)	1-18yrs (13.1yrs)	57 (66)	8:49	51 (77.3)	8 (12.1)	4 (6.1)	3 (4.5)
Lugo-Vicente et al (1998)[85] (Thyroid)	9-18yrs (14.9yrs)	24	4:20	19 (79.2)	0 (0.00)	5 (20.8)	0 (0.0)
Khurana et al (1999)[86] (Thyroid)	9-20yrs	57	11:46	36 (63.2)	14 (24.6)	7 (12.3)	0 (0.0)
Corrias et al (2001)[87] (Thyroid)	8.6-17.9yrs (13.1)	42	8:34	22 (52.4)	0 (0.0)	20 (47.6)	0 (o.0)
Al-Shaikh et al (2001) [79] (Thyroid)	0.3-17.9yr(13.1yrs)	41	6:35	30 (73.2)	6 (14.6)	2 (4.9)	3 (7.3)
Amrikachi et al (2005)[88] (Thyroid)	10-21 (17yrs)	185 (218)	23:162	119 (54.6)	20 (9.2)	17 (7.8)	62 (28.4)
Chang et al (2006) [78] (Thyroid)	2-21yrs (17yrs)	51 (60)	13:38	45 (75.0)	5 (8.3)	6 (10.0)	4 (6.7)
Hosler et al (2006)[83] (Thyroid)	8-18yrs (14.6yrs)	82 (101)	19:63	48 (47.5)	18 (17.8)	22 (21.8)	13 (12.9)
Total (Head & neck)	1d-18yrs	240 (253)	-	202 (79.8)	2 (0.8)	37 (14.6)	12 (4.7)
Total (Thyroid)	0.3-21yrs	539 (609)	92: 447	370 (60.8)	71 (11.7)	83 (13.6)	85 (14.0)

D= day, m= month, yrs= years.

Table 5. Head and Neck Malignancy in Children and Adolescents: Efficacy of Fine Needle Aspiration (FNA) Cytology

Authors and year (Sites of FNA)	Age range (mean/median)	No of patients (FNAs)	Male: female	Diagnostic efficacy in percentages		
				Sensitivity	Specificity	Accuracy
Mobley et al (1991)[70] (Head and neck)	≤16yrs	89	44:45	94.4	97.1	96.6
Rapkiewicz et al (2007)[72] (Head & neck)	4m-18yrs	85	59:26	100	93	-
Lugo-Vicente et al (1998)[85] (Thyroid)	9-18yrs (14.9yrs)	24	4:20	60	90	80
Al-Shaikh et al (2001)[79] (Thyroid)	0.3-17.9yrs (13.3yrs)	41	6:35	100	86	87
Corrias et al (2001)[87] (Thyroid)	8.6-17.9yrs (13.1yrs)	42	8:34	95	86.3	90.4
Amrikachi et al (2005)[88] (Thyroid)	10-21yrs	185 (218)	23:162	100	65	-
Chang et al (2005)[78] (Thyroid)	2-21yrs (17yrs)	51 (60)	13:38	100	63	81
Hosler et al (2006)[83] (Thyroid)	8-18yrs (14.6yrs)	82	19:63	87	92	-
Total (Head &neck*)		174	103:71	97.2± 3.96	95.1± 2.90	-
Total (Thyroid)	0.3-21	425 (467)	73:352	90.3± 15.71	80.4± 12.91	84.6± 4.95

*Head and neck sites excluding thyroid.

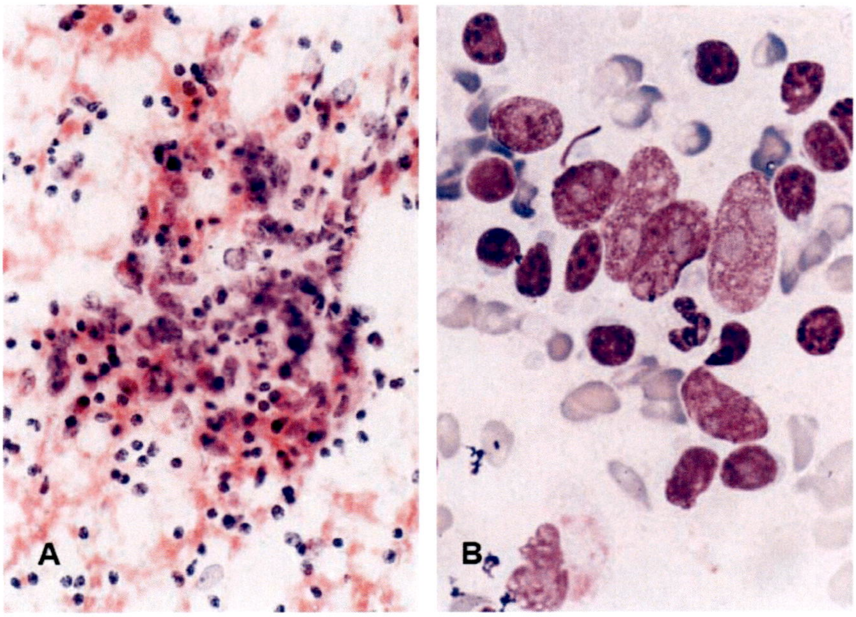

Figure 1. Metastatic nasopharyngeal carcinoma (NPC): FNA smears from left cervical lymph node in a 12-year-old girl. A. Cellular smear shows neoplastic cells in small loose cohesive clusters among lymphoid cells (Papanicolaou x 200). B: The neoplastic cells have oval elongated vesicular nuclei with prominent nucleoli (MGG x 1000).

The average sensitivity and specificity of FNA cytology for pediatric head and neck masses were 93.7% and 98.6%, respectively (table 5).[70, 72] Among primary and metastatic head and neck lesions in children, Dave et al [69] were able to offer an overall accuracy of diagnosis in 79.3%, a working broad diagnosis in 16.3% and misdiagnosis in remaining 4.4%.

Thyroid Cancers

The thyroid tumor represents 0.5% of all tumors and of these 10% is observed in patients younger than 21 years old.[77] In India, the frequency of thyroid cancers in adolescent females of 15-19 years age group was 4.9% of all malignancies[48] and was very close to that observed in adolescent females in England.[7] In France the incidence of thyroid cancer was 13.1 per million adolescent females,[1] which was lower than that observed in white females aged 15-19 years in USA (3.0 per 100,000).[9]

A number of studies [78-80] indicate that the thyroid nodules are uncommon in children compared to adults, but the risk of malignancy much higher in children (14-40%) than in adults (5%). Thyroid carcinomas in the children and adolescents can be quite aggressive.[81] Of the 23 children and adolescents with thyroid carcinoma reported by Pazaitou-Panayiotou et al,[81] there was cervical lymph node matastasis in 18 (78.2%), mediastinal metastasis in 2 (8.7%) and pulmonary metastasis in 3 (13%). Because of the higher prevalence of local lymph node metastasis in children and adolescents, a more radical treatment is recommended in this group than in adults, despite more favorable outcome of cases in less than 21 years age group. Since the extent of primary surgical treatment is closely related to overall prognosis, a preoperative diagnostic protocol including FNA cytodiagnosis as the initial test becomes essential in the management of thyroid neoplasms in young patients.[82]

According to Hosler et al,[83] the clinical utility of thyroid FNA in the pediatric patients has not been adequately addressed since this diagnostic technique is seldom performed in pediatric population. The frequency of malignany in thyroid FNAs from children and adolescents range from 4.9 to 47.6% (table 4) with an average of 13.3% [78, 79, 83-88] and the frequency of cases suspicious of malignancy also show a wide range (0-24.6%, average 12.1%). Papillary thyroid carcinoma (PTC) is the most common thyroid malignancy detected in FNA smears (figure 2) and in thyroidectomy specimens from adolescents. Of the 17 malignant aspirates from thyroid described by Amrikachi et al, [88] sixteen were PTC and one medullary carcinoma. Of the 20 suspicious aspirates reported by these authors, [88] seven were characterized as follicular neoplasm, 6 as PTC and one as follicular variant of PTC/follicular neoplasm. Of the malignant thyroid nodules from children and adolescents examined by histopathology following FNA in four studies, papillary thyroid carcinoma (PTC) was the most common (average 81.5%), followed by follicular carcinoma (11.1%), medullary carcinoma (2.8%), lymphoma (1.9%), Hürthle cell carcinoma (0.9%), mucoepidermoid carcinoma (0.9%), and sarcoma (0.9%).[83, 84, 87, 89]

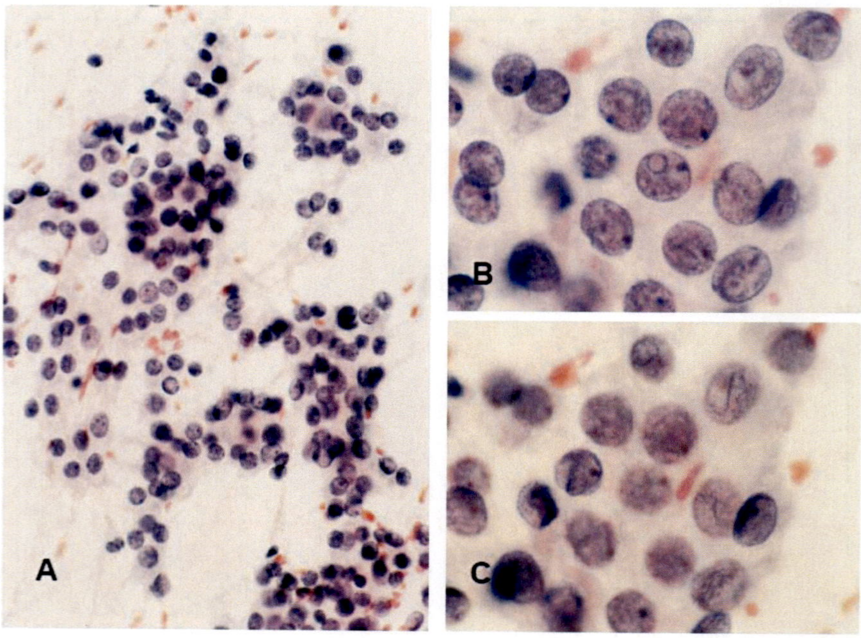

Figure 2. Papillary thyroid carcinoma (Follicular variant): FNA smears from the solitary nodule in the right lobe of thyroid in a 21-year-old woman. A. Microfollicular formation by follicular cells (Papanicolaou x 400). B. The neolastic follicular cells have fine chromatin and one intranuclear cytoplasmic inclusion (Papanicolaou x 1000). C. Same field as B shows nuclear grooves in a different plane (Papanicolaou x 1000).

FNAB is a safe and highly accurate method in the evaluation of thyroid nodules in children and adolescents.[79] Based on six FNA studies of thyroid, followed by histopathological examination of the nodules, [78, 79, 83, 85, 87, 88] the range and averages of sensitivity, specificity, and diagnostic accuracy of FNA were 60-100% (average 90.3%), 63-92% (average 80.4%), 80-90.4% (average 84.6%), respectively. FNA cytology was found to be superior to other preoperative diagnostic procedures in evaluation of thyroid nodules in children and adolescents. Corrias et al [87] reported 95% sensitivity, 86.3% specificity, and 90.4% accuracy of cytological examination as opposed to very low values of these parameters by clinically palpable nodule (e.g. 80%, 13.6%, and 45.2%, respectively) and imaging parameters (e.g. 70%, 40.9%, and 54.7%, respectively by US of solitary nodule). The sensitivity, specificity, and diagnostic accuracy of FNAB were 60%, 90%, and 80%, respectively in a study by Lugo-Vicente and Ortíz.[85] U-S achieved 80% sensitivity, 88% specificity, and 86% accuracy and radionucleotide scan (RNS) had success rate of 80%, 11%, and 26%, respectively for these parameters in this study.[85] According to Raab et al,[84] FNAB is useful in the management of pediatric thyroid nodules because of its high diagnostic accuracy and minimal invasiveness. Amrikachi et al[88] are of opinion that the acceptance of FNAB in the routine evaluation of young patients' thyroid nodules should reduce the number of unnecessary surgeries for benign thyroid disease.

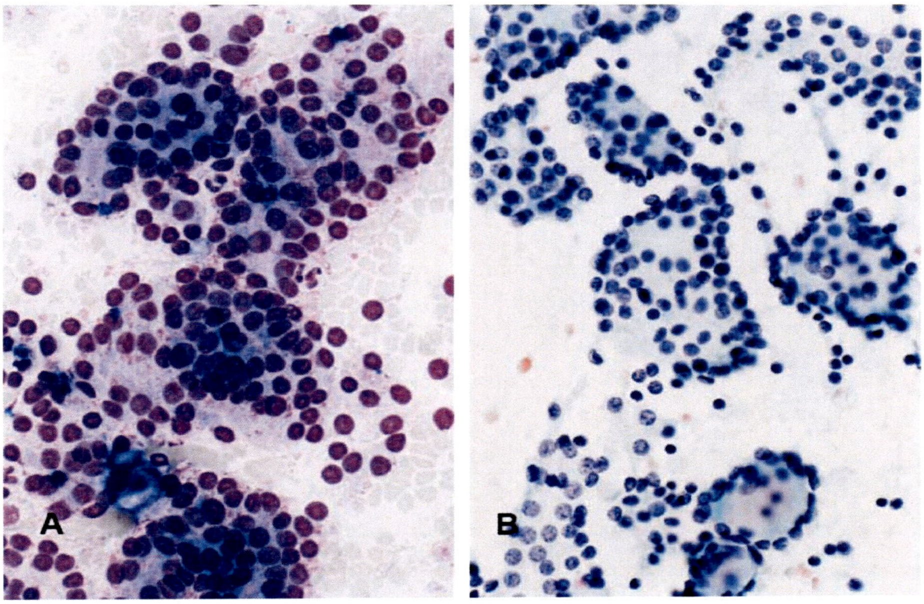

Figure 3. FNA smears from a 3x 3 cm nodule in the right lobe of thyroid in a 17-year-old adolescent female: A. Follicular cells are arranged as microfollicles (MGG x 400). B. Follicular cells arranged as microfollicles and macrofollicles (Papanicolaou x 400).

Limitations of FNA cytology in thyroid lesions includes failure/difficulty in differentiating diagnosis of follicular carcinoma from follicular adenoma since histologic criteria of capsular and vascular invasion can not be appreciated in FNA smears. Therefore, the term follicular neoplasm (figure 3) is utilized in cytology instead of adenoma or carcinoma. Further, follicular neoplasm has to be differentiated from hyperplastic nodule on one hand and follicular variant of papillary carcinoma on the other. Presence of occult/microscopic papillary thyroid carcinoma in colloid goiter and papillary carcinoma with cystic degeneration also adds to the diagnostic difficulty in cytology. According to Khurana et al, [90] solitary papillary hyperplastic thyroid nodules (SPHTNs), which are frequently encountered in children and adolescents, are likely to be misdiagnosed as papillary thyroid carcinoma. In all the three cases described by these authors, [90] the possibility of PTC was considered in FNA smears. Willgerodt et al [91] observed low sensitivity, specificity, and diagnostic accuracy of FNA biopsy of thyroid (78.9%, 63.6%, and 77.2%, respectively) and suggested a more aggressive diagnostic and therapeutic approach in children and adolescents than for adults.

Lymphadenopathy

Lymphadenopathy is a common problem in children and adolescents and its diagnosis by FNA is an easy, safe, and reliable procedure.[92] In a review of 6 studies (table 6) on FNA cytology diagnosis of lymphadenopathy in children and adolescents, [65, 92-96] malignancy was detected in 1.3 to 35.6% (average 5.6%) and the benign conditions including infections, inflammation, and reactive lymphadenopathy was diagnosed in 47.9 to 93.9% with an average of 87.7%. In four of the six studies, benign picture was observed in more than 80% cases. According to Ponder et al, [94] the percentage of suspicious or malignant diagnoses is greater in near adolescent and adolescent patients, comared to children. Since most lymphadenopathy cases subjected to FNA in children and adolescents reveal benign reactive conditions that fail to respond to antibiotics rather than proving to be malignant; the use of FNA can direct further testing, save time, expense, and morbidity for the patient, and reduce anxiety for the parents.[94]

The lymphoreticular malignancy dominates the malignant lymph node aspirates in children and adolescents and the metastatic lesions (figure 4) are rare. Of the 15 malignancy cases diagnosed by Chen et al [92] in FNA of lymph nodes, 9 were Hodgkin's lymphoma, 4 NHL or leukemic infiltrate and 2 metastatic tumors. Buchino and Jones [65] diagnosed 5 malignancies consisting of 2 Hodgkin's lymphaoma, I NHL, 1 leukemic infiltration, and 1 rhabdomyosarcoma. Handa et al, [96] observed 9 cases of malignancies in lymph node aspirates, which included 7 lymphomas, and 2 metastatic lesions.

Review of three studies on lymphadenopathy in children, adolescents, and young adults (table 7) revealed that the averages of sensitivity and specificity were high (92.8% and 94.5%, respectively).[65, 95, 97]

Table 6. Fine Needle Aspiration (FNA) of Lymph Nodes in Children and Adolescents

Author (s) and year	Age range (mean/median)	No of patients (No of FNAs)	Male: female	FNA cytodiagnosis			
				Benign	Suspicious	Malignant	Inadequate
Buchino and Jones (1994)[65]	10m-20yrs	119 (123)	76:43	103 (83.7)	2 (1.6)	5 (4.1)	13 (10.6)
Rios and Otoya (1999)[93]	3m-19yrs	90	-	83 (92.2)	0 (0.0)	5 (5.6)	2 (2.2)
Ponder et al (2000)[94]	≤ 21yrs	103 (106)	-	88 (83.0)	3 (2.8)	5 (4.7)	10 (9.4)
Van de Schoot et al (2001)[95]	15m-20yrs (9yrs)	64 (73)	35:29	35 (47.9)	0 (0.0)	26 (35.6)	12 (16.4)
Chen et al (2002)[92]	8m-19yrs	71	-	54 (76.1)	0 (0.0)	15 (21.1)	2 (2.8)
Handa et al (2003)[96]	≤14yrs	692	415:277	650 (93.9)	1 (0.1)	9 (1.3)	32 (4.6)
Total	3m-20yrs	1139 (1155)	-	1013 (87.7)	6 (0.5)	65 (5.6)	71 (6.1)

m= months, yrs= years.

Table 7. Efficacy of Fine Needle Aspiration (FNA) Cytology in Diagnosis of Lymphadenopathy in Children, Adolescents, and Youg Adults

Authors and year (Sites of FNA)	Age range (mean/median)	No of patients (FNAs)	Male: female	Diagnostic efficacy in percentages		
				Sensitivity	Specificity	Accuracy
Buchino and Jones (1994)[65]	10m-20yrs	119 (123)	76:43	100	97	98
Kardos et al (1989)[97]	≤30yrs	126 (127)	67:59	93	95	-
Van de Schoot et al (2001)[95]	15m-20yrs	64 (73)	35:29	*86	96	-
				†92	90	-
Total	10m-30yrs	309 (323)	178:131	92.8± 5.74	94.5± 3.11	-

M= months, yrs= years, * based on 39 cases of de novo lymphadenopathy with adequate material, ** based on 23 cases lymphadenopathy in cases with previous history of malignancy and adequate FNA material.

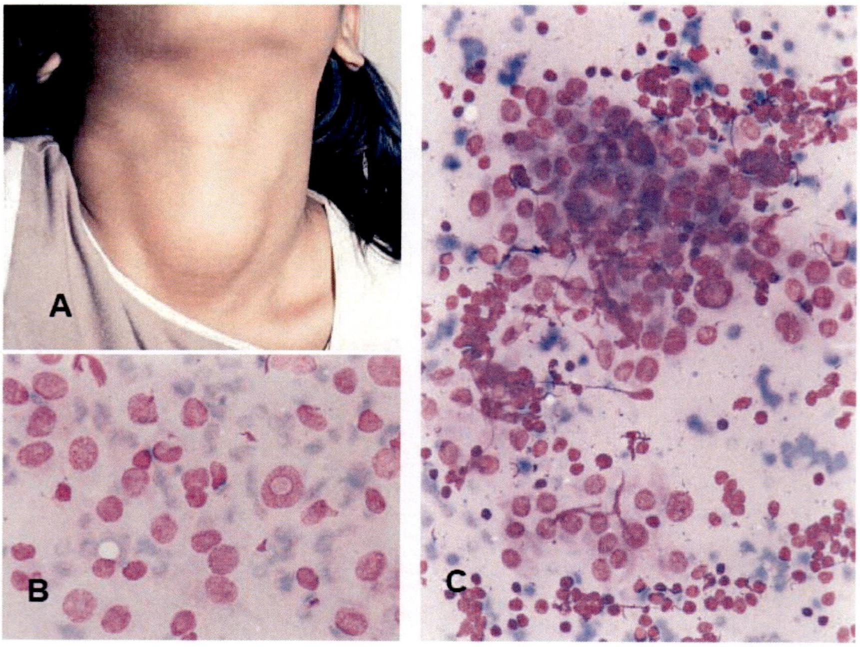

Figure 4. Papillary thyroid carcinoma with cervical lymph node metastasis in a 9-year-old-girl: A. Diffuse swelling of thyroid and left cervical lymphadenopathy. B. FNA smears from thyroid swelling shows tumor cells in dispersed form and an intranuclear cytoplasmic inclusion (MGG x 500). C. FNA smear from the lymph node shows lymphoid cells and groups of neoplastic cells, one of them having an intranuclear cytoplasmic inclusion (MGG x 480).

Lymphomas and Leukemias

Lymphomas are the most frequent cancers in western industrialized countries of the northern hemisphere and in Middle East, and occurred in substantial numbers in all other regions. Hodgkin lymphoma outnumbered non-Hodgkin's lymphomas in western industrialized countries, and leukemias were the most frequent diagnostic group among adolescents in India, East Asia and Latin America. [43] Data from population based cancer registries in India [48] revealed that lymphomas and leukemias were the most common malignancy (34.1%) in females aged 10-19 years; the frequencies among 10-14 yrs and 15-19 yrs-old females were 39.6 and 29.7%, respectively.

FNA cytology remains the first line of investigations (screening test) used in cases of lymphadenopathy. Besides initial diagnosis of lymphoma and its subtyping, it helps in detection of residual disease, recurrences and progression of low-grade to high-grade lymphoma, and helps in staging of the disease. [98] In a study of 56 NHL in childhood and adolescence by Mann et al [62] the common non-Hodgkin lymphoma types observed were Burkitt lymphoma (23 cases), lymphoblastic lymphoma (22), and large cell lymphomas (11 cases) consisting of 3 ALCL and 8 diffuse large B-cell lymphoma. Burkitt-lymphoma is predominantly a tumor of childhood and adolescence. Among 213 African Burkitt lymphoma patients, the ages ranged from 3-45 years (median= 9 yrs) at diagnosis and male-female ratio was1.8: 1.[99] The Indian Burkitt-type lymphoma patients were, however, older than the

African counter part with ages ranging from 2 to 80 years (median= 22 years) and male to female ratio of 4:1.[100] Although younger age of the patients and tumors involving jaw bone is the commonest presentation in African patients,[101] involvement of abdominal viscera is most common in American (56.2% to 76.7%)[102, 103] and Indian cases (48.5%).[100] Massive bilateral breast tumors have been described as a characteristic feature of Burkitt's lymphoma in females of child bearing age, particularly women during pregnancy and lactation.[104] Diagnosis of Burkitt's lymphoma is based on fine needle aspiration cytology of easily accessible mass in a large majority of patients.[99] The exclusive sites in an adolescent female in which FNA cytologic feature can help to arrive at a diagnosis of Burkitt type lymphoma rather than an epithelial malignancy are ovary (figure 5) and breast.[105]

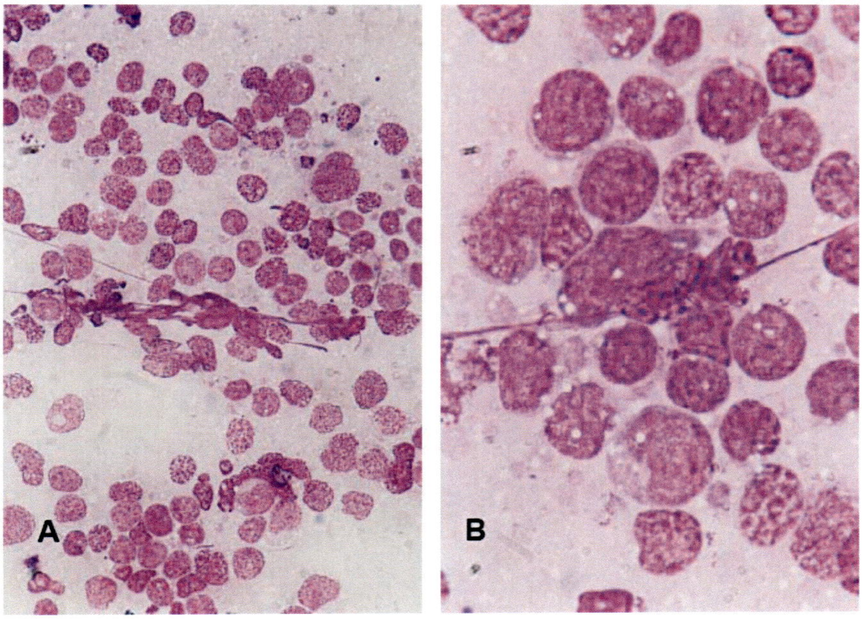

Figure 5. Non-Hodgkin lymphoma (Burkitt-type): FNA smear from ovarian mass in a 20-year-old-woman. A. Lymphoma cells along with a few lymphoglandular bodies in the background (MGG x 400). B. Higher magnification of the lymphoma cells reveals small non-cleaved type cells with cytoplasmic vacuolations due to neutral lipids (MGG x 1000).

Besides Bukitt's lymphoma, the other lymphoreticular malignancies which commonly affect adolescents and young adults are lymphoblastic lymphoma and anaplastic large cell lymphoma (ALCL). Wakely and Kornstein [106] reported 8 lymphoblastic lymphomas and 6 lymphoblastic leukemias and two aspirates from lymphoblastic transformation of CML in children aged 10 months to 15 years (mean age 10.5 years). These cases were diagnosed by superficial FNA from sites such as lymph nodes (9 cases), soft tissues of neck (four), parotid gland (one), buttock (one) and forehead (one). The age of the 31 cases lymphoblastic lymphoma patients reported by Das et al [107] ranged from 5 to 70 years (median= 24 years) and male to female ratio was 25:6. Anaplastic large cell lymphoma (ALCL), especially its small cell variant is also frequent in childhood and adolescence. Ng et al [108] detected 6 common and 2 small cell variant of ALCL among 8 patients including 2 adolescent cases

(13-year-old male and 17-year-old female). In a study of 9 patients of small cell variant of ALCL, [109] the age ranged from 0.3-40 years (median 14 years). In contrast to classic type of ALCL, which is sometimes mistaken for carcinoma or sarcoma, the small cell variant may be misdiagnosed as a reactive lesion without a high index of suspicion.[110]

Hodgkin lymphoma can be diagnosed by FNA cytology based on characeteristic cytologic features (figure 6). A wide variation is observed in age and sex distribution in Hodgkin lymphoma cases. Of the nine Hodgkin lymphoma cases diagnosed or suspected in FNA smears from children by Chen et al, [92] six were adolescent female patients with ages ranging from 16 to 19 years. In the study by Das et al,[111] the age of the patients ranged from 4 to 85 years with a median of 25 years and male to female ratio was 6.7:1, indicating that more than half of the patients were children, adolescents and young adults. In a recent study on WHO classification of Hodgkin's lymphoma, a bimodal age distribution with a young adult age group of 18 to 44 years (median, 25 years) and an older patient group, from 45 to 64 years (median 58 years) was reported.[112]

Analysis of cyto- and histological discrepant cases revealed that the common lesions which can create confusion in the diagnosis of NHL in FNA smears are Hodgkin's disease, small cell anaplastic carcinoma, reactive hyperplasia of lymph node, and some soft tissue tumors.[113] Of the 43 discrepant cases described by Das et al,[113] eight were observed in the age group ≤ 21 years.

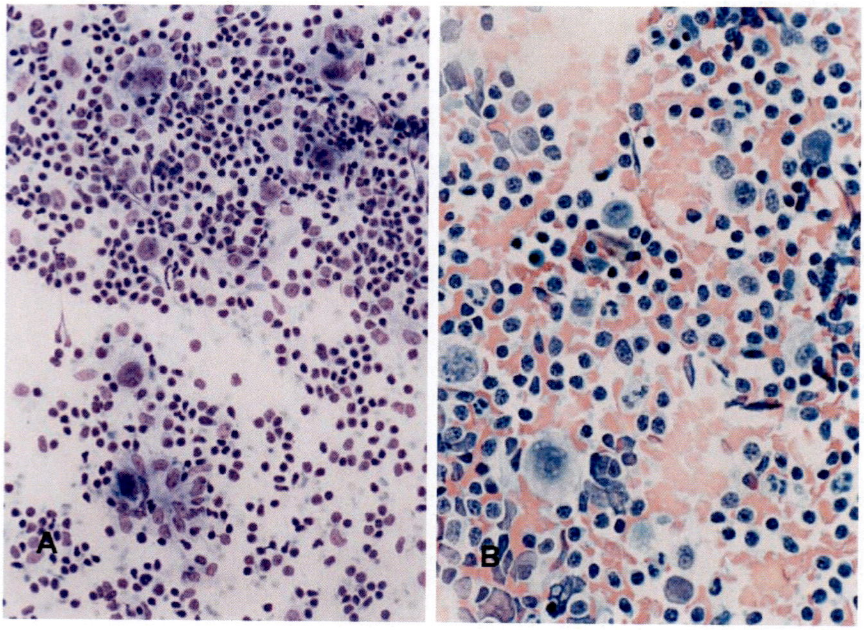

Figure 6. Hodgkin lymphoma: FNA smear from left cervical lymph node in a 21-year-old woman. A. Hodgkin cells and one R-S cell among reactive lymphoid cells (MGG x 200). B. Hodgkin and RS cells have prominent nucleoli (Papanicolaou x 400).

Breast Cancers

According to Neinstein, [114] breast cancer cases are rare in women less than 20 years old and uncommon in women less than 30 years old. In the data from population based cancer registries of India (1991-96), breast cancers constituted 4.1% of all cancers in the 15-19 year age group among females.[48] In England breast cancer among adolescent females (15-19 age group) was 0.89% of all cancers[7] but no case of breast cancer was recorded among adolescent females in this age group in the report by Desandes et al.[1] West et al[115] also did not observe any breast cancer cases among 74 children and adolescents referred for surgical evaluation of breast masses. Although breast cancer is rare in childhood and adolescence, breast concerns among patients in this age group are common.[116]

According to De Silva and Brandt, [117] primary carcinoma of the breast has been reported in 39 children (3-19 years of age) and over 80% of these patients were diagnosed with juvenile secretory carcinoma, the remainder having intraductal carcinoma. However, in another review of literature, published between 1888 and 1972, there were 74 cases of breast cancer in children[118] and majority of them were secretary (juvenile) type but other adult types of cancer have also been described. A 40-year single-institution experience of all breast cancer patients reported by Corpron et al, [119] revealed 16 adolescent breast cancer cases including 10 adenocarcinomas, 4 cystosarcoma phyllodes, and 2 metastatic lesions. These 10 adenocarcinomas included invasive ductal, invasive lobular, signet ring and secretory adenocarcinoma. Rivera-Hueto et al[120] found four cases of adolescent females (< 20 years) with breast cancer from their records over a period of 24 years, which included an invasive ductal carcinoma associated with fibroadenoma, 2 secretory carcinomas, and one invasive lobular-type carcinoma.

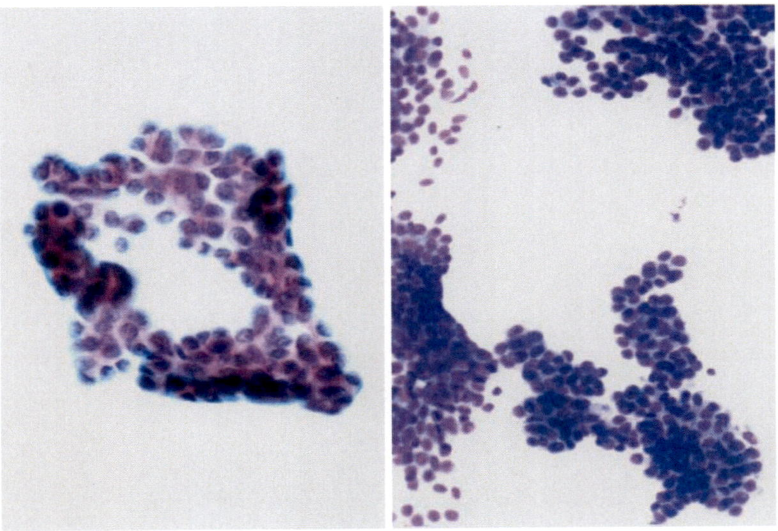

Figure 7. Duct papilloma with cytologic features suspicious of malignancy in a 12-year-old girl, who presented with serosanguinous nipple discharge and a 3 x 3 x 2 cm subareolar mobile lump. A. Nipple discharge shows a cluster of ductal cells with vague papillary formation and cytologic atypia (Papanicolaou x 400). B. FNA smear from the sub-areolar lump shows a sheet of benign duct cells and papillary clusters with atypical epithelial hyperplasia (MGG X 200).

Reports on FNA cytologic diagnosis of breast cancer in adolescent females are rare. Occasional cases of secretory carcinomas have been described in FNA smears from breasts of children and adolescent females.[121-123] The differential diagnosis of secretory carcinoma in children includes abnormal thelarche.[121] A case described by Nonomura et al [123] was associated with juvenile papillomatosis. According to Rosen [118] about 10% of patients with juvenile papillomatosis are associated with breast carcinoma, the histlogical types being intraductal carcinoma, lobular carcinoma in situ, infiltrating ductal carcinoma, and secretary carcinoma. We suspected malignancy in a duct papilloma case with atypical hyperplasia in a 12-year-old girl (figure 7). However, the histology of the resected mass turned out to be a papilloma with florid epithelial proliferation.

Primary sarcoma of the breast is rare and constitutes 0.5 to 1% of all mammary malignancies.[124] Ninteen of breast sarcoma cases studied by Pandey et al[124] revealed two cases in adolescent females aged 12 years, which were diagnosed as spindle cell sarcoma and embryonal rhabdomyosarcoma, respectively. Diagnosis of bilateral rhabdomyosarcoma in an adolescent girl by FNA cytology has been reported by Torres and Ferrer.[125] Like primary sarcomas, primary breast lymphoma is a rare form of localized extranodal lymphoma, which constitutes 0.18% of breast malignancies and is usually of large B-cell type.[126] Rare cases of Burkitt-type lymphomas affecting adolescent females have been reported in the literature[127-129] and the report on cytodiagnosis of this neoplasm in adolescent females is also extremely rare (figure 8).[105]

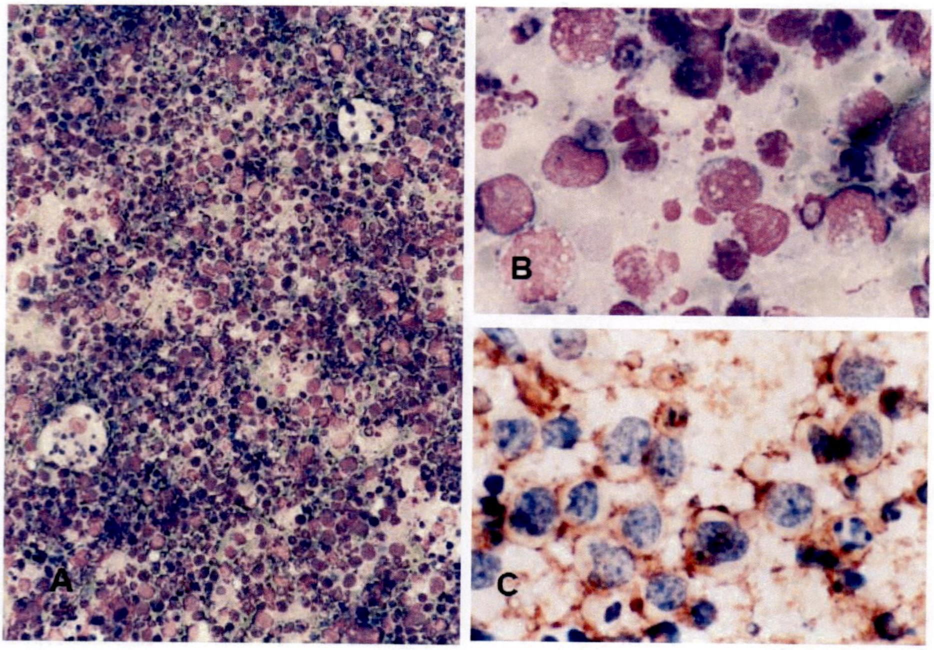

Figure 8. Burkitt-type lymphoma: A. FNA smear from a left breast mass in a 20-year-old woman. A: lymphoma cells are interspersed with non-neoplastic histiocytes containing cell debris (MGG x 200). B. Tumor cells have cytoplasmic vacuoles due to neutral lipids (MGG x 400). C: The lymphoma cells are positive for B-cell marker (L 26 x 1000).

Metastatic malignancies in breasts of children and adolescent females have been reported with primary hepatocellular carcinoma, Hodgkin's lymphoma, non-Hodgkin's lymphoma, neuroblastoma, and rhabdomyosarcoma, particularly the alveolar variant.[117] Shukla et al[130] described 15 cases of metastatic breast neoplasms, which constituted 1.47% of all malignant tumors of the breast diagnosed by FNA. Included among these 15 cases were 4 adolescent females with rhabdomyosarcomas (three embryonal and one alveolar) aged 13 to 16 years (median 15 years) and a 10-year-old girl with acute myeloid leukemia. Tamiolakis et al [131] reported the touch imprint cytology of bilateral metastatic rhabdomyosarcoma to the breast in an adolescent female.

Body Cavities

Most of the publications on cytodiagnosis of body cavity mass lesions are on adult patients. A few reports are based on all age groups including children and adolescents[132-135] and exclusive reports on FNA cytodiagnosis of body cavity (thorax, abdomen, and pelvis) lesions in children and adolescents are relatively rare (table 8).[136-138] The frequency of malignancies in these studies varies widely. Cahill et al [137] detected malignancy in 18.7% of aspirates from the lungs and Shabb et al [132] found 81.0% mediastinal aspirates to be malignant. The frequency of malignancy from abdominal visceras like liver and spleen ranged from 33.3% to 65.5%. [133-135,138] Shabb et al [132] described 34 malignant tumors from the mediastinum, which included 4 male patients aged 10 to 17 years (median 14.5 years) with the diagnosis of nonHodgkin lymphoma (3 cases) and Hodgkin lymphoma (1 case) but the youngest female with a malignant tumor (Hodgkin lymphoma) in this study was 22 years old. Nagakawa et al, [56] reported a basaloid squamous cell carcinoma in an 18-year-old woman (youngest patient), diagnosed by transbronchial FNA cytology as primary suamous cell carcinoma. Das et al, [136] reported malignancy in 32.2% of FNAs from the thoracic and abdominal visceras. The 39 pediatric and adolescent cancers of thorax and abdomen diagnosed by these authors[136] included 27 small round cell tumors, 7 malignant germ cell tumors, and 5 miscellaneous malignancies. The malignant neoplasms in the adolescent age groups (15-19 years) were Ewing's sarcoma, non-Hodgkin's lymphoma, germ cell tumors, Hodgkin's disease, and hepatocellular carcinoma but no bronchogenic carcinoma was observed. Fifteen malignant pediatric abdominal masses diagnosed by Obers and Phillip [139] included 9 nephroblastomas, and single examples of neuroblastoma, hepatoblastoma, NHL, rhabdomyosarcoma, renal carcinoma, and malignant rhabdoid tumor. Baksi et al,[138] diagnosed hepatic lesions in pediatric patient diagnosed by FNA cytology, which included hepatoblastoma (7 cases), hepatocellular carcinoma (4), undifferentiated embryonal sarcoma of liver (3), and metastasis (6). In children aged 1 to 14 years, Radhika et al [140] described 32 renal lesions with both FNA cytology and histopathology, and the diagnoses were Wilms' tumor (25 cases), clear cell sarcoma of kidney (4), and one case each of renal cell carcinoma, rhabdoid tumor, and yolk sac tumor. The sensitivity, specificity, and diagnostic accuracy of FNA cytology in body cavity lesions (table 9) range from 90.2-95.1%, 100%, and 93.7-96.9%, respectively.[133,134,138]

Table 8. FNA Cytology Diagnosis of Thoracic, Abdominal, and Pelvic Organs in Children, Adolescents, and Adults

Author (s) and year	Site	Age range (Mean/median)	No of patients (FNAs)	Male: Female	Cytodiagnosis: No (%)			
					Benign	Suspicious	Malignancy	Inadequate
Shabb et al (1998)[132]	Med	10-70yrs* (41yrs)	42	25:17	5 (11.9)	0 (0.0)	34 (81.0)	3 (7.1)
Cahill et al (2004)[137]	Lung	6-20yrs (10.8yrs)	64** (75)	32:32	50 (66.7)	5 (6.7)	14 (18.7)	6 (8.0)
Guo et al (2002)[134]	Liver	1-85 yrs (61yrs)	114 (119)	65:49	32 (26.9)	8 (6.7)	78 (65.5)	1 (0.8)
Baksi et al (2006)[138]	Liver	9d-14yrs	36 (41)	29:7	12 (29.3)	0 (0.0)	20 (48.8)	9 (22.0)
Kumar et al (2007)[135]	Spleen	3-71yrs	48	25:23	32 (66.7)	0 (0.0)	16 (33.3)	0 (0.0)
Guo et al (2001)[133]	Pelvis, RP	2-79yrs (55)	64 (68)	24:40	22 (32.4)	7 (10.3)	37 (54.4)	2 (2.9)
Das et al (1993)[136]	Abd, thorax	20d- 18yrs	121	73:48	53 (43.8)	1 (0.8)	39 (32.2)	28 (23.1)
Total		20d-85yrs	489 (514)	273:216	206 (40.1)	21 (4.1)	238 (46.3)	49 (9.5)

*Included 4 males <20yrs (1 HD, 3 NHL) but youngest female was 22 yrs (HD), Med= mediastinum, RP= retroperitoneum, Abd= abdomen

** Core biopsy in 56, FNA in 15, and both in 4.

Table 9. Efficacy of Fine Needle Aspiration (FNA) in Diagnosis of Abdominal Visceras in Children, Adolescents, and Adults

Authors and year	Site of FNA	Age range (mean/median)	No of patients (FNAs)	Male: female	Diagnostic efficacy in percentages		
					Sensitivity	Specificity	Diagn accuracy
Baksi et al (2006)[138]	Liver	9d-14yrs	36 (41)	29:7	95.0	100	96.9
Guo et al (2002)[134]	Liver	1-85yrs (66yrs)	114(119)	65:49	95.1	100	96.4
Guo et al (2001)[133]	Pelvis and RP	2-79yrs (55yrs)	64 (68)	24:40	90.2	100	93.7
Total	-	9d-85yrs	214 (228)	118:96	93.4±2.80	100.0±0.00	95.7±1.72

D=days, yrs=years. RP= retroperitoneum

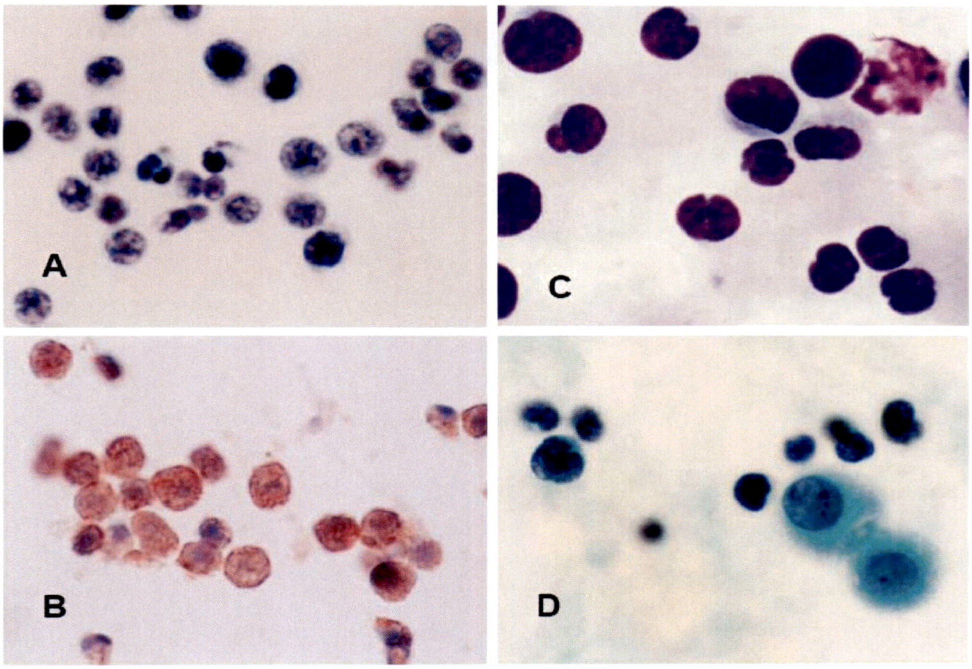

Figure 9. NHL in pleural effusion: A. Lymphoblastic lymphoma: Pleural effusion smear from a 6-year-old boy already diagnosed as a case of NHL from lymph node FNA. Smear shows lymphoblasts with lobulated nuclei (Papanicolaou x 1000). B. Diffuse positive reaction for CD3 in most of the lymphoblasts shown in figure 8A (x 1000). C. 15-year-old female presented pleural effusion and an anterior mediastinal mass, diagnosed as NHL by FNA cytology. Neoplastic lymphoid cells were mostly cleaved and a few with lobulated nuclei (MGG x 1000). D. Lymphoma cells and two mesothelial cells in the case shown in Figure 8C (Papanicolaou x 1000).

Like FNA cytology, exfoliative cytology has been utilized for diagnosis of malignancies inchildren and adolescents. According to Hallman and Geisinger [141] almost all pediatric effusions were benign but a few malignant pediatric effusions were caused by neoplasms of small cell type, mostly lymphoreticular. Of the 32 ascitic fluid, 45 pleural effusions, and 4 pericardial fluids studied by these authors, [141] malignancies were detected in 13 samples (11 patients) and these included 8 lymphoreticular malignancies, 1 neuroblastoma, 1 Wilms' tumor, and 1 malignant mesothelioma. In a study of 21 pleural effusions in lymphoma patients reported by Das et al [142] from India, the age of the patients ranged from 5-60 years, with a median of 23 years and male to female ratio of 6:1. Positive cytology reports in 17 cases included lymphoblastic lymphoma in 12 cases, follicular center cell lymphoma (FCC) in three and leukemias in two. The adolescent females included among positive cases were an 18-year-old with lymphoblastic lymphoma and and a 15-year-old girl with small cleaved cell type of FCC lymphoma. In another report on 22 lymphomatous effusions by Das et al [143] from Kuwait, the lymphoblastic lymphoma cases (figure 9) were very few (2 cases). The age of these 22 patients ranged from 5-83 years (median 46 years and male to female ratio of 13:9) and among them, there were 3 male children aged 5-11 years and an adolescent female aged 15 years. Since brain and testes are considered pharmacological sanctuaries for leukemic lymphoblasts during hematological remission of childhood ALL, bone marrow biopsy, spinal fluid sampling, and testicular FNA are performed as part of end therapy evaluation in these cases.[144] Salzburg et al,[145] found 6% childhood/adolescent NHL patients with CNS positive status and CNS disease was the strongest predictor of relapse in Burkitt lymphoma (BL) and B-ALL patients with advanced-stage disease.

Female Genital Cancer

As per the data of the Department of Defense Tumor Registry (USA), the most common primary gynecological site in women aged 25 years or younger was ovary (46%), followed by cervix (43%) and the most common histologic types were germ cell tumors for ovary, squamous cell carcinoma for cervix, choriocarcinoma for uterus, and squamous cell carcinoma for vulva/vagina.[146]

In a study of 10, 296 pediatric and adolescent Papanicolaou smears in patients from northern New England with age ranging from 10 to 19 years, the cytologic diagnoses were atypical squamous cells of undetermined significance (ASCUS) in 9.75%, squamous intraepithelial lesion (SIL) in 3.77% (LSIL 2.5%, HSIL 0.7%, and SIL undetermined 0.6%), and atypical glandular cells of undetermined significance (AGUS) in 0.06% but no case of malignancy was found.[63] Case et al[12] observed that the rate of CIN 2/3 in histology in adolescent patients with ASCUS, LSIL, and HSIL was 35%, 36%, and 50%, respectively but no patients were diagnosed with cervical carcinoma. Of the 501 cytologically deteced cervical dysplasia cases subjected to biopsy and histology, 324 (65%) had CIN I or less, and 177 (35%) had $\geq$ CIN 2. With or without treatment, 5% patients progressed with no cancer.[147] The afore said studies [12, 63, 147] give an impression that cervical lesion upto high-grade SIL may be found in adolescent females but frank invasive cancer does not occur. In extremely rare instances, however, primary or metastatic adenocarcinoma of the cervix has been diagnosed by cytology in adolescent females.[148, 149] In the Department of Defense tumor registry data, there were 8 cases of cervical carcinoma (5 squamous, 3 adeno) in patients younger than 20 years of age, with an additional 12 histologically unspecified cases in the ACTUR (Automated Central Tumor Registry) database.[146]

Human papillomavirus (HPV) infection is a sexual transmitted disease associated with cervical dysplasia and cancer. In a study conducted at three urban adolescent clinics administered by the Denver Departments of Health and Hospital, predominantly on low-income adolescent females aged 12-18 years (mean 16.8 years) cervical HPV was the most prevalent STD in the population, detected in 15.6% subjects, followed by infection with C. tracomatis (11.0%), N. gonorrhoea (7.1%), and T. vaginalis. Most prevalent were the higher-risk HPV types 16/18 (7.3%), followed by 31/33/35 (4.7%) and 6/11 (3.5%).[10] Vetrano et al [15] observed that the sites most frequently affected by HPV lesions in adolescent females were vulva, perianus and perineum, and the cervix. A few studies relate HPV infection to cervical precancerous lesions in adolescent female population. When genital wart on examination, LSIL in cytology or HPV DNA was considered as indicators of HPV infection by Jamison et al,[10] 24% had any manifestations of genital HPV infections. Kahn et al[13] observed 51% HPV positive status and 23% with an abnormal Pap test among 100 adolescent females. Fifteen percent of adolescent patients with ASCUS and known high-risk HPV infection were found to have CIN 2 or 3 in histology of colposcopic directed biopsy and these high-grade lesions among adolescents were small and single.[64]

The SEER incidence of ovarian malignancies was about 6 per 1000,000 in the age group 16-20 years and the mortality rates were 0.1 per 100,000 for patients aged 15-19 years. The high survival rates are likely attributable to the preponderance of germ cell and borderline tumors in this age group.[146] Malignant ovarian tumors accounts for 4.2 to 11.4% of all ovarian neoplasms in children and/or adolescents.[150-152] Of the neoplastic lesion reported by Deligeoroglou et al, [150] germ cell tumors were most frequent (62.5%) followed by epithelial (20.8%) anf sex cord-stromal tumors (16.7%). In an exclusive study of 109 germ cell tumors in young and adolescent girls,[153] mature cystic teratoma, gonadoblastoma, and malignant tumors accounted for 92, 4, and 13 cases, respectively. The 13 malignant germ cell tumors comprised 7 dysgerminoma, 3 immature teratomas, 2 endodermal sinus tumors (EST), and one embryonal carcinoma.

The sensitivity, specificity, and diagnostic accuracy of FNA cytology for diagnosis of gynecological malignancies ranged from 65-100%, 92-100%, and 73-95.2%, respectively.[154-156] Ganjei et al,[157] achieved sensitivity, specificity, and diagnostic accuracy of 75%, 100%, and 96%, respectively for malignant cysts in a study of neoplastic and non-neoplastic ovarian cysts by aspiration cytology.

Bone and Soft Tissue Sarcomas

In France the incidence of soft tissue sarcoma (STS) in adolescent females (15-19 years) was 12.1 per million individuals.[1] The incidence was 1.8 per 100,000 among black adolescent females in USA.[9] In England soft tissue sarcomas constituted 6.1% of all cancers in adolescent females, and these included fibrosarcoma (1.3%), rhabdomyosarcoma (1.8%) and other STS (3.0%).[7] In India bone and soft tissue tumors were 16.7% of all malignancies among adolescent females.[48]

FNA biopsy of bone lesions is a reliable and easily performed diagnostic test for metastatic and primary bone tumors.[158] However, exclusive studies on FNA diagnosis of bone and soft tissue malignancies in children, adolescents and young adults are very few.[159-164] In most of the studies, children and adolescents form only part of the patients from all age groups.[158, 165-167] There is a wide variation in frequency of malignancy in fine needle aspirates from bone and soft tissues (table 10); [158, 159, 161, 165-167] the values ranged from 30.3% to 88.7% (average, 58%). There is also a wide variation in frequency of primary versus metastatic lesion in FNA diagnosis of bone tumors. Bommer et al[158] observed 18.6% primary and 81.4% metaststaic carcinomas but the ratio of primary to metastatic lesions was 3:2 in a report by Handa et al.[167]

Table 10. Fine Needle Aspiration (FNA) Cytodiagnosis of Bone and Soft Tissue Tumors in Children, Adolescents, and Adults

Author (s) and year	Site	Age range (Mean /median)	No of patients (FNAs)	Male: Female	Cytodiagnosis: Nos and (%)			
					Benign	Suspicious	Malignancy	Inadequate
Bomer et al (1997)[158]	Bone	5-95yrs	427 (450)	237:190	157(34.9)	11 (2.4)	215 (47.8)	67 (14.9)
Wakely et al (1990)[159]	Soft tissue	2m-29yrs (16yrs)	22 (28)	11:10¶	7 (25.0)	1 (3.6)	20 (71.4)	0 (0.0)
Wakely and Kneisl (2000)[165]	Soft tissue	12-88yrs (50yrs)	77 (82)	46: 31	32 (39.0)	2 (2.4)	42 (51.2)	6 (7.3)
Treaba et al (2002)[166]	Bone*	14-86yrs (64yrs)	187	114:73	12 (6.4)	0 (0.0)	166 (88.7)	9 (4.8)
Handa et al (2005)[167]	Bone	5-70yrs	66	33:33	34 (51.5)	0 (0.0)	20 (30.3)	12 (18.2)
Kilpatrick et al (1998)[161]	Bone and soft tissue	≤19yrs	32 (33)	20:12	2 (6.1)	0 (0.0)	28 (84.8)	3 (9.1)
Total			811 (846)	461:349¶	244 (28.8)	14 (1.7)	491 (58.0)	97 (11.5)

*In case with previous history of malignancy, ¶Information about sex was not available in one case.

In a study of 33 consecutive FNA biopsies of bone and soft tissue tumors in children (≤ 19 years age), there were 28 primary and 5 metastatic lesions, including osteosarcoma (8 patients), rhabdomyosarcoma (5), neuroblastoma (5), Ewing's sarcoma/ PNET (4), Langerhans cell histiocytosis (3), and one each case of synovial sarcoma, undifferentiated sarcoma, infantile myofibromatosis, fibroma, chondroblastoma, chondromyxoid fibroma, and desmoplastic small round-cell tumor.[161] Skoog et al[168] diagnosed soft issue tumors and osteo/chondrosarcoma in 14 females and 14 males patients (age range, 2-84 years) and among them, there were five females in their childhood and adolescence with age ranging from 2 to 18 years (median 17 years). The cytodiagnosis in these five cases included malignant schwannoma, osteosarcoma, chondrosarcoma, cranial fascitis, and fibromatosis in one case each.

Among bone tumors, Ewing's sarcoma appears to be primarily a tumor of childhood and adolescence. Udayakumar et al, [169] performed FNA on 57 Ewing's sarcoma cases (34 males and 23 females), which included 70.6% of males and 69.6% of females in their childhood and adolescence (≤ 19 years). Fröstad et al, [164] diagnosed Ewing family of tumors (EFT) in 22 patients and EFT/neuroblastoma in one patient by FNA cytology. The age of the patients ranged from 0.7 to 20.2 years (median 14.4 yrs). Histopathology performed in 17 of these cases revealed EFT in 13, necrosis in 3 and osteosarcoma in one. The findings indicate the superiority of aspirates in sampling this neoplasm. Among 15 skeletal osteosarcoma patients, aged 10 to 58 yrs, diagnosed by FNA cytology, Nicol et al [170] observed 4 male children aged 10- 14 yrs (median 12 yrs) and two females aged 10 and 16 yrs. Domanski and Åkerman [171] studied the FNA reports of 59 hisologically proved osteosarcomas (57 high-grade and 2 low-grade), which included osteosarcoma in 28, suspicious of osteosarcoma in 16, sarcoma NOS in 4, metastatic carcinoma in one and inconclusive results in the remaining 10. These included 33 male and 26 female patients with age ranging from 3 to 84 years.

Wakely et al, [159] studied metachronous soft-tissue masses in 22 children and young adults, and diagnosed malignancies in 20 out of 28 fine needle aspirates, comprising sarcomas (13 cases), seminoma (2), lymphoma/leukemia (2), melanoma (1), neuroblastoma (1), and undifferentiated neoplasm (1). In a subsequent report on FNA diagnosis of soft tissue masses in all age groups by Wakely and Kneisl, [165] the malignant aspirates comprised 24 sarcomas (57.1%), 9 carcinomas (21.4%), 6 malignant lymphoma (14.3%), and 3 melanomas (7.1%). Rhabdomyosarcoma (RMS) is the most common soft tissue sarcoma of children under 15 years of age, adolescents and young adults.[162] Atahan et al,[162] could diagnose 43 rhabdomyosarcomas by fine needle aspiration (37 cases) and touch imprints (6 cases), and could subtype these tumors into alveolar RMS (n=21), embryonal RMS (n=15), and botryoid RMS (n=7) by characteristic cytomorphological features alone. Synovial sarcoma (SS) is also a well defined neoplastic disease of adolescents and young adults.[163] Viguer et al,[163] studied the cytologic material in 11 histologically proven synovial sarcoma cases aged 11-68 years (mean 28.1 years) and male to female ratio of 3:8. The cytodiagnosis in these cases was synovial sarcoma in 9 cases, spindle cell sarcoma in one and low-grade sarcoma in one. Included in this group were 4 adolescent females aged 11-21 years (mean 15.7 years).

Table 11. Efficacy of Fine Needle Aspiration (FNA) Cytology in Diagnosis of Bone and Soft Tissue Tumors in Children, Adolescents, and Adults

Authors and year	Site of FNA	Age range (mean/median)	No of patients (FNAs)	Male: female	Diagnostic efficacy in percentages		
					Sensitivity	Specificity	Diagn accuracy
Wakely et al (1990)[159]	Soft tissue	2m-29yrs (16yrs)	22 (28)	11:10¶	100	88	96
Bomer et al (1997)[158]	Bone	5-95yrs	427 (450)	237:190	95.7	99.3	97.1
Wakely and Kneisl (2000)[165]	Soft tissue	12-88yrs (50yrs)	77 (82)	46:31	100	97	-
Dodd et al (2002)[178]	Bone	10-86yrs	40	26:14	65	-	95
Total		2m-95yrs	566 (600)	320:245¶	90.2±16.91	94.8±5.97	96.0±1.05

¶ Information about sex was not available in ine patient, m= months, yrs= years.

Besides rhabomyosarcoma and synovial sarcoma, the other malignant soft tissue sarcoma of children is the malignant peripheral nerve sheath tumor (malignant schwannoma).[160] However, there are only occasional cases of this malignancy diagnosed cytologically.[168] Soft tissue sarcomas like malignant fibrous histiocytoma (MFH), liposarcoma (LS), and leiomyosarcoma (LMS) are largely tumors of adult individuals but a few cases belong to adolescent age group, the age range in cytologically diagnosed cases being 17-85 years for LMS, [172] 15-88 and 8-92 years, respectively in two studies on MFH[173,174] and 15 to 90 years for LS.[175] FNA cytodiagnosis of rare cases of recurrent leimyosarcoma in children and adolescents [176,177] appear to be easy but the primary tumor may give rise to diagnostic difficulty in FNA smears. Of the 96 histologically proven leimyosarcomas from 68 patients, only 23 were diagnosed as LMS by FNA cytology by Klijanienko et al [172] the other cytodignostic labels being sarcoma NOS (44 cases), fibrosarcoma (13), fibromyxosarcoma (5), malignant fibrous histiocytoma (3), miscellaneous types of sarcomas (4), and supicious/unsatisfactory (4). Similarly, of the 44 primary MFH reported by Klijanienko et al, [174] only 6 were diagnosed as MFH at original cytodiagnosis and the remaining were diagnosed as sarcoma NOS and miscellaneous sarcomas.

According to Kilpatrick et al, [161] the use of FNA biopsy in the initial evaluation of bone and soft tissue tumors is controvertial. However, FNA is sufficient to provide the diagnosis of osteosarcoma prior to definitive treatment when interpreted in conjunction with imaging studies and clinical findings. [178] With adequate FNAB specimens from bone and soft tissue tumors in children and adolescents, a histogenetic specific diagnosis was rendered in 27 (93%) of 29 cases by Kilpatrick et al [161] and all were correctly recognized as either benign or malignant. The aspirates correctly identified malignancy in 49 (83%) of osteogenic sarcomas in a study by Domanski and Åkerman.[171] For bone and soft issue tumors, the sensitivity, specificity, and diagnostic accuracy range from 65-100%, 88-100%, and 95-97.1%, respectively (table 11).[158, 159, 165, 178]

'Melanoma

Melanona is the commonest cancer among adolescents in Australia and Newzealand and moderately frequent in many other, predominantly white populations but rarely seen elsewhere.[43] Bütter et al[179] reported 12 cases of cutaneous melanomas in children aged 0.3 to 17.9 years (mean age 8.5 years); the site distribution in these cases was extremity (7 cases), trunk (4), and head and neck (1). In a study by Roaten et al, [180] sentinel lymph node biopsy was successful in all the 20 cases of melanomas in adolescent patients younger than 21 years, and 8 (40%) were found to have metastasis within sentinel lymph node. FNA with US aid has been utilized to get a quick diagnosis and select patients for sentinel lymph node biopsy in melanoma patients. A review by van Rijk et al[181] shows that the results of most FNA studies on this subject are far from encouraging, with sensitivity ranging from 6% to 39% and specificity from 99.8% to 100%, and the tumor positive nodes 18 to 27%. In their own material, van Rijk et al, [181] however, observed higher sensitivity of FNAC and specificity (71% and 100%, respectively), and 12% patients were spared sentinel lymph node biopsy because of FNA.

Small Round Cell Tumors

Small round cell tumors (SRCTs) are a group of malignancies (non-Hodgkin lymphoma, neuroblastoma, retinoblastoma, hepatoblastoma, nephroblastoma, rhabdomyosarcoma, small cell anaplastic carcinoma, Ewing sarcoma/peripheral neuroectodermal tumor, and desmoplastic small round cell tumor), characterized cytologically and histologically by a predominantly small round to oval, and relatively undifferentiated cells, and form an overwhelming majority (frequency varying from 69-94%) among the childhood malignancies.[74] In a study of intra-abdominal and intra-thoracic malignancies, the frequency of SRCTs among pediatric cases (78.1%) was significantly higher ($p<0.001$) than that of adults (13.2%).[182] FNA cytology of SRCTs of childhood can be diagnostic in majority of cases, aiding the surgeon in planning the extent of surgery in resectable malignant neoplasm, allowing specific therapy to be given to patients with unresectable SRCTs without a tissue biopsy and documenting recurrent and/or metastatic disease. [59,183]

A review of seven studies on FNA cytology diagnosis of SRCTs in children and adolescents (table 12), showed that NHL and leukemia were the most frequent neoplasm (38.5%), followed by neuroblastoma (18.6%), Ewing sarcoma/PNET (15.9%), rhabdomyosarcoma (10.3%), nephroblastoma (8.6%), retinoblastoma (4.2%), hepatoblastoma (3.0%), and medulloblastoma (0.9%).[67, 69, 136, 184-187] Of the SRCTs, small cell anaplastic carcinoma and desmoplastic SRCTs are neoplasms of adult age group; NHL occurs in both children and adults; and remaining are predominantly neoplasms of childhood. Ravindra and Kini [188] reported FNA cytodiagnosis in 21 cases of Wilms' tumor but all were in pediatric age group 2-6 years. Fröstad et al, [164] reported FNA cytology diagnosis of 24 Ewing's sarcoma and PNET in children and adolescents aged 0.7 to 20.2 years (median 14.1 years and male to female 17:7), which included 6 adolescents, with age ranging from 16 to 20 years.

Because of their morphological similarities, the small round cell tumors may pose a differential diagnostic problem in the practice of clinical cytology, especially when they are poorly differentiated.[74] Cytomorphologic features along with results of one or more ancillary studies can increase the FNA diagnostic accuracy of SRCTs in such situations.

Table 12. Fine-Needle Aspiration (FNA) Cytology Diagnosis of Specific Small Round Cell Tumors (SRCT) Types in Children and Adolescents

Authors and Year	No of cases	FNA cytodiagnosis: Nos (percentages)							
		NB	HB	WT	RB	MB	EFT	NHL	RMS
Akhtar et al (1985)[184]	58	8 (13.8)	0 (0.0)	3 (5.2)	3 (5.2)	0 (0.0)	12 (20.7)	29 (50.0)	3 (5.2)
Rajwanshi et al (1989)[185]	145	32 (22.1)	4 (2.8)	17 (11.7)	4 (2.8)	2 (1.4)	10 (6.9)	61 (42.1)	15 (10.3)
Layfield et al (1991)[67]	39	7 (17.9)	2 (5.1)	4 (10.3)	0 (0.0)	0 (0.0)	2 (5.1)	18 (46.2)	6 (15.4)
McGahey et al (1992)[186]	40	3 (7.5)	0 (0.0)	2 (5.0)	1 (2.5)	2 (5.0)	7 (17.5)	22 (55.0)	3 (7.5)
Das et al (1993) [136]*	25	6 (24.0)	7 (28.0)	3 (12.0)	0 (0.0)	0 (0.0)	1 (4.0)	8 (32.0)	0 (0.0)
Brahmi et al (2001)[187]	51	12 (23.5)	0 (0.0)	8 (15.7)	2 (3.9)	0 (0.0)	19 (37.3)	5 (9.8)	5 (9.8)
Dave et al (2006)[69†]	71	12 (16.9)	0 (0.0)	0 (0.0)	8 (11.3)	0 (0.0)	17 (23.9)	22 (31.0)	12 (16.9)
Total	429	80 (18.6)	13 (3.0)	37 (8.6)	18 (4.2)	4 (0.9)	68 (15.9)	165 (38.5)	44 (10.3)

* FNA of abdomen and thorax only. †From head and neck region only, NB= neuroblastoma, HB= hepatoblastoma, WT= Wilms' tumor (nephroblastoma), RB= retinoblastoma, MB= medulloblastoma, EFT= Ewing family of tumors (Ewing sarcoma and peripheral neuroectodermal tumor or PNET), NHL= nonHodgkin lymphoma including leukemia cases, RMS= rhabdomyosarcoma.

Role of Ancillary Studies

Ancillary studies, including immunocytochemistry (ICC), electron microscopy, microbiologic culture, cytogenetic studies, and flowcytometry performed on pediatric FNA material, enable a more specific diagnosis or supply additional information in many cases [59]. In ancillary studies performed on pediatric FNA biopsies by Gurley et al, [189] ICC data helped to narrow the differential diagnosis or classify the disease process in 42.1%, confirmed the cytologic impression in 47.4%, and gave contradictory results in 10.5%. The ultrastructural studies were diagnostic, or helped classify the disease process in 35.7%, confirmed the cytologic impression in 28.6%, helped diagnostic considerations in 21.4%, and were adjudged noncontributory in 14.3%.

Rossi et al, [190] observed that immunostaining with a combined panel of antibodies (RET, HMB-1, and Galectin-3) and the nuclear pleomorphism of follicular cells were effective in distinguishing between thyroid nodules requiring surgery from those requiring just follow-up. According to Khurana et al [90] negative immunostaining for cytokeratin 19 in FNA smears of solitary papillary hyperplastic thyroid nodule (SPHTN) in adolescents is useful in excluding a diagnosis of PTC.

According to Chen et al [92] FNA is an easy, safe, and reliable procedure in the diagnosis of lymphadenopathy in children. However, in difficult cases, flow cytometry immunophenotying (FCI) can be used to exclude NHL. Of the 69 cases reported by these authors, [92] 25 cases (38%) were diagnosed based on cytomorphology alone, and 30 (43%) by combined cytomorphology and flow cytometric immunophenotyping. A recent study by Laane et al [191] reveals that malignant B-cells have a higher Bcl-2 expression than did reactive B and T cells, indicating that Bcl-2 staining by flow cytometry can be recommended for primary differentiation between reactive hyperplasia and NHL. Characterization of ALL or lymphoblastic lymphoma diagnosed by FNA into T- cell or B-cell type or their precursors, which is of prognostic significance, is possible by ICC studies and T-cell beta gene/ concomitant JH gene rearrangements.[106, 192] The ICC markers in FNA smears, cytogenetic studies, and B-cell receptor gene rearrangements by polymerase chain reaction have been utilized in the diagnosis of ALCL [108] and blastoid variant of mantle cell lymphoma [193] in childhood and adolescence, respectively. A diagnosis of Hodgkin lymphoma is dependent on the recognition of Reed-Sternberg cells or Hodgkin's cells. However, other cells types including the large cells found in infectious mononucleosis, anaplastic large lymphoma, T-cell-rich B-cell lymphoma, peripheral T-cell lymphoma of mixed type, Burkitt-type lymphoma, metastatic carcinoma, melanoma, sarcoma, germ cell tumor, and reactive lymphoid hyperplasia can mimic the morphology of these cells.[100, 112, 194] Immunocytochemical studies on FNA smear can contribute to the specific diagnosis of these lesions (figure 10).

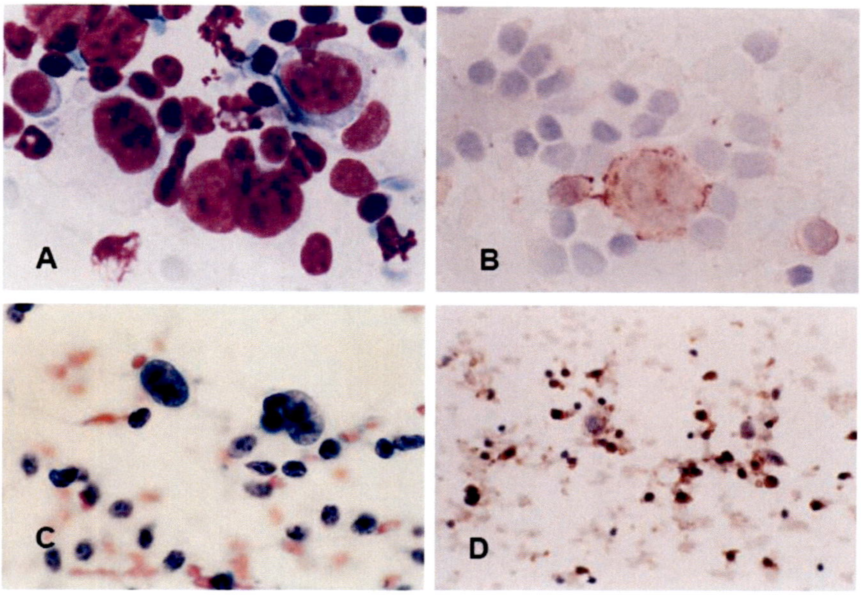

Figure 10. T-cell-rich B-cell lymphoma (TCRBCL): FNA smears from 6x6 cm right inguinal lymph node in a 16-year-old adolescent female. A. Large mono- and bi-nucleated atypical cells along with small lymphoid cells (May-Grünwald-Giemsa x 1000). B. The large atypical cells have prominent nucleoli (Papanicolaou x 1000). C. The large atypical cells and occasional small lymphoid cells show positive reaction for B-cell marker (CD-20 x 1000). D. Most small lymphoid cells are positive for T-cell marker but large atypical cells are negative (CD-3 x 400).

Cytologic recognition triphagic cellular components of Wilms' tumor (blastemal cells, spindle cells, and epithelial cells), which are helpful for correct diagnosis may not be always present. Of the 8 cases of WT described by Ellison et al, [195] only blastemal component was present in 5 cases but in these cases immunocytochemical stain (Ck+, Vim +) and electron microscopy proved useful in arriving at a correct FNAB diagnosis of WT. Fröstad et al, [164] observed that FNAC together with immunocytochemistry is a rapid, physically atraumatic and accurate method in diagnosing Ewing sarcoma family of tumors (EFT). Important immunocytochemical studies by these athors [164] in FNA smears of Ewing's sarcoma/PNETs included MIC2+ (15/15), NSE+ (12/18), and NFP+ (7/7). Chromosomal analysis revealing t(11;22)(q24;q12) characterizes EFT.[169, 196, 197] In cytogenetic study of 46 Ewing's sarcoma and 12 PNET based on FNA material, Udayakumar et al[169] observed t(11;22)(q24;q12) in 87.9% and abnormalities other than t(11;22) in another 6.8%. Torres and Ferrer [125] suspected rhabdomyosarcoma in FNA smears from bilateral breast masses in an 11-year-old adolescent girl and confirmed it by immunohistochemical staining for intracellular myoglobin. Fulciniti et al, [53] described the cytologic findings of a case of alveolar rhabdomyosarcoma (ARMS) of the perineum in a 13-year-old girl and highlighted the importance of immunohistochemical staining for markers of myogenic differentiation.

Although FNA has emerged as a cost effective tool for initial diagnosis of both neoplastic and non-neoplastic lesions of the bone, the diagnosis of primary bone tumors is limited by precise sub-typing of the tumors.[167] Inconclusive FNA cytologic diagnoses of osteosarcoma (30% cases) are likely to be due to insufficient sample cellularity or the presence of variants of osteosarcoma.[178] When the chondroblastic and fibroblastic variants create confusion with chondrosarcoma and fibrosarcoma, respectively or small cell variant give rise to differential diagnostic problem with some small round cell umors, cytochemical staining showing intense alkaline phosphatase positivity (figure 11) may be of help to arrive at a diagnosis of osteosarcoma. In a study of 22 high-grade soft tissue sarcomas diagnosed by FNA biopsy, Sápi et al [197] detected 3 female adolescent patients aged 18-21 years (mean 20years). The case positive for desmin turned out to be rhabdomyosarcoma, the case showing vimentin and keratin positivity was an epithelioid sarcoma and the third one positive for s-100 was a malignant peripheral nerve sheath tumor in histology. These authors [197] could also decide precise histogenetic origin in 16 soft tissue sarcomas by cytogenetic studies and these included 3 adolescent female cases aged 18-21 years (Median 19 years). Two of these cases, which proved to be grade III synovial sarcoma in histology, revealed t(X;18) by FISH and Vim+, Ker+, EMA+ in immunocytochemistry. The remaining case, which turned out to be a Ewing/PNET in histology showed t(11;22) and Vim+, CD-99+,Ker- by immunocytochemistry. Kilpatrick et al, [196] were successful in cytogenetic analysis in 10 cases of sarcomas. Five of these were children and adolescents including 2 Ewing's sarcoma cases (5M, 6F) with cytogenetic abnormality of t(11;22)(q24;q12), 2 synovial sarcomas (15F, 18M) with cytogenetic abnormality t(X;18)(p11;q11), and an alveolar sarcoma in a 14-year-old boy with t(2;13)(q35;q14). Thus, with a multidisciplinary approach and judicious use of ancillary studies, FNAB represents a highly accurate and cost-effective technique for the diagnosis of pediatric bone and soft tissue tumors, especially sarcomas, and should be considered as a viable diagnostic technique for pediatric therapeutic protocols.[161]

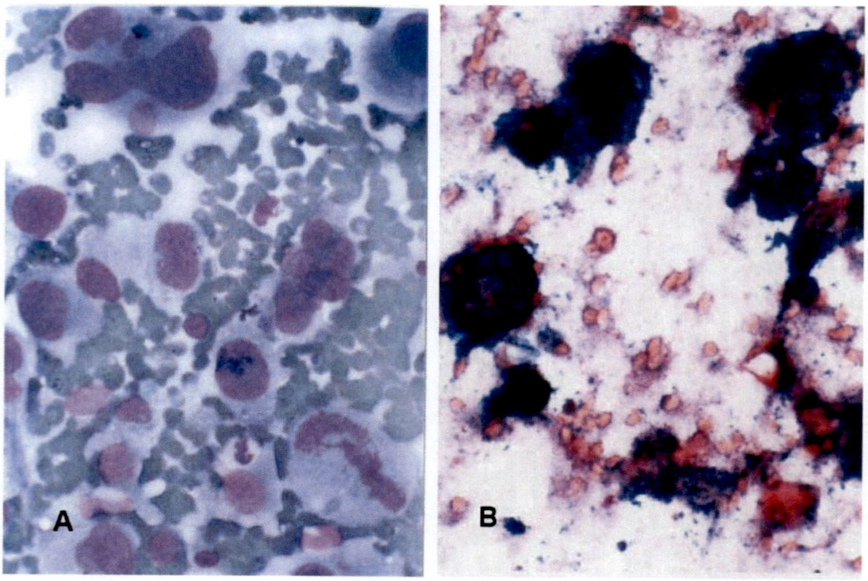

Figure 11. FNA from a painful lesion in the upper part of left arm in a 19-year-old adolescent male with osteosclerotic and osteolytic lesions in left humerus: A. Highly pleomorphic tumor cells with abnormal mitotic activity (MGG X 400). B. Tumor cells were intensely positive for alkaline phosphatase (X 400).

Conclusion

The overall rate of cancer incidence in adolescents has been rising at an average of 0.9% per year, the greatest annual increases being displayed by melanoma (5%), NHL (2%), and testicular carcinoma (2%).[45] The Europe average annual percentage change (AAPC) was significant in adolescents (1.5%, p<0.0001) between 1970s and 1990s and so also the specific increase (p<0.0001) in AAPC rates in adolescents for carcinomas (3.9%), lymphomas (2.4%) , germ cell tumors (1.7%), soft tissue sarcomas (2.6%), and CNS tumors (1.4%).[8] The two major cytodiagnostic tools, viz., exfoliative and fine needle aspiration cytology, have major diagnostic role, which guide the clinicians and oncologists in management of patients. Cancer of the uterine cervix is the second most cancer among women worldwide, with 70% of this cancer caused by HPV-16 and -18. Precancerous lesions and the presence of HPV, which is linked to sexual activity in adolescent females [10], can be effectively detected with the use of exfoliative cytology (Pap test) and molecular techniques on cytologic material leading to their regular followup and management at appropriate time. To control this cancer, the primary target population for HPV vaccination should be females aged 11-12 years.[198] Definitive diagnosis of mass lesions throughout the body by FNA biopsy in pediatric patients enables radiation therapy and/or chemotherapy to be administered for unresectable malignant neoplasms, provide material for culture of infectious lesions, identifies benign lesions not needing surgery, and aids the surgeon in planning of the extent of surgery in respectable malignant neoplasms.[59]

References

[1] Desandes E, Lacour B, Sommelet D, Buemi A, Danzon A, Delafosse P, Grosclaude P, Mace-Lecesh J, Raverdy-Bourdon N, Trettare B, Velten M, Brugieres L. Cancer incidence among adolescents in France. *Pediatr. Blood Cancer.* 2004; 43: 742- 748.

[2] Missouri adolescent deaths (age 15-19) by race and gender. In: *Focus. Missouri Department of Health and Senior Services,* Missouri, 2003.

[3] The Adolescent Health and Development (AHD) unit-Investing in a health sector response to Adolescents and Young People. WHO/SEARO Home. *WHO Regional Office for South-East Asia,* 2007.

[4] Barr RD. The adolescent with cancer. *Eur. J. Cancer.* 2001; 37: 1523-1527.

[5] Hollis R, Morgan S. The adolescent with cancer-at the edge of no-man's land. *Lancet Oncol.* 2001; 2; 43-48.

[6] Stiller C. Epidemiology of cancer in adolescents. *Med. Pediatr. Oncol.* 2002; 39: 149-155.

[7] Birch JM, Alston RD, Kelsey AM, Quinn MJ, Babb P, McNally RJQ. Classification and incidence of cancers in adolescents and young adults in England 1979-1997. *Br. J. Cancer.* 2002; 87: 1267- 1274.

[8] Steliarova-Foucher E, Stiller C, Kaatsch P, Berrino F, Coebergh J-W, Lacour B, Parkin M. Geographical patterns and time trends of cancer incidence and survival among children and adolescents in Europe since the 1970s (the ACCIS project): an epidemiological study. *Lancet.* 2004; 364: 2097- 2105.

[9] Wu X, Groves FD, McLaughlin CC, Jemal A, Martin J, Chen VW. Cancer incidence patterns among adolescents and young adults in the United States. *Cancer Causes Control.* 2005; 16: 309- 320.

[10] Jamison JH, Kaplan DW, Hamman R, Eagar R, Beach R, Douglas JM Jr. Spectrum of genital human papillomavirus infection in a female adolescent population. *Sex Transm. Dis.* 1995; 22: 236- 243.

[11] Jones GL, Taylor PR, Windebank KP, Hoye NA, Lucraft H, Wood K, Angus B, Proctor SJ. Outcome of a risk-related therapeutic strategy used prospectively in a population-based study of Hodgkin's lymphoma in adolescents. *Br. J. Cancer.* 2007; 97: 29- 36.

[12] Case AS, Rocconi RP, Straughn JM, Wang W, Roark K, Waltman EE, Huh WK. Cervical intraepithelial neoplasia in adolescent women. Incidence and treatment outcomes. *Obstet. Gynecol.* 2006; 108: 1369-1374.

[13] Kahn JA, Slap GB, Bernstein DI, Tissot AM, Kollar LM, Hillard PA, Rosenthal SL. Personal meaning of human papillomavirus and Pap test results in adolescent and young adult women. *Health Psychol.* 2007; 26: 192- 200.

[14] Patte C, Ribrag V, Brugières L. NonHodgkin's lymphoma in adolescents. *Bull. Cancer.* 2007; 94: 339-348.

[15] Vetrano G, Lombardi G, Di Leone G, Parisi A, Scardaaglia P, Pate G, Verrico M, Corosu R. Cervical intraepithelial neoplasia: risk factors, persistence, and recurrence in adolescents. *Eur. J. Gynecol. Oncol.* 2007; 28: 189- 192.

[16] Puberty: Adolescent female. In: Adolescent Medicine, UVa Health.com, 2004. Http://www.healthsystem.virginia.edu/uvahealth/peds_adolescent/paf.cfm

[17] Singh UR, Gupta K, Arora VK, Gupta S, Bhatia A. Cytomorphology of some uncommon tumors of childhood and adolescence. *Indian J. Pediatr.* 1996; 63: 539-547.

[18] Dehner LP. The evolution of the diagnosis and understanding of primitive and embryonic neoplasms in children: living through an epoch. *Mod. Pathol.* 1998; 11: 669-685.

[19] Craft AW. Childhood cancer-mainly curable. So where next? *Acta Pediatr.* 2000; 89: 386- 392.

[20] Friedmann AM, Weinstein HJ. The role of prognostic features in the treatment of childhood acute lymphoblastic leukemia. *Oncologist.* 2000; 5: 321- 328.

[21] Haas RJ, Schmidt P, Göbel U, Harms D. Testicular germ cell tumors, an update. Results of the German Cooperative studies 1982-1997. *Klin. Pediatr.*1999; 211: 300-304.

[22] Défachelles AS, Martin Delassalle E, Boutard P, Nelken B, Schneider P, Patte C. Pancreatoblastoma in childhood: clinical course and therapeutic management of seven cases. *Med. Pediatr. Oncol.* 2001; 37: 47- 52.

[23] Bisogno G, Pilz T, Perilogno G, Ferrari A, Harms D, Ninfo V, Treuner J, Carli M. Undifferentiated sarcoma of the liver in childhood: a curable disease. *Cancer.* 2002; 94: 252- 257.

[24] Terenźiani M, Massimino M, Casanova M, Cefalo G, Fernari A, Luksch R, Spreafico F, Polastri D, Fontanelli D, Piva L, Fossati-Bellani F. Childhood malignant germ cell tumors: a monoinstitutional experience. *Gynecol. Oncol.* 2001; 81: 436- 440.

[25] Magné N, Haie-Meder C. Brachytherapy of genital-tract rhabdomyosarcoma in girls: technical aspects, reports, and perspectives. *Lancet Oncol.* 2007; 8: 725- 729.

[26] Calaminus G, Weinspach S, Teske C, Göbel U. Quality of survival in children and adolescents after treatment for childhood cancer: the influence of reported late effects on health related quality of life. *Klin. Padiatr.* 2007; 219: 152-157.

[27] Forrest G, Plumb C, Zeibland S, Stein A. Breast cancer in the family—children's perceptions of their mother's cancer and its initial treatment:qualitative study. *BMJ.* 2006; 332: 998- 1003.

[28] Zahlis EH. The child's worries about the mother's breast cancer: sources of distress in school-age children. *Oncol. Nurs. Forum.* 2001; 28: 1019- 1025.

[29] Tercyak KP, Peshkin BN, Streisand R, Lerman C. Psychological issues among children of hereditary breast cancer gene (BRCA1/2) testing participants. *Psychooncology.* 2001; 10: 336- 346.

[30] McInerney-Leo A, Biesecker BB, Hadley DW, Kase RG, Giambarresi TR, Johnson E, Lerman C, Struewing JP. BRCA 1/2 testing in hereditary breast and ovarian cancer families II: impact on relationships. *Am. J. Med. Genet. A.* 2005; 133: 165- 169.

[31] Kumar A. Poverty and adolescent girl health. The Bihar Times: A Passage to Bihar. (www.bihartimes.com/poverty/anant_pandey.html)

[32] Nour NM. Health consequences of child marriage in Africa. *Emerg. Infect. Dis.* 2006; 12: 1644- 1649.

[33] Adolescent health: Risky behavior in adolescence contributes to 6 in 10 premature deaths in adulthood. Disease Control and Priorities Project. Fogarty International Center of the U.S. National Institute of Health, The World Bank, World Health Organization, Population Reference Bureau, and Bill and Melinda Gates Foundation, 2006.

[34] Kreuzer M, Kreienbrock L, Gerken M, Heinrich J, Brusche-Hohlfeld I, Muller KM, Wichmann HE. Risk factors for lung cancer in young adults. *Am. J. Epidemiol.* 1998; 147: 1028- 1037.

[35] Boffetta P, Kreuzer M, Benhamou S, Agudo A, Wichmann HE, Gaborieau V, Simonato L. Risk of lung cancer from tobacco smoking among young women from Europe. *Int. J. Cancer.* 2001; 91: 745- 746.

[36] Jemal A, Chu KC, Tarone RE. Recent trends in lung cancer mortality in the United States. *J. Natl. Cancer Inst.* 2001; 93: 277- 283.

[37] Strand T-E, Malayeri C, Eskonsipo PKJ, Grimsrud TK, Norstein J, Grotmol T. Adolescent smoking and trends in lung cancer incidence among young adults in Norway 1954-1998. *Cancer Causes Control.* 2004; 15: 27- 33.

[38] Current trends premarital sexual experience among adolescent women—United States, 1970-1988. *MMWR.* (Weekly) 1991; 39: 929-932.

[39] Bunnell RE, Dahlberg L, Rolfs R, Ransom R, Gershman K, Farshy C, Newhall WJ, Schmid S, Stone K, St. Louis M. High prevalence and incidence of sexually transmitted diseases in urban adolescent females despite moderate risk behaviors. *J. Infect. Dis.* 1999; 180: 1624-1631.

[40] HIV/AIDS and adolescents: Young people- a window of hope in the HIV/AIDS pandemic. Child and Adolescent Health and Development. World Health Organization (Home Page), 2000- 2004.

[41] Brown DR, Shew ML, Qadadri B, Neptune N, Vagas M, Tu W, Juliar BE, Breen TE, Fortenberry JD. A longitudinal study of genetial human papillomavirus in a cohort study in closely followed adolescent women. *J. Infect. Dis.* 2005; 191: 182- 192.

[42] Brogly SB, Watts DH, Ylitalo N, Franco EL, Seage GR 3rd, Oleske J, Eagle M, Van Dyke R. Reproductive health of adolescent girls perinatally infected with HIV. *Am. J. Public Health.* 2007; 97: 1047-1052.

[43] Stiller CA. International patterns of cancer incidence in adolescents. *Cancer Treat. Rev.* 2007; 33: 631- 645.

[44] Alston RD, Rowan S, Eden TO, Moran A, Birch JM. Cancer incidence patterns by region and socioeconomic deprivation in teenagers and young adults in England. *Br. J. Cancer.* 2007; 96: 1760- 1766.

[45] Pentheroudakis G, Pavlidis N. Juvenile cancer: improving care for adolescents and young adults within the frame of medical oncology. *Ann. Oncol.* 2005; 16: 181- 188.

[46] McNally RJ, Kelsey AM, Cairns DP, Taylor GM, Eden OB, Birch JM. Temporal increases in the incidence of childhood solid tumors seen in Northwest England (1954-1988) are likely to be real. *Cancer.* 2001; 92: 1967- 1976.

[47] McNally RJ, Cairns DP, Eden OB, Kelsey AM, Taylor GM, Birch JM. Examination of temporal trends in the incidence of childhood leukemias and lymphomas provides aetiological clues. *Leukemia.* 2001; 15: 1612- 1618.

[48] National cancer registry programme: consolidated report of the population based cancer registries 1990-1996. Indian Council of Medical Research, New Delhi, 2001.

[49] Eisenhut CC, King DE, Nelson WA, Olson LC, Wall RW, Glant MD. Fine-needle biopsy of pediatric lesions: a three-year study in an outpatient biopsy clinic. *Diagn. Cytopathol.* 1996; 14: 43- 50.

[50] Cohen MB, Bottles K, Ablin AR, Miller TR. The use of fine-needle aspiration biopsy in children. *West J. Med.* 1989; 150: 665- 667.

[51] Martin S, Ulrich C, Munsell MGG, Taylor S, Lange G, Bleyer A. Delays in cancer diagnosis in underinsured young adults and older adolescents. *Oncologist.* 2007; 12: 816- 824.

[52] Klein-Geltink J, Pogany L, Mary LS, Barr RD, Greenberg ML. Impact of age and diagnosis of waiting times between important health care events among children 0-19 years cared for in pediatric units: the Canadian Childhood Cancer Surveilance and Control Program. *J. Pediatr. Hematol. Oncol.* 2006; 28: 433- 439.

[53] Fulciniti F, Botti G, De Chiara A, Parlato V, Russo S, Vosa L, Nappi MM. Fine needle aspiration cytology of perineal alveolar rhabdomyosarcoma: cytohistopathologic and immunocytochemical correlations. *Acta Cytol.* 2007; 51: 385-389.

[54] Yusuf K, Reyes-Mugica M, Carpenter TO. Insular carcinoma of the thyroid in an adolescent: a case report and review of literature. *Curr. Opin. Pediatr.* 2003; 15: 512-515.

[55] Siklar Z, Ocal G, Berberoğlu M, Adiyaman P, Ergür AT, Evliyaoğlu O, Sak SD. Importance of thyroglobulin levels for diagnosis and monitoring of follicular thyroid carcinoma in an adolescent with severe iodine deficiency. *J. Pediatr. Endocrinol. Metab.* 2006; 19: 1175-1178.

[56] Nagakawa H, Hiroshima K, Takiguchi Y, Yatomi M, Takahashi Y, Mikami M, Nakatani Y, Kuriyama T. Basaloid squamous-cell carcinoma of the lung in a young woman. *Int. J. Clin. Oncol.* 2006; 11: 66-68.

[57] Taylor SR, Nunez C. Fine-needle aspiration biopsy in a pediatric population: Report of 64 consecutive cases. *Cancer.* 1984; 54: 1449- 1453.

[58] Wakely PE Jr, Kardos TF, Frable WJ. Application of fine needle aspiration biopsy to pediatrics. *Human Pathol.* 1988; 19:1383-1386.

[59] Silverman JF, Gurley AM, Holbrook CT, Joshi VV. Pediatric fine needle aspiration biopsy. *Am. J. Clin. Pathol.* 1991; 95: 653-659.

[60] Almeida MM, Mendonça ME, Sousinha M, Martins AG, de Sousa JV, Soares J. Application of aspiration cytology in the diagnosis of tumor lesions in children. *Acta Med. Port.* 1991; 4: 71- 75.

[61] Drut R, Drut RM, Pollono D, Tomarchio S, Ibáñez O, Urrutia A, Ripoll MC. Fine-needle aspiration biopsy in pediatric oncology patients: a review of experience with 829 patients (899 biopsies). *J. Pediatr. Hematol. Oncol.* 2005; 27: 370-376.

[62] Mann G, Attarbaschi A, Steiner M, Simonitsch I, Strobl H, Urban C, Meister B, Haas O, Dworzak M, Gadner H: Austrian Berlin-Frankfurt-Münster (BFM) Group. Early and reliable diagnosis of non-Hodgkin lymphoma in childhood and adolescence: contribution of cytomorphology and flow cytometric immunophenotyping. *Pediatr. Hematol. Oncol.* 2006; 23: 167- 176.

[63] Mount SL, Papillo JL. A study of 10 296 pediatric and adolescent Papanicolaou smear diagnoses in Northern New England. *Pediatrics.* 1999; 103: 539- 545.

[64] Boardman LA, Weitzen S, Stanko C. Atypical squamous cells of undetermined significance, human papillomavirus, and cervical intraepithelial neoplasia 2 or 3 in adolescents: ASC-US, age, and high-grade cervical neoplasia. *J. Low Genit. Tract. Dis.* 2006; 10: 140-145.

[65] Buchino JJ, Jones VF. Fine needle aspiration in the evaluation of children with lymphadenopathy. *Arch. Pediatr. Adolesc. Med.* 1994; 148: 1327-1330.

[66] Dickson PV, Davidoff AM. Malignant neoplasms of the head and neck. *Semin. Pediatr. Surg.* 2006; 15: 92- 98.

[67] Layfield LJ, Glasgow B, Ostrzega N, Reynolds CP. Fine-needle aspiration cytology and diagnosis of neoplasms in pediatric age group. *Diagn. Cytopathol.* 1991; 7: 451-461.

[68] Liu ES, Bernstein JM, Sculerati N, Wu HC. Fine needle aspiration biopsy of pediatric head and neck masses. *Int. J. Pediatr. Otorhinolaryngol.* 2001; 60: 135-140.

[69] Dave B, Shet T, Ramadwar M, Kane S. Cytological evaluation of head and neck tumors in children-a pattern analysis. *Diagn. Cytopathol.* 2006; 34: 434-446.

[70] Mobley DL, Wakely PE Jr, Frable MA. Fine needle aspiration biopsy: application to pediatric head and neck masses. *Laryngoscope.* 1991; 101: 469-472.

[71] Ramadan HH, Wax MK, Boyd CB. Fine-needle aspiration of head and neck masses in children. *Am. J. Otolaryngol.* 1997; 18: 400- 404.

[72] Rapkiewicz A, Thuy B, Simsir A, Cangiarella J, Levine P. Spectrum of head and neck lesions diagnosed by fine-needle aspiration cytology in the pediatric population. *Cancer.* (Cancer Cytopathol) 2007; 111: 242- 251.

[73] Kollur SM, El-Hag IA. Fine-needle aspiration cytology of metastatic nasopharyngeal carcinoma in cervical lymph nodes: Comparision with metastatic squamous-cell carcinoma, and Hodgkin's and non-Hodgkin's lymphoma. *Diagn. Cytopathol.* 2003; 28: 18- 22.

[74] Das DK. Fine-needle aspiration (FNA) cytology diagnosis of small round cell tumors: value and limitations. *Indian J. Pathol. Microbiol.* 2004; 47: 309- 318.

[75] Salomão DR, Sigman JD, Greenebaum E, Cohen MB. Rhabdomyosarcoma presenting as a parotid gland mass in pediatric patients: fine-needle aspiration biopsy findings. *Cancer.* 1998; 25: 245- 251.

[76] Mathew S, Ali SZ. Parotid fine-needle aspiration: A cytologic study of pediatric lesions. *Diagn. Cytopathol.* 1997; 17: 8-13.

[77] Cerdá J, Rodríguez A, Molina E, Peligros MI, Navascués JA, Rodríguez Arnao D, Barrientos G, Sánchez R, Romero R, Vázquez J. Thyroid tumors in childhood. *Cir. Pediatr.* 1999; 12: 65- 70.

[78] Chang SH, Joo M, Kim H. Fine needle aspiration biopsy of thyroid nodules in children and adolescents. *J. Korean Med. Sci.* 2006; 21: 469- 473.

[79] Al-Shaikh A, Ngan B, Daneman A, Daneman D. Fine-needle aspiration biopsy in the management of thyroid nodules in children and adolescents. *J. Pediatr.* 2001; 138: 140- 142.

[80] Millman B, Pellitteri PK. Nodular thyroid disease in children and adolescents. *Otolaryngol. Head Neck. Surg.* 1997; 116: 604- 609.

[81] Pazaitou-Panayiotou K, Kaprara A, Boudina M, Georgiou E, Drimonitis A, Vainas I, Raptou E, Galactidou G. Thyroid carcinoma in children and adolescents: presentation, clinical course, and outcome of therapy in 23 children and adolescents in Northern Greece. *Hormones.* (Athens) 2005; 4: 213-220.

[82] Ardito G, Pintus C, Revelli L, Grottesi A, Modugno R, Vincenzoni C, Fadda G, Perrelli L. Thyroid tumors in children and adolescents: preoperative study. *Eur. J. Pediatr. Surg.* 2001; 11: 154- 157.

[83] Hosler GA, Clark I, Zakowski MF, Westra WH, Ali SZ. Cytopathologic analysis of thyroid lesions in the pediatric population. *Diagn. Cytopathol.* 2006; 34: 101- 105.

[84] Raab SS, Silverman JF, Elsheikh TM, Thomas PA, Wakely PE. Pediatric thyroid nodules: disease demographics and clinical management as determined by fine needle aspiration biopsy. *Pediatrics.* 1995; 95: 46- 49.

[85] Lugo-Vicente H, Ortíz VN, Irizarri H, Camps JI, Pagán V. Pediatric thyroid nodules: management in the era of fine needle aspiration. *J. Pediatr. Surg.* 1998; 33: 1302-1305.

[86] Khurana KK, Labrador E, Izquierdo R, Mesonero CE, Pisharodi LR. The role of fine-needle aspiration biopsy in the management of thyroid nodules in children, adolescents, and young adults: a multi-institutional study. *Thyroid.* 1999; 9: 383- 386.

[87] Corrias A, Einaudi S, Chiorboli E, Weber G, CrinòA, Andreo M, Cesaretti G, de Sanctis L, Messina MF, Segni M, Cicchetti M, Vigone M, Pasquino AM, Spera S, de Luca F, Mussa GC, Bona G. Accuracy of fine needle aspiration biopsy of thyroid nodules in detecting malignancy in childhood: comparision with conventional clinical, laboratory, and imaging approaches. *J. Clin. Endocrinol. Metab.* 2001; 86: 4644- 4648.

[88] Amrikachi M, Ponder TB, Wheeler TM, Smith D, Ramzy I. Thyroid fine-needle aspiration biopsy in children and adolescents: experience with 218 aspirates. *Diagn. Cytopathol.* 2005; 32: 189- 192.

[89] Fassina AS, Rupolo M, Pelizzo MR, Casara D. Thyroid cancer in children and adolescents.*Tumori.* 1994; 80: 257- 262.

[90] Khurana KK, Baloch ZW, LiVolsi VA. Aspiration cytology of pediatric solitary papillary hyperplastic thyroid nodule. *Arch. Pathol. Lab. Med.* 2001; 125: 1575-1578.

[91] Willgerodt H, Keller E, Bennek J, Emmrich P. Diagnostic value of fine-needle aspiration biopsy of thyroid nodules in children and adolescents. *J. Pediatr. Endocrinol. Metab.* 2006; 19: 507- 515.

[92] Chen Y, Savargaonkar P, Fuchs A, Wasserman P. Role of flow cytometry in the diagnosis of lymphadenopathy in children. *Diagn. Cytopathol.* 2002; 26: 5-9.

[93] Ríos E, Otoya L. Diagnosis of lymphadenopathy in children: role of fine needle aspiration biopsy. *Rev. Med. Chil.* 1999; 127: 323- 328.

[94] Ponder TB, Smith D, Ramzy I. Lymphadenopathy in children and adolescents: role of fine needle aspiration in management. *Cancer Detect. Prev.* 2000; 24: 228- 233.

[95] van de Schoot L, Aronson DC, Behrendt H, Bras J. The role of fine-needle aspiration cytology in children with persistent or suspicious lymphadenopathy. *J. Pediatr. Surg.* 2001; 36: 7-11.

[96] Handa U, Mohan H, Bal A. Role of fine needle aspiration cytology in evaluation of pediatric lymphadenopathy. *Cytopathology.* 2003; 14: 66-69.

[97] Kardos TF, Maygarden SJ, Blumberg AK, Wakely PE Jr, Frable WJ. Fine needle aspiration biopsy in the management of children and young adults with peripheral lymphadenopathy. *Cancer.* 1989; 63: 703-707.

[98] Das DK. Value and limitations of fine-needle aspiration cytology in diagnosis and classification of lymphomas: A review. *Diagn. Cytopathol.* 1999; 21: 240- 249.

[99] Kagu BM, Durosinmi, Adeodu OO, Akinola NO, Adediran IA, Salawu L. Determinants of survival in Nigerians with Burkitt's lymphoma. *Afr. J. Med. Med. Sci.* 2004; 33: 195-200.

[100] Das DK, Gupta SK, Pathak IC, Sharma SC, Datta BN. Burkitt-type lymphoma: Diagnosis by fine needle aspiration cytology. *Acta Cytol.* 1987; 31: 1-7.

[101] Wright DH. Microscopic features, histochemistry, histogenesis and diagnosis. In: Burkitt's lymphoma. Edited by DP Burkitt and DH Wright. E and S Livingstone, Edinburgh. 1970. pp 82-102.

[102] Levine PH, Kamaraju LS, Cannelly RR, Berard CW, Dorfman RF, Magrath I, Easton JM. The American Burkitts lymphoma registry: Eight years experience. *Cancer.* 1982; 1016-1022.

[103] Arseneau JC, Canellos GP, Banks PM, Berard CW, Gralnick HR, De Vita VT. American Burkitt's lymphoma: A clinical factor relating to prolonged survival. *Am. J. Med.* 1975; 58: 314-321.

[104] Shepherd JJ, Wright DH. Burkitt's tumor presenting as bilateral swelling of the breast in women of child bearing age. *Br. J. Surg.* 1967; 54: 76-780.

[105] Das DK, Sheikh ZA, Jassar AK, Jarallah MA. Burkitt-type lymphoma of the breast: diagnosis by fine-needle aspiration cytology. *Diagn. Cytopathol.* 2002; 27: 60-62.

[106] Wakely PE Jr, Kornstein MJ. Aspiration cytopathology of lymphoblastic lymphoma and leukemia: the MCV experience. *Pediatr. Pathol. Lab. Med.* 1996; 16: 243-252.

[107] Das DK, Gupta SK, Datta U, Sharma SC, Datta BN. Malignant lymphoma of convoluted lymphocytes: Diagnosis by fine-needle aspiration cytology and cytochemistry. *Diagn. Cytopathol.* 1986; 2: 307-311.

[108] Ng W-K, Ip P, Choy C, Collins RJ. Cytologic and immunocytochemical findings of anaplastic large cell lymphoma: Analysis of ten fine-needle aspiration specimens over a 9-year period. *Cancer.* (Cancer Cytopathol) 2003; 99: 33-43.

[109] Kinney MC, Collins RD, Greer JP, Whitlock JA, Sioutos N, Kadin ME. A small-cell predominant variant of primary Ki-1 (CD30)+ T-cell lymphoma. *Am. J. Surg. Pathol.* 1993; 17: 859-868.

[110] Kim SE, Kim SH, Lim BJ, Hong SW, Yang WI. Fine needle aspiration cytology of small cell variant of anaplastic large cell lymphoma: A case report. *Acta Cytol.* 2004; 48: 254- 258.

[111] Das DK, Gupta SK, Datta BN, Sharma SC. Fine needle aspiration cytodiagnosis of Hodgkin's disease and its subtypes: I. Scope and limitations. *Acta Cytol.* 1990; 34: 329-336.

[112] Zhang J-R, Raza AS, Greaves TS, Cobb CJ. Fine-needle aspiration diagnosis of Hodgkin lymphoma using current WHO classification-Re-evaluation of cases from 1999-2004 with new proposals. *Diagn. Cytopathol.* 2006; 34:397-402.

[113] Das DK, Gupta SK, Datta BN, Sharma SC. FNA cytodiagnosis of nonHodgkin's lymphoma and its subtyping under working formulation of 175 cases. *Diagn. Cytopathol.* 1991; 7: 487-498.

[114] Neinstein LS. Breast disease in adolescent and young women. *Pediatr. Clin. North Am.* 1999; 46: 607- 629.

[115] West KW, Rescorla FJ, Scherer LR 3rd, Grosfeld JL. Diagnosis and treatment of symptomatic breast masses in the pediatric population. *J. Pediatr. Surg.* 1995; 30: 182- 186.

[116] Arca MJ, Caniano DA. Breast disorders in the adolescent patient. *Adolesc. Med. Clin.* 2004; 15: 473- 485.

[117] De Silva NK, Brandt ML. Disorders of the breast in children and adolescents, part 2: Breast masses. *J. Pediatr. Adolesc. Gynecol.* 2006; 19: 415- 418.

[118] Rosen PP. In *Rosen's Breast Pathology*. Lippincott-Raven Publishers. Philadelphia, 1997, pp: 633-650.

[119] Corpron CA, Black CT, Singletary SE, Andrassy RJ, West K. Breast cancer in adolescent females. Discussion. *J. Pediatr. Surg.* 1995; 30: 322-324.

[120] Rivera-Hueto F, Hevia-Vázquez A, Utrilla-Alcolea JC, Galera-Davidson H. Long-term prognosis of teenagers with breast cancer. *Int. J. Surg. Pathol.* 2002; 10: 273-279.

[121] Noh WC, Paik NS, Cho KJ, Chung JH, Kim MS, Moon NM. Breast mass in a 3-year-old girl: Differentiation of secretory carcinoma versus abnormal thelarche by fine needle aspiration biopsy. *Surgery.* 2005; 137: 109-110.

[122] Buchino JJ. Moore GD, Bond SJ. Secretory carcinoma in a 9-year-old girl. *Diagn. Cytopathol.* 2004; 31: 430- 431.

[123] Nonomura A, Kimura A, Mizukami Y, Nakamura S, Ohmura K, Watanabe Y, Tanimoto K, Ikegaki S. Secretory carcinoma of the breast associated with juvenile papillomatosis in a 12-year-old girl. A cases report. *Acta Cytol.* 1995; 39: 569- 576.

[124] Pandey M, Mathew A, Abraham EK, Rajan B. Primary sarcoma of the breast. *J. Surg. Oncol.* 2004; 87: 121- 125.

[125] Torres V, Ferrer R. Cytology of fine needle aspiration biopsy of primary breast rhabdomyosarcoma in an adolescent girl. *Acta Cytol.* 1985: 29: 430- 434.

[126] Khalbuss W, Villas B, Bakhshandeh M. Cytomorphology and immunophenotyping of Burkitt's lymphoma presenting as a breast mass. *Breast J.* 2006; 12: 177- 178.

[127] Plantaz D, Bachelot C, Dyon JF, Frappat P, Schaerer R, Bost M. Massive breast involvement in Burkitt's lymphoma. *Arch. Fr. Pediatr.* 1987; 44: 199- 200.

[128] Fahmy JL, Wood BP, Miller JH. Bilateral breast involvement in a teenage girl with Burkitt lymphoma. *Pediatr. Radiol.* 1995; 25: 56- 57.

[129] Mukhtar AU, Francisco CC. Burkitt's lymphoma involving the breast in a 15-year-old girl. *Trop. Doct.* 2001; 31: 236.

[130] Shukla R, Pooja B, Radhika S, Nijhawan R, Rajwanshi A. Fine-needle aspiration cytology of extramammary neoplasms metastatic to the breast. *Diagn. Cytopathol.* 2005; 32: 193- 197.

[131] Tamiolakis D, Venizelos I, Nikolaidou S, Prassopoulos P, Alexiadis G, Simopoulos C, Papadopoulos N. Bilateral metastatic rhabdomyosarcoma to the breast in an adolescent female: touch imprint cytology and implication of myoD1 nuclear antigen. *Onkologie.* 2004; 27: 469- 471.

[132] Shabb NS, Fahl M, Shabb B, Haswani P, Zaatari G. Fine-needle aspiration of the mediastinum: A clinical, radiologic, cytologic, and histologic study of 42 cases. *Diagn. Cytopathol.* 1998; 19: 428- 436.

[133] Guo Z, Kurtycz DFI, De Las Casas LE, Hoerl HD. Radiologically guided fine-needle aspiration biopsy of pelvic and retroperitoneal masses: A retrospective study of 68 cases. *Diagn. Cytopathol.* 2001; 25: 43- 49.

[134] Guo Z, Kurtycz DFI, Salem R, De Las casas LE, Caya JG, Hoerl HD. Radiologically guided percutaneous fine-needle aspiration biopsy of the liver: Retrospective study of 119 cases evaluating diagnostic effectiveness and clinical complications. *Diagn. Cytopathol.* 2002; 26: 283- 289.

[135] Kumar PV, Monabati A, Raseki AR, Arshadi C, Malek-Hosseini SA, Talei AR, Sadeghi E. Splenic lesions: FNA findings in 48 cases. *Cytopathology.* 2007; 18: 151-156.

[136] Das DK, Pant CS, Rath B, Parkash S, James T, Sodhani P. Fine needle aspiration diagnosis of intrathoracic and intra-abdominal lesions: Review of experience in the pediatric age group. *Diagn. Cytopathol.* 1993; 9: 383-393.

[137] Cahill AM, Baskin KM, Kaye RD, Fitz CR, Towbin RB. CT-guided percutaneous lung biopsy in children. *J. Vasc. Interv. Radiol.* 2004; 15: 955- 960.

[138] Baksi P, Srinivasan R, Rao KL, Marwaha RK, Gupta N, Das A, Nijhawan R, Rajwanshi A. Fine needle aspiration biopsy in pediatric space-occupying lesions of liver: a retrospective study evaluating its role and diagnostic efficacy. *J. Pediatr. Surg.* 2006; 41: 1903- 1908.

[139] Obers VJ, Phillips JI. Fine needle aspiration of pediatric abdominal masses. Cytologic and electron microscopic diagnosis. *Acta Cytol.* 1991; 35: 165- 170.

[140] Radhika S, Baksi A, Rajwanshi A, Nijhawan R, Das A, Kakkar N, Joshi K, Marwaha RK, Rao KLN. Cytopathology of uncommon malignant renal neoplasms in the pediatric age group. *Diagn. Cytopathol.* 2005; 32: 281- 286.

[141] Hallman JR, Geisinger KR. Cytology of fluids from pleural, peritoneal and pericardial cavities in children: a comprehensive survey. *Acta Cytol.* 1994; 38: 209-217.

[142] Das DK, Gupta SK, Ayyagari S, Bambery PK, Datta BN, Datta U. Pleural effusions in non-Hodgkin's lymphoma: A cytomorphologic, cytochemical and immunologic study. *Acta Cytol.* 1987; 31: 119-124.

[143] Das DK, Juwaiser A, George SS, Francis IM, Sathar SS, Sheikh ZA, Shaheen A, Pathan SK, Haji BE, George J, Kapila K. Cytomorphological and immunocytochemical study of non-Hodgkin's lymphoma in pleural effusion and ascitic fluid. *Cytopathology.* 2007; 18: 157- 167.

[144] Hayder S, Das DK, Björk O, Löwhagen T. Fine needle aspiration cytology (FNAC) of the testes in childhood acute lymphoblastic leukemia and non-Hodgkin's lymphoma: Preliminary report. *Pediatr. Hematol. Oncol.* 1988; 5: 29- 34.

[145] Salzburg J, Burkhardt B, Zimmermann M, Wachowski O, Woessmann W, Oschlies I, Klapper W, Wacker HH, Ludwig WD, Niggli F, Mann G, Gadner H, Riehm H, Schrappe M, Reiter A. Prevalence, clinical pattern, and outcome of CNS involvement in childhood and adolescent non-Hodgkin's lymphoma differ by non-Hodgkin's lymphoma subtype: A Berlin-Frankfurt-Munster Report. *J. Clin. Oncol.* 2007; 25: 3915- 3922.

[146] You W, Dainty LA, Rose GS, Krivak T, McHale MT, Olsen CH, Elkas JC. Gynecologic malignancies in women aged less than 25 years. *Obstet. Gynecol.* 2005; 105: 1405-1409.

[147] Moore K, Cofer A, Elliot L, Lanneau G, Walker J, Gold MA. Adolescent cervical dysplasia: Histologic evaluation, treatment, and outcomes. *Am. J. Obstet. Gynecol.* 2007; 197: 141- 146.

[148] Hirokawa M, Shimizu M, Nakamura E, Kanahara T, Yamauchi H, Fujiwara K, Kohno I, Manabe T. Basement membrane material and tigroid background in a fine needle aspirate of clear cell adenocarcinoma of the cervix. A case report. *Acta Cytol.* 2000; 44: 251-254.

[149] Sozen I, Small L, Kowalski M, Mayo SW, Hurwitz CA. Adenocarcinoma of the cervix metastatic from a colon primary and diagnosed from a routine Pap smear in a 17-year-old woman: a case report. *J. Reprod. Med.* 2005; 50: 793-795.

[150] Deligeoroglou E, Eleftheriades M, Shiadoes V, Botsis D, Hasiakos D, Kontoravdis A, Creatsas G. Ovarian masses during adolescence: clinical, ultrasonographic and pathologic findings, serum tumor markers and endocrinological profile. *Gynecol. Endocrinol.* 2004; 19: 1-8.

[151] Skiadas VT, Koutoulidis V, Eleytheriades M, Gouliamos A, Moulopoulos LA, Deligeoroglou E, Vlachos L, Kreatsas G. Ovarian masses in young adolescents: imaging findings with surgical confirmation. Eur J Gynaecol Oncol 2004; 25: 201-206.

[152] de Silva KS, Kanumakala S, Grover SR, Chow CW, Warne GL. Ovarian lesions in children and adolescents—an 11-year review. *J. Pediatr. Endocrinol. Metab.* 2004; 17: 951- 957.

[153] Rzepka-Górska I, Błogowska A, Zajaczek S, Zielińska D. Germinal cell tumors in young and adolescent girls. *Ginecol. Pol.* 2003; 74: 840- 846.

[154] Layfield LJ, Heaps JM, Berek JS. Fine-needle aspiration cytology accuracy with palpable gynecologic neoplasms. *Gynecol. Oncol.* 1991; 40: 70- 73.

[155] Imachi M, Tsukamoto N, Shigematsu T, Saito T, Kamura T, Nakano H. Fine-needle aspiration cytology in patients with gynecologic malignancies. *Gynecol. Oncol.* 1992; 46: 309- 312.

[156] Malmström H. Fine-needle aspiration cytology versus core biopsies in the evaluation of recurrent gynecologic malignancies. *Gynecol. Oncol.* 1997; 65: 69- 73.

[157] Ganjei P, Dickinson B, Harrison T, Nassiri M, Lu Y. Aspiration cytology of neoplastic and non-neoplastic ovarian cysts: is it accurate? *Int. J. Gynecol. Pathol.* 1996; 15: 94- 101.

[158] Bommer KK, Ramzy I, Mody D. Fine-needle aspiration biopsy in the diagnosis and management of bone lesions: A study of 450 cases. *Cancer.* (Cancer Cytopathol) 1997; 81:148-156.

[159] Wakely PE Jr, Powers CN, Frable WJ. Metachronous soft-tissue masses in children and young adults with cancer: correlation of histology and aspiration cytology. *Hum. Pathol.* 1990; 21: 669- 677.

[160] Meis JM, Enzinger FM, Martz KL, Neal JA. Malignant peripheral nerve sheath tumors (malignant schwannomas) in children. *Am. J. Surg. Pathol.* 1992; 16: 694-707.

[161] Kilpatrick SE, Ward WG, Chauvenet AR, Pettenati MJ. The role of fine needle aspiration biopsy in the initial diagnosis of pediatric bone and soft tissue tumors: an institutional experience. *Mod. Pathol.* 1998; 11: 923-928.

[162] Atahan Ş, Aksu Ö, Ekinci C. Cytologic diagnosis and subtyping of rhabdomyosarcoma. *Cytopathology.* 1998; 9: 389- 397.

[163] Viguer JM, Jiménez-Heffernan JA, Vicandi B, López-Ferrer P, Gamallo C. Cytologic features of synovial sarcoma with special emphasis on the monophasic fibrous variant: A morphologic and immnocytochemical analysis of bcl-2 protein expression. *Cancer.* (Cancer Cytopathol) 1998; 84: 50-56.

[164] Fröstad B, Tani E, Brosjö O, Skog L, Kogner P. Fine needle aspiration cytology in the diagnosis and management of children and adolescents with Ewing sarcoma and peripheral neuroectdermal tumor. *Med. Pediatr. Oncol.* 2002; 38: 33-40.

[165] Wakely Jr PE, Kneisl J. Soft tissue aspiration cytopathology: Diagnostic accuracy and limitations. *Cancer.* (Cancer Cytopathol) 2000; 90: 292-298.

[166] Treaba D, Assad L, Govil H, Sariya D, Reddy VB, Kluskens L, Green L, Selvaggi SM, Gattuso P. Diagnostic role of fine-needle aspiration of bone lesions in patients with previous history of malignancy. *Diagn. Cytopathol.* 2002; 26: 380- 383.

[167] Handa U, Bal A, Mohan H, Bhardwaj S. Fine needle aspiration cytology in the diagnosis of bone lesions. *Cytopathology.* 2005; 16: 59- 64.

[168] Skoog L, Pereira ST, Tani E. Fine-needle aspiration cytology and immunocytochemistry of soft-tissue tumors and osteo/chondrosarcomas of the head and neck. *Diagn. Cytopathol.* 1999; 20: 131- 136.

[169] Udayakumar AM, Sundareshan TS, Goud TM, Devi MG, Biswas S, Appaji L, Arunakumari BS, Rajan KR, Prabhakaran PS. Cytogenetic characterization of Ewing tumors using fine needle aspiration samples: a 10-year experience and review of literature. *Cancer Genet. Cytogenet.* 2001; 127: 42-48.

[170] Nicol KK, Ward WG, Savage PD, Kilpatrick SE. Fine-needle aspiration biopsy of skeletal versus extraskeletal osteosarcoma. *Cancer.* (Cancer Cytopathol) 1998; 84: 176- 185.

[171] Domanski HA, Åkerman M. Fine-needle aspiration of primary osteosarcoma: A cytological-histological study. *Diagn. Cytopathol.* 2005; 32: 269- 275.

[172] Klijanienko J, Caillaud J-M, Lagacé R, Vielh P. Fine-needle aspiration of leiomyosarcoma: A correlative cytohistopathological study of 96 tumos in 68 patients. *Diagn. Cytopathol.* 2003; 28: 119- 125.

[173] Berardo MD, Powers CN, Wakely Jr PE, Almeida MO, Frable WJ. Fine-needle aspiration cytopathology of malignant fibrous histiocytoma. *Cancer.* (Cancer Cytopathol) 1997; 81: 228- 237.

[174] Klijanienko J, Cailaud J-M, Lagacé R, Viehl P. Comparative fine-needle aspiration and pathologic study of malignant fibrous histiocytoma: Cytodiagnostic features of 95 tumors in 71 patients. *Diagn. Cytopathol.* 2003; 29: 320- 326.

[175] Klianienko J, Cailaud J-M, Lagacé R. Fine-needle aspiration in liposarcoma: Cytohistologic correlative study including well-differentiated, myxoid, and pleomorphic variants. *Diagn. Cytopathol.* 2004; 30: 307- 312.

[176] Das DK, Das JC, Kumar D, Bhatt NC, Banot K, Natarajan R. Leiomyosarcoma of the orbit: Diagnosis of its recurrence by fine needle aspiration cytology. *Diagn. Cytopathol.* 1992; 8: 609- 613.

[177] Das DK, Grover RK, Anand VJ, Mandal AK, Jain S, Jain J, Bhat NC, Chowdhury V. Oral leiomyosarcoma in childhood: Report of a case with fine needle aspiration cytology. *Acta Cytol.* 1999; 43: 1150- 1154.

[178] Dodd LG, Scully SP, Cothran RL, Harrelson JM. Utility of fine-needle aspiration in the diagnosis of primary osteosarcoma. *Diagn. Cytopathol.* 2002; 27: 350- 353.

[179] Bütter A, Hui T, Chapdelaine J, Beaunoyer M, Flageole H, Bouchard S. Melanoma in children and the use of sentinel lymph node biopsy. *J. Pediatr. Surg.* 2005; 40: 797-800.

[180] Roaten JB, Partrick DA, Pearlman N, Gonzalez RJ, Gonzalez R, McCarter MD. Sentinel lymph node biopsy for melanoma and other melanocytic tumors in adolescents. *J. Pediatr. Surg.* 2005; 40: 232- 235.

[181] van Rijk MC, Teertstra HJ, Peterse JL, Nieweg OE, Valdés Olmos RA, Hoefnagel CA, Kroon BBR. Ultrasonography and fine needle aspiration cytology in the preoperative evaluation of melanoma patients eligible for sentinel node biopsy. *Ann. Surg. Oncol.* 2006; 13: 1511-1516.

[182] Das DK, Bhambhani S, Chachra KL, Murthy NS, Tripathi RP. Small round cell tumors of abdomen and thorax: Role of fine needle aspiration cytologic features in the diagnosis and differential diagnosis. *Acta Cytol.* 1997; 41:1035-1047.

[183] Silverman JF, Joshi VV. FNA biopsy of small round cell tumors of childhood: cytomorphologic features and the role of ancillary studies. *Diagn. Cytopathol.* 1994; 10: 245- 255.

[184] Akhtar M, Ali MA, Sabbah R, Bakry M, Nash JE. Fine-needle aspiration biopsy diagnosis of round cell malignant tumors of childhood. A combined light and electron microscopic approach. *Cancer.* 1985; 55: 1805-1817.

[185] Rajwanshi A, Rao KL, Marwaha RK, Nijhawan VS, Gupta SK. Role of fine-needle aspiration cytology in childhood malignancies. *Diagn. Cytopathol.* 1989; 5: 378- 382.

[186] McGahey BE, Moriarty AT, Nelson WA, Hull MT. Fine-needle aspiration biopsy of small round blue cell tumors of childhood. *Cancer.* 1992; 69: 1067-1073.

[187] Brahmi U, Rajwanshi A, Joshi K, Ganguly NK, Vohra H, Gupta SK, Dey P. Role of immunocytochemistry and DNA flow cytometry in the fine-needle aspiration diagnosis diagnosis of malignant small round-cell tumors. *Diagn. Cytopathol.* 2001; 24: 233- 239.

[188] Ravindra S, Kini U. Cytomorphology and morphometry of small round-cell tumors in the region of the kidney. *Diagn. Cytopathol.* 2005; 32: 211-216.

[189] Gurley AM, Silverman JF, Lassaletta MM, Wiley JE, Holbrook CT, Joshi VV. The utility of ancillary studies in pediatric FNA cytology. *Diagn. Cytopathol.* 1992; 8: 137- 146.

[190] Rossi ED, Raffaelli M, Minimo C, Mule A, Lombardi CP, Vecchio FM, Fadda G. Immunocytochemical evaluation of thyroid neoplasms on thin-layer smears from fine-needle aspiration biopsies. *Cancer.* 2005; 105: 87- 95.

[191] Laane E, Tani E, Björklund E, Elmberger G, Everaus H, Skoog L, Porwit-MacDonald A. Flow cytometric immunophenotyping including Bcl-2 detection on fine needle aspirates in the diagnosis of reactive lymphadenopathy and non-Hodgkin's lymphoma. *Cytometry B. Clin. Cytom.* 2005; 64:34-42.

[192] Jacobs JC, Katz RL, Shabb N, el-Naggar A, Ordonez NG, Pugh W. Fine needle aspiration of lymphoblastic lymphoma. A multiparameter diagnostic approach. *Acta Cytol.* 1992; 36: 887-894.

[193] Smock KJ, Yaish HM, Cairo MS, Lones MA, Willmore-Payne C, Perkins SL. Mantle cell lymphoma presenting with unusual morohology in an adolescent female: A case report and review of literature. *Pediatr. Dev. Pathol.* 2007; 10: 403- 408.

[194] Aljajeh IA, Das DK, Krajci D. Ki-1-positive anaplastic large cell lymphoma initially diagnosed as Hodgkin's disease by fine needle aspiration (FNA) cytology. *Cytopathology.* 1995; 6: 226- 235.

[195] Ellison DA, Silverman JF, Strausbauch PH, Wakely PE, Holbrook CT, Joshi VV. Role of immunocytochemistry, electron microscopy, and DNA analysis in fine-needle aspiration biopsy diagnosis of Wilms' tumor. *Diagn. Cytopathol.* 1996; 14: 101-107.

[196] Kilpatrick SE, Bergman S, Pettenati MJ, Gulley ML. The usefulness of cytogenetic analysis in fine needle aspirates for the histologic subtyping of sarcomas. *Mod. Pathol.* 2006; 19: 815- 819.

[197] Sápi Z, Antal I, Pápai Z,Szendröi M, Mayer A, Jakab K, Pajor L, Bodó M. Diagnosis of soft issue tumors by fine-needle aspiration with combined cytopathology and ancillary techniques. *Diagn. Cytopathol.* 2002; 26: 232- 242.

[198] Ljubojević S. The human papillomavirus vaccines. *Acta Dermatovenerol. Croat.* 2006; 14: 208.

In: Cancer in Female Adolescents
Editor: Margarite T. Moorland
ISBN: 978-1-60456-421-1

Chapter II

Cancers Related to Human Papillomavirus in Adolescent Females

Yasmin Jayasinghe[1,2,3,4,5] ***and Suzanne Garland***[1,3,4]
[1]Department of Microbiology and Infectious Diseases, Royal Women's Hospital,
[2]Departments of Pediatrics and [3]Obstetrics & Gynaecology, University of Melbourne,
[4]Murdoch Children's Research Institute, Department of Gynaecology,
[5]Royal Children's Hospital, Melbourne, Australia.

Abstract

Persistent anogenital infection with oncogenic human papillomaviruses (HPVs) is a prerequisite for HPV related squamous and adenocarcinoma anogenital malignancies of the cervix, vulva, vagina and anus of the female anogenital tract. Integration of the E6 and E7 HPV genes of the oncogenic HPVs into the host genome in the presence of co-carcinogens may result in cellular proliferation, and malignant transformation. Ano-genital HPV infection is primarily sexually transmitted and very common after sexual debut, yet anogenital malignancies are very rare in adolescents. This is largely due to high clearance rates of initial HPV infection, plus the fact that development of neoplasias from the precancerous lesions of high-grade dysplasia (such as cervical intraepithelial neoplasia grade 2 or 3 [CIN2/3]) takes around 15-20 years. In adolescents, apart from genital warts (caused largely by low risk genotypes 6/11) HPV infection is asymptomatic. Both high and low risk genotype infection may cause cell abnormality, otherwise recognized on cytology as low-grade dysplasia, although these really just represent manifestations of cellular infection. They are highly prevalent within a couple of years of initial HPV infection, but generally have a high chance of regression, not requiring treatment. Furthermore there is good evidence that excisional biopsy is associated with future adverse obstetric outcome, such as preterm labour. Therefore national organisations in the UK and USA have recently revised their protocols for young women, recommending cervical screening to commence at a later age, with more conservative management of early stage dysplasias. However while overall rates of cervical cancer have significantly declined with the introduction of well-organized nationalized Pap screening programmes, a trend of increasing rates in young women has been seen in some countries, with cervix cancer being second in incidence in genital tract cancers for the age group 20-24 years.

Whilst various risk factors predisposing to anogenital carcinomas are recognized, it is unclear if those cancers occurring in adolescents represent infection with more virulent types of HPV (a particular variant) or if they are due to other risk factors in childhood, such as immunosuppression or a result of earlier acquisition of HPV due to sexual abuse.

American Pap screening guidelines have suggested that earlier screening may be required in those who have been sexually abused or are immunosuppressed, although other national organizations have not made these recommendations. There have been significant recent advances in the treatment of early stage cervical carcinomas in young women, meaning that fertility sparing surgery may be offered to a larger number of young women with invasive cervical cancer without compromising survival. The introduction of prophylactic HPV vaccines has been a monumental step in the fight against anogenital carcinomas, with the distinct possibility that these cancers can be largely prevented in the future with wide coverage of such vaccines. However as immunity is largely type specific a successful vaccine programme at best will be 70% preventative for cervical cancer. Australia is the first country that has introduced the quadrivalent HPV vaccine as part of a widespread federally funded school-based public health initiative, with a current uptake of around 80% in the target age, compared to a other countries using family physician based reimbursable schemes where uptake is more in the order of 30%. Moreover with the extremely high cost of the current vaccines HPV infection and anogenital cancer, particularly cervical cancer will continue to be a problem worldwide for decades to come, with maximal burden of disease occurring in developing nations. Vertical transmission from the maternal genital tract of low risk HPV genotypes 6/11 is also known to play an aetiological role in the rare, but recalcitrant to treatment, juvenile onset recurrent respiratory papillomatosis (JORRP). JORRP usually presents within the first 5 years of life and runs a protracted course, with malignant transformation occurring rarely. This review will therefore also discuss the implications for adolescents who have this rare but debilitating condition.

Introduction

Human papillomavirus (HPV) is a common sexually transmitted infection with up to 80% of sexually active individuals acquiring HPV sometime during their life [1]. Persistent infection with oncogenic HPVs are established as causing 99.7% of cervical cancer, [2] 20-50% of vulvar cancer, 60-65% of vaginal cancer, and 83-92% of anal cancer [3]. Necessary steps for carcinogenesis include HPV transmission, viral persistence, progression of a clone of infected cells to precancer (also known as dysplasia or intraepithelial neoplasia), and finally invasion [4].

Adolescence is a unique period between childhood and adulthood, during which young women are establishing patterns of behavior and making lifestyle choices that form the foundation for their future health. Therefore adolescence provides a unique window of opportunity for positive evidence based health interventions. WHO clearly defines adolescence as the period of life between 10-19 years, youth as the period between 15- 24 years and young people, as those between 10-24 years. The health of both groups, youth and adolescents are often taken together, as biological and sociocultural conditions force these stages of life to be dynamic and interchanging [5].

Sexually active women under 25 years of age have the highest rates of HPV infection, due to high rates of partner change, as well as cervical factors [6]. In 14-26 year olds, the overall cross-sectional prevalence of genital HPV infection ranges from 20-46%, and oncogenic types have been reported in 18% - 30% [7-11]. Therefore high rates of viral clearance and a long latent phase from high-grade intraepithelial neoplasia to cancers ensure that carcinomas are uncommon in this age group.

This chapter will discuss the natural history of genital HPV in adolescents, and clinical presentation and management of HPV related anogenital cancers and pre-cancers specific to the young. Vulval, vaginal and anal carcinomas are exceedingly rare in adolescence; therefore, the chapter will concentrate on cervical dysplasia and carcinoma in adolescents, including recommended preventative strategies such as cervical cancer screening and prophylactic HPV vaccination strategies. The latter part of this chapter will discuss juvenile onset recurrent respiratory papillomatosis, (JORRP) which is due to laryngeal HPV infection acquired during birth from the maternal genital tract. The condition may have a prolonged and debilitating course in adolescence, occasionally associated with malignant transformation.

Human Papillomavirus

Virology

HPV is a DNA virus which has a circular genome of 8000 base pairs of double stranded DNA. The HPV genome has evolved over around 200 000 years, and can be classified into 5 major phylogenetic clusters worldwide according to ethnicity and area of origin (European, Asian, Asian-American, African 1 and African 2) [12,13]. The genome is divided into eight open reading frames (ORF's) coding for six early proteins (E1,E2,E4,E5,E6, E7) involved in DNA replication and cellular proliferation; and two late proteins (L1 and L2) which encode for the L1 and L2 outer capsid structural proteins [13]. HPV types are further classified according to their L1 nucleotide sequence: at least 10% dissimilarity from any other type, defines a new HPV type; <10 and >2% dissimilarity defines a new subtype; and <2% dissimilarity defines an intratypic variant[14].

There are around 40 types of HPV which specifically infect the genital tract, and they are divided into high risk (HR) and low risk (LR), depending on their oncogenic potential [15]. Fifteen HR-HPV types may cause cervical cancer (HPV 16, 18, 31, 33, 35, 39, 45, 51, 52, 56, 58, 59, 68, 73, 82). The most carcinogenic types are HPV 16 and 18 which consistently cause 70% of cervical cancer and 50% of cervical intraepithelial neoplasia 3 (CIN 3) worldwide[16,17]. Fifty per cent of squamous cell carcinomas are due to HPV 16 and 20% due to HPV 18. HPV 16 is also found more frequently in adenocarcinoma or its precursor lesion adenocarcinoma *in situ* (ACIS) as in squamous cell carcinoma, but there is a relatively higher prevalence of HPV 18 (around 39 % of positives worldwide, with detection in women under 50 years being around 46%) [18-20].

Transmission

Genital HPV's are largely sexually transmitted, and in adolescents first infection has been detected as soon as one month after sexual debut [21,22]. Penetrative intercourse is not strictly necessary and transmission to the cervix may occur via introital contact alone [22]. HPV first infects the parabasal cells in the squamous epithelium through micro-abrasions in the skin and results in a productive infection in 6-12 weeks, where infectious viral particles are shed within desquamated squamous cells[15]. Following infection, the virus may also exist in a non-productive state without complete virion production, detected by molecular methods only (known as latent infection). The extent to which this occurs is currently unknown.

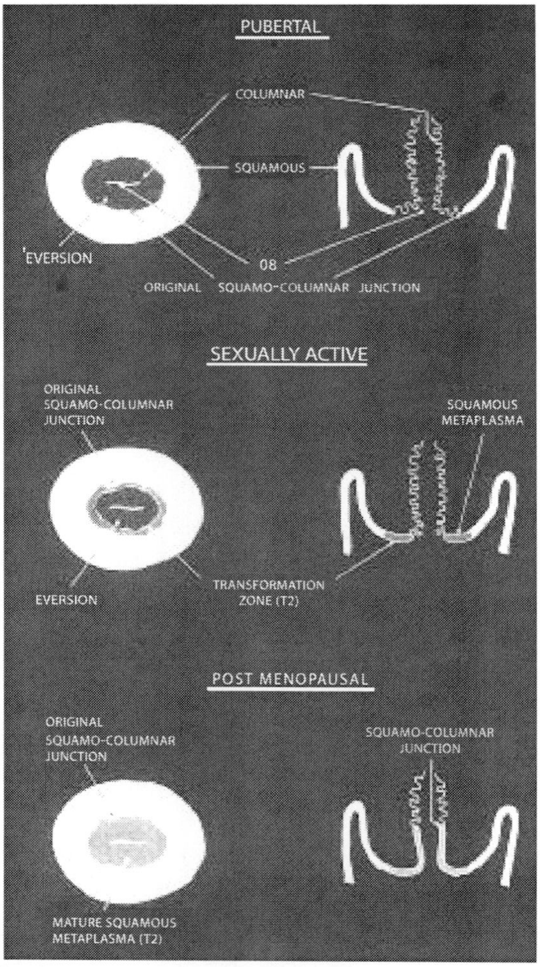

Awaiting permission, Garland S et al, MJA 1992;156(3):204-212.

Figure 1. Migration of the transformation zone up the endocervical canal from puberty to menopause.

The majority of cancers of the cervix and anus arise in the local transformation zone (TZ),[3] and may arise in the squamous or glandular cells resulting in squamous cell carcinomas or adenocarcinomas respectively. In the cervix the epithelial lining is undergoing constant change. In adolescents under the influence of oestrogen, the glandular epithelium lining the endocervix is everted onto the ectocervix and the squamocolumnar junction (SCJ) is found on the ectocervix. The SCJ migrates towards the endocervical canal over time. The TZ is a vulnerable area of intervening tissue between the old and new SCJ, where the columnar epithelium is undergoing metaplasia to immature squamous epithelium which then undergoes a process of maturation. Adolescents who are likely to have a wider cervical ectropion and larger area of exposed TZ are more vulnerable to HPV infection (Figure 1) [23,24] [25].

Clearance and Persistence

The average length of time for detectable cervical HPV infection which is newly acquired in an adolescent is 8-13 months, with most cervical HPV infections cleared by a cell mediated immune response within 2 years of exposure[7,26]. Average duration of carriage of LR-HPV types is 4-6 months, with total clearance in over 90% of young women. HR-HPV types may persist for longer (average duration of carriage almost 2 years for HPV 16), with eventual clearance in over 70% of young women[9,26,27]. It is still unclear to what extent there is complete viral clearance or whether the infection remains in a latent state in copy numbers, so low that it is undetectable by molecular methods, but reactivate many years later.

Progression

When there is impaired cellular immunity, there may be persistent carriage of HPV [15]. Chronic infection with HR-HPV is the most significant risk factor for development of cervical carcinoma. E6 and E7 are the two primary oncoproteins of HR-HPV. Integration of E6 and E7 genes into the host genome results in unregulated over expression of E6 and E7 proteins which inactivate and degrade tumour suppressor proteins p53 and retinoblastoma protein respectively, causing disruption of the cell cycle[28]. In the presence of co-carcinogens such as smoking, cellular proliferation and progression to dysplasia and malignancy may eventually occur.

Cervical Carcinoma in Adolescents

Preinvasive Disease

Terminology

Cervical dysplasia or intraepithelial neoplasia refers to preinvasive changes of the cervical epithelium which are often asymptomatic. They may be predicted on cytology (conventional cervical cytology Papanicolaou smears or liquid based cytology such as Thin-prep), colposcopy or detected on cervical biopsy. Cervical cytological abnormalities are described according to the 2001 Bethesda System (Table 1) [29]. The new terminology reflects our new understanding that low-grade changes on Pap or biopsy are merely cytopathic changes induced by HPV infection alone, are likely to undergo regression, and are therefore not regarded as precancerous lesions. Furthermore distinction between HPV and CIN 1 on cytology or CIN 2 and CIN 3 on cytology is poorly reproducible.

In Australia, cytological abnormalities are classified according to the Australian Modified Bethesda System (AMBS), which is similar to the 2001 Bethesda System, apart from the ASCUS and ASC-H being classified as 'possible LSIL' and 'possible HSIL' respectively[31].

Histological nomenclature of biopsy material is still described according to CIN terminology. CIN 1 and CIN2 refer to mild and moderate dysplasia involving the lower third and the lower two thirds of the cervical squamous epithelium, respectively. CIN 3 refers to severe dysplasia which extends into the upper third of the cervical epithelium. Carcinoma *in situ* is a category of CIN 3 where the abnormal undifferentiated cells have replaced the full thickness of the cervical epithelium. Invasive cervical cancer occurs when the abnormal cells have penetrated deeper into the cervix after penetrating the basement membrane. Rather than a continuum of progression from CIN1 to CIN 2 to CIN 3, CIN 1 is likely to undergo spontaneous regression and is not regarded as precancerous, while CIN 2 is heterogeneous and may regress. CIN 3 is regarded as the true precursor to cervical cancer. It is thought that CIN 2/3 can arise *de novo* without having to go through CIN 1 as once believed.

Table 1. 2001 Bethesda System for classification of cervical epithelial abnormalities

Squamous Cell Abnormalities	
Low-grade intraepithelial lesion (LSIL)	Early changes in size, shape and number of abnormal cells. Encompasses previous nomenclature of CIN 1 or HPV on Pap smear
High-grade intraepithelial lesion (HSIL)	Significant changes in size and shape of abnormal cells Encompasses previous nomenclature of CIN 2 and CIN 3 on Pap smear
Squamous Cell Carcinoma	Invasive SCC
Atypical squamous cells (ASC) ASC-US ASC –H	 Atypical squamous cells of undetermined significance. Prevalence of invasive cancer is low (0.1-0.2 %) [30] Atypical squamous cells cannot exclude HSIL Prevalence of CIN 2 or 3 is higher in this group than with ASC-US, therefore investigate as per HSIL
Glandular Abnormalities	
AGC	Atypical glandular cells either specified as endocervical, endometrial, or not otherwise specified (NOS)
AGC favour neoplastic	Endocervical or NOS
AIS	Endocervical adenocarcinoma *in situ*
Adenocarcinoma	Invasive adenocarcinoma

Prevalence of High- and Low-Grade Squamous Intraepithelial Lesions in Adolescents

Mean age of diagnosis of low and high grade squamous intraepithelial lesions is decreasing, with increasing prevalence among adolescents and women under 30 [32]. This is thought to reflect the reducing mean age of first sexual intercourse. Cross-sectional prevalence of both LSIL and HSIL combined was reported to be around 3.7% in sexually active adolescents aged 10-19 in the USA [33]. However more recent international multicenter trials in a slightly older population aged 15-26 years reveal baseline prevalence to lie between 10-12% [11, 34, 35].

Rates of ASCUS in adolescents can reach 9% [33]. Prevalence of LSIL is around 5-6% in adolescents[21, 36, 37], while prevalence of HSIL is around 0.5-0.7% in multicentre international studies[34, 37]. Much higher incidence rates of HSIL have been found in high risk areas, for example an HSIL prevalence of 3% in adolescents aged 12-19 years has been seen in a clinic base population in Rio de Janeiro[21]. The prevalence of glandular abnormalities on cytology in adolescents is <0.1% [33, 37].

Cytological LSIL or HSIL do not always correspond to similar rates of CIN on biopsy. Combined rates of HPV 16 or 18 positive CIN 2 or CIN 3 are around 0.3-0.9% and AIS <0.1% on histology[11, 37].

Natural History of SIL and CIN in Adolescents

Longitudinal studies of college students, where screening techniques are performed at very frequent intervals have picked up high cumulative prevalence rates of dysplasia in adolescents, which have developed reasonably rapidly, but also show high rates of spontaneous resolution. This is a reflection of the fact that adolescents have high rates of HPV infection, which can be detected mostly as LSIL or CIN 1 (a manifestation of viral infection), most of which clears within 2 years after infection.

Cumulative prevalence of LSIL ranges from 28-50% by 2-3 years after HPV infection, with spontaneous resolution rates of 62-95%. In adolescents, resolution of CIN 1 is greater than 85%. Cumulative prevalence of HSIL, 3 years after onset of sexual activity is much lower (2.6%), although interval between onset of sexual activity and median time to diagnosis is around 36 months. For those positive for HPV 16 or 18, median time from detection of these HR-HPV types and HSIL may be more rapid, and CIN2 or 3 may be detected by 2 years [7, 9, 26, 27, 38-40]. Resolution of CIN 2 may occur in 50% of patients and may take years [41-43].

Malignant potential of HSIL is not uniform. In the general population, median time from HSIL to microinvasive carcinoma is around 15 years, and about 20% of histologically proven CIN 3 progress to carcinoma over 10 years and 36% at 20 years ie 1% per annum risk if left untreated, although progression may take as little as 12-18 months [44-47]. The natural history of CIN 3 in adolescents is unknown as the standard of care is to treat on diagnosis.

Risk Factors for HPV Infection and Progression to Cervical Carcinoma

While risk factors for the acquisition of HPV infection and cervical carcinoma are well known (Table 7), risk factors for development of cervical carcinoma, particularly early in life during adolescence are less well known.

Persistent HR-HPV Infection

The most important and necessary risk factor for development of cervical carcinoma is persistent infection with oncogenic HPV types which increases the risk several hundred-fold [27,48].

Sexual Activity

Risk is also increased with earlier sexual activity, increased sexual partners (for the woman as well as of her partner), new partners within the last 5-8months, increased parity and younger age of first full term pregnancy. [38, 49-51] A study of Brazilian adolescents demonstrated that risk of HSIL and cervical carcinoma increased 2-fold with each year of age and each successive pregnancy. These factors increase the risk of exposure and acquisition of a new HPV infection, while parity may reflect non-utilisation of condoms [21], as well as hormonal factors. A randomised controlled trial demonstrated that correct and persistent use of condoms reduce the risk of genital HPV infection by 70%[52], while a meta-analysis demonstrated a reduced risk of genital warts, SIL and cervical cancer with condom use[53]. Unwanted sexual encounters after drinking, and illegal drug use have also been shown to be independent risk factors, and can form the basis of important preventative messages during the adolescent consultation [8].

In developed countries, sexual debut is occurring at increasingly earlier ages providing a window of opportunity of many years between contact with HPV and onset of screening. In Finland there has been a doubling of cervical cancer incidence in women aged 25-49 years, thought to be due in part to changes in sexual behaviour [54, 55]. In the USA, a nationwide survey of high school females in grades 9 to 12, revealed that 43% reported having had sexual intercourse, (29% in grade 9, and 60% in grade 12). Furthermore, 11% reported ≥ 4 sexual partners, and 4% had initiated sexual intercourse before 13 years [56]. In Australia, average age of coitarche has declined to 16 years, compared to 19 years 40 years previously [57] and is contributing to the increasing prevalence of CIN and ACIS in younger women [18].

Sexual Abuse

While there have been calls for earlier cervical screening in adolescents who have been sexually abused [58], risk for development of cervical carcinoma at an earlier age (which may warrant earlier screening prior to recommended national guidelines) is unknown. Children who have been sexually abused have been shown to have HPV DNA or abnormal cervical cytology in 3.4-33% [59], however these cytological changes may represent transient viral infection alone, and long-term outcome studies are required before introduction of special cervical screening or vaccination protocols in these young women.

Special Risk Factors in Developing Countries

Young women in developing countries face specific cultural practices and economic barriers that increase their risk of cervical carcinoma. In a case control study of 200 participants in Mali Africa, with and without cervical cancer, among whom the mean age was 15 years, risk factors were child marriage (marriage prior to 18 years of age), high parity (>10 children), polygamous husbands (>2 wives), poor genital hygiene, no tap water available and reuse of sanitary napkins [60]. Similar risk factors were seen in a Moroccan population [61]. In 2002, approximately 52 million girls less than 18 years were married worldwide, the majority in south Asia. By 2012 the cumulative estimate will reach 100 million [62]. Furthermore, marriage by age 20 is a risk factor for HIV infection for girls [63].

HIV and Immunosuppression

The Centers for Disease Control (CDC) defined cervical cancer as an AIDS defining malignancy in 1993 [64]. While it is the most common AIDS related cancer in women [65], the association between HIV and cervical cancer is currently under scrutiny due to recent reports from developing countries failing to demonstrate a strong link [66]. Some have argued that this may be due to the long latency of disease, with increased chance of subjects dying from AIDS before development of cancer. In the era of highly active antiretroviral therapy (HAART), an AIDS defining illness should still remain a surrogate marker for immunosuppression. Criteria for an AIDS defining illness therefore includes increased risk of disease in the HIV population, increased risk as the CD4 count decreases, and a decline in incidence and improved survival with the introduction of HAART [67]. International meta-analyses have demonstrated a 4-6 fold increase in incidence of cervical cancer with HIV positivity [68, 69]. While disease progression and recurrence after treatment may sometimes be affected by HIV status, and CD4 count [70,71] there is no clear relationship. Furthermore there has been no decline in the incidence of cervical cancer in the era of HAART [72], and there is no clear benefit of antiretroviral therapy in incidence or regression of pre-invasive lesions [65].

Cervical cancer has been reported in association with HIV infection in adolescents [73]. HIV positivity in female adolescents is associated with a 3.3 fold risk of HPV infection, (including higher relative risk of HR-HPV carriage and multiple infections), and 4.7 fold risk of abnormal cytology (mainly ASCUS and LSIL) compared with matched HIV negative controls. CD4 count and viral load were not associated with risk of HPV infection or abnormal cytology in this group of 133 adolescents, however only 9 girls had a CD4 count $<0.2 \times 10^9/l$ [74].

It has been recommended by some that adolescents with suppressed immunity have earlier cytological screening [58]. In 1997, the CDC and the US Public Health Service (USPHS) have recommended that 2 Pap smears be obtained within 12 months of diagnosis of HIV infection, and the CDC, USPHS and the American Cancer Society (ACS) recommend indefinite yearly screening for those who are immunosuppressed or HIV positive [75,76]. The American Society for Colposcopy & Cervical Pathology (ASCCP) have recommended that immunosupressed women with ASC-US be managed the same as the rest of the general population, rather than being referred for immediate colposcopy, as ASC-US has been found to be common and only has a low association with the presence of CIN2,3 in these women[77,78]. In Australia, immunosuppression is defined according to a CD4 count of <400 in HIV positive women, or transplantation with immunosuppressive therapy greater than 3 years [79]. Yearly indefinite screening is recommended according to National Health and Medical Research Council (NHMRC) guidelines, with referral for colposcopy with any degree of screen detected abnormality[31].

Cervical Factors in Young Women

Young women may be prone to HPV infection and SIL due to their immature cervical epithelium. Squamous metaplasia at the transformation zone of the cervix is a pivotal process in development of cervical neoplasia, and is largely initiated at puberty. Young women have wider areas of exposed cervical ectopy [46]. Later age of onset of menarche, a reduced menarche –sexual debut interval, and wider areas of cervical ectopy are significantly associated with HPV infection and SIL, suggesting vulnerability of the immature transformation zone to HPV infection [23, 24, 27].

Oral Contraceptive Pill (OCP)

Some studies in college students have shown a reduced association between HPV infection and OCP use; most likely reflecting contraceptive use associated with stable relationships hence reduced risk of new HPV infection [80]. However there is an increased association between ever use of the OCP and cervical adenocarcinoma [81], and ACIS (3.2 fold risk, independent of interval since last Pap smear). There is a dose-response effect, with risk of ACIS increasing to 5.5 fold in women who have used OCPs for 12 or more years, relative to nonusers[18]. This may be due to increased cervical ectopy, thereby increasing the area of vulnerable epithelium which may be infected by HR HPV, or may be due to a direct carcinogenic effect of the OCP on the metaplastic cervical epithelium. This does not justify cessation of the OCP in those at risk for pregnancy, as pregnancy itself poses some difficulty in effective management of these lesions [82].

Risk of Cervical Carcinoma in Women in Same-Sex Relationships

A large study of Danish women found the rate of invasive cervical cancer in women in same-sex relationships to be the same as the general population, however there was a significantly reduced risk of carcinoma in situ, possibly reflecting poorer participation of lesbian women in cervical screening [83,84]. Importantly, 22% of women in the Danish study had been involved in previous heterosexual encounters. Many who have not been in heterosexual relationships still have high carriage of HPV [84]. Therefore cervical screening is still recommended according to national guidelines, regardless of sexual preference.

Smoking

Smoking increases the risk of HPV infection and SIL in adolescents [27]. Women with HR-HPV infection with minimally abnormal smears who smoke are 3 times more likely to progress to CIN 3 or cervical cancer [85]. Interestingly, smoking has not been associated with an increased risk of ACIS, possibly due to the fact that smoking decreases cervical ectopy [86].

Low Education

HPV infection, premalignant and malignant disease is found more commonly in women of lower socioeconomic groups, reflecting poorer access to care and lower education [87]. Also once age, lifetime number of sexual partners and smoking history are taken into account, this association is less clear. The ASCUS-LSIL triage (ALTS) trial demonstrated that in those positive for oncogenic HPV, risk of CIN 3 increased 2.4 fold in those with less than high school education versus those who had completed college. Therefore low education may serve as surrogate marker for some other risk factor that influences progression to CIN 3 [88].

Co-infections

Genital infections with *Chlamydia trachomatis,* and herpes simplex virus independently increase the risk of HPV infection, although the mechanisms of action are unknown [89].

Prevention of Cervical Carcinoma

Cervical Screening

National cervical screening programs have been highly successful in detecting preinvasive changes that may be monitored or treated to prevent cervical cancer incidence and mortality. However, screening of adolescents is likely to pick up high rates of low grade changes that are likely to either undergo spontaneous resolution or be picked up later before invasion to carcinoma. Mass screening of adolescents may lead to overtreatment, and high recurrence rates of low grade changes due to new incident HPV infection, and adverse obstetric outcome [90-93]. Therefore, there is an international trend towards later onset of screening, and less aggressive management of low grade changes.

However the issue of screening in adolescents and young women will continue to be a focus of further investigation for some years to come. In the United Kingdom where age of onset of screening was recently changed from 20 to 25 years, a small increase in cervical cancer incidence is expected in women aged 20-25 years; however a policy of routine screening in this age group is predicted to have minimal impact on the cumulative lifetime incidence of cervical cancer, decreasing it from 0.63 to 0.61% [94]. An upsurge in numbers of cancers around 35 years of age has already been seen however [95]. In Wales, the National cervical screening program has contributed to a 58% reduction of cervical cancer incidence in women aged 20-24 years (from 4.2 per 100 000 women per year in 1981-1988, to 2.2 per 100 000 per women per year in 1989 to 2003); therefore, cervical screening will still be offered in this age group [96]. A recent study of cervical cancer incidence in the USA using the ACTUR registry, found that 20% of cervical cancers in those under 25 years occurred in those under 21 years or age [97], and SEER data suggest that the figures are around 13% [48,98]. Targeted screening may be the best solution. Some have suggested that those young women with immunosuppression and those who have been sexually abused may require earlier screening and intervention[58]. To shed further light on this issue, studies assessing specific characteristics of those who develop carcinoma at a very young age are underway.

Readers should follow their own national guidelines for cervical screening, which are set according to local natural history of disease and resource constraints. Finland has the lowest rate of cervical cancer amongst countries with comparable screening programs, with 100% cervical screening coverage in 44-55 year olds, demonstrating that population coverage is more important than screening interval in reducing the burden of cervical cancer[99].

Cytological screening may be performed by conventional Pap smear testing or Liquid based cytology. If it is decided that it should be performed in an adolescent, ideally the consultation should take place in a youth friendly environment that ensures privacy and confidentiality. Providers must be aware that Pap testing may lead to further investigation or even treatment in the event of a high grade abnormality. In Australia like some other countries, if the patient is under 18, parental consent is not required where the young person is deemed competent and mature. Specifically they should understand the nature of the specific condition for which they seek medical attention, the nature of any treatment being proposed, (including treatment options), possible outcomes of treatment and likely outcomes if the treatment is not performed. In Australia, competence and maturity for one examination or treatment (such as a Pap smear) does not necessarily guarantee the same for any new procedure (such as proceeding to cone biopsy), and assessment would need to be made on an individual basis. Therefore while parental consent is sometimes preferred for specific procedures, it is not mandatory. In some states in the USA, the law allows the health provider to disclose information to parents if it is necessary to protect the minors health [101-103].

Table 2. International Guidelines for Age of Onset of Cervical Screening [31, 58, 90, 99, 100]

Country	Age of onset of screening	Screening Interval
USA	3 years after sexual debut or no later than 21 years	Annual or 2 yearly if liquid-based.
Australia	2 years after sexual debut or 18 years of age, whichever is later	2 yearly
New Zealand	20 years	3 yearly
UK	25 years	3-5 yearly
Finland	30 years	5 yearly

Cervical Cytology Screening

Whilst a case-control study was never performed, quite clearly Pap test screening has been effective in reducing cervical cancer incidence and mortality in those countries where it has had wider coverage and high-quality methodology. Its overall sensitivity is 50-70% at best, with the strength of the Pap lying in the fact that pre-invasive disease is slowly progressive, and repeat interval examinations therefore likely to pick up disease eventually. Seventy percent of false-negatives (where the slide is free of abnormal cells yet disease is present) are due to inadequate specimen collection, and 30% are due to laboratory error. Nevertheless the biggest cause of missed cases of cervical cancer is due to absent or inadequate screening [58].

Prior to specimen collection, the patient should avoid tampons, any intravaginal preparations, or intercourse for 48 hours. If she has any evidence of vaginal or cervical infection it is best to treat this prior to the smear collection. Samples should not be collected during menstruation, although abnormal bleeding such as post-coital bleeding warrants further investigation. During collection, avoid lubricants apart from saline, wipe away any excess mucus with a cotton swab, and avoid washing the cervix which may cause a hypo cellular smear [58]. The best time to take the smear is mid-cycle, but in the young compliance issues may necessitate taking the smear when possible. The ectocervical specimen can be collected with an Ayres spatula or "Cervex" brush via rotation of 360 degrees at on the ectocervix, and gently smeared onto the slide. The endocervical brush may be rotated 90-180 degrees and rolled onto the slide. The specimens must be fixed immediately after collection and not allowed to air dry. Despite the best technique, 80% of the cellular sample may not be transferred to the slide.

Liquid based Cytology (LBC)

The most widely researched of these techniques is the *ThinPrep* method [Cyte Corporation, Boxborough, MA]. The sample is taken in the conventional way and is rinsed in a vial of buffered alcohol liquid preservative. The cells are then transferred to the slide in a monolayer, after excess blood, mucus and inflammatory debris has been removed. This technique reduces the percentage of inflammatory and unsatisfactory smears. Trials have shown LBC to increase the sensitivity of both LSIL and HSIL[46,104], although data regarding sensitivity is conflicting [105]. A recent multicenter randomised controlled trial of 45, 000 women demonstrated that LBC did not increase sensitivity of detection of ≥ CIN 2 and had reduced positive predictive value for ≥ CIN 2, compared to conventional smears [106]. Another trial of 55,164 split sample pairs demonstrated that the Thin prep image reader detected more cases of HSIL than conventional cytology. [107]. In 2007, the National Institute of Health and Clinical Excellence in the UK concluded that LBC was as sensitive as conventional cytology [108], and endorsed its use, with the desired end-points of reducing the number of inconclusive smears, and increasing screening capacity.

HR-HPV DNA Testing

In adolescents there is no role for the use of HR-HPV DNA testing in primary screening for cervical cancer. Adolescents have high rates of transient HPV infection, and a positive HR-HPV result has low correlation with disease. In the USA, testing for HR-HPV types using Hybrid Capture 2 (HC 2) is FDA approved for primary screening of women over 30 years only. This is because a positive result in such a woman is likely to indicate chronic carriage of HPV and has a high negative predictive value for high grade dysplasia [78,109]. Furthermore the American Society for Colposcopy and Cervical Pathology (ASCCP) have stated that it is unacceptable to perform such testing in adolescents at all, including as a secondary screen, (or reflex test), in the triage of ASCUS or LSIL in adolescents due to its low specificity for disease, and if testing is accidentally performed, it should not influence results [78, 110]. However 2006 guidelines from the American College of Obstetricians and Gynaecologists (ACOG) have not yet made such modifications [103]. In Australia, HR-HPV DNA testing is only approved for post-treatment follow up of women with HSIL with reviews showing excellent negative predictive value for recurrence. The further role of HPV DNA testing as a primary screen or for triage is currently under review [31, 111].

Colposcopy

Colposcopy is the examination of the cervical and anogenital epithelium under magnification, performed as a diagnostic test after abnormal cervical screening. Abnormal epithelium has an increased nuclear:cytoplasmic ratio, therefore staining with 3-5% acetic acid causes protein coagulation, and turns the abnormal epithelium white (termed acetowhite epithelium). Characteristic capillary abnormalities within the acetowhite epithelium, (known as mosaicism and punctuation), as well as neovascularisation, may be seen. Application of Lugols iodine stains the normal glycogen-containing vaginal epithelium a brown colour, while normal columnar, metaplastic and dysplastic epithelium remain white. The Reid colposcopic index is used to assess the severity of these features and has good correlation with severity of disease. During examination it is important that the upper limit of the lesion is adequately visualised (otherwise the colposcopy is deemed unsatisfactory, as there may be a more significant lesion further inside the endocervical canal), and biopsies are taken of the most severely affect area [46].

Management of Abnormal Cervical Cytology in Adolescents

There is some variability in national guidelines (Table 3), although there is general agreement that aggressive screening and management of benign lesions should be avoided, and that compliant adolescents may undergo monitored observation. Clinical judgement should be used for individual cases. ACOG and ACCP have introduced adolescent specific guidelines, while in Australia National Health and Medical Research Council (NHMRC) guidelines are currently under review.

Table 3. Comparison of guidelines for abnormal cervical cytology in adolescents

	ACOG 2006 [103]	ASCCP 2006 [78]	NHMRC 2005 [31]
ASCUS & LSIL	Do HR-HPV test If HR-HPV negative, repeat pap in 12 months If HR-HPV positive repeat HPV in 12 months, or perform cytology at 6 and 12 months. If any abnormality refer for colposcopy	Repeat Pap at 12 and 24 months If repeat at 12 months is ≥ HSIL, refer for colposcopy If repeat at 24 months is ≥ ASCUS, refer for colposcopy	Repeat Pap at 12 months If repeat is ≥ possible LSIL, refer for colposcopy

	ACOG 2006 [103]	ASCCP 2006 [78]	NHMRC 2005 [31]
ASC=H	Colposcopy	Colposcopy If no evidence of CIN2/3: HR HPV DNA in 12 months , or repeat Pap at 6 and 12 months. Refer for colposcopy if HPV DNA positive or ≥ ASCUS on smear	Colposcopy
HSIL	Colposcopy and endocervical assessment 'See and treat' in one step is unacceptable as a large proportion will have CIN 2 which may regress	Colposcopy and endocervical assessment "See and treat" unacceptable If there is failure to detect CIN 2 or 3 and colposcopy is adequate repeat Pap for 2 years at 6 monthly intervals, and excise TZ if HSIL present at 12 or 24 months, or if lesion seen at 12 months Also excise if any CIN on endocervical assessment, or unsatisfactory colposcopy	Colposcopy
AGC of any sort	Colposcopy and endocervical sampling	Colposcopy and endocervical sampling	Colposcopy

Management of CIN in an Adolescent

Surgical management of CIN may involve ablative techniques (such as cryotherapy, laser ablation, electrofulguration) or excision techniques (such as cold-knife cone, laser cone, large loop excision of the transformation zone, also known as LLETZ or LOOP). Ablative and excisional techniques have similar efficacy in reducing the risk of future cervical cancer [112]. Excisional procedures allow histological evaluation, and assessment of excision margins, and are favoured for CIN 3 where there is risk of microinvasive or occult invasive carcinoma especially in larger lesions [113]. LLETZ in particular is highly popular for treatment of preinvasive disease, as it can be performed rapidly as a day procedure and is of low cost.

A meta-analysis of 27 studies has confirmed that cone biopsy and LLETZ are associated with around a 2-fold risk of preterm delivery and low birth weight. Cone biopsy is also associated with 3 fold risk of caesarean section, and LLETZ associated with a greater than 2 fold risk of preterm rupture of membranes. Depth of the cone beyond 10 mm appears to increase the risk. Therefore more conservative management to minimize destruction of cervical architecture prior to child-bearing is the recommended management in the young (Table 4) [92, 93].

Table 4. Comparison of guidelines for management of histologically confirmed CIN in adolescents

	ACOG 2006[103]	ASCCP 2006[116]	NHMRC 2005[31]
CIN 1	Perform repeat Pap in 6 and 12 months Or repeat HR-HPV at 12 months Refer for colposcopy if abnormalities detected	Annual cytology at 12 and 24 months If ≥ HSIL at 12 months, refer for colposcopy If ≥ ASCUS at 24 months , refer for colposcopy	Repeat cytology at 12 and 24 months If either show ≤ LSIL, repeat smears annually until 2 consecutive negatives, then routine cytology
CIN 2	If compliant, reliable, adequate colposcopy, then cytology and colposcopy at 4-6 month intervals If risk of loss to follow-up, then surgical excision	Cytology and colposcopy at 6 monthly intervals If HSIL cytology or CIN2 persists for 1 year, perform surgical treatment	Surgical treatment
CIN 2/3		Surgical treatment acceptable Or observation with 6 monthly colposcopy and cytology If HSIL or CIN 2 persists for one year, perform surgical treatment	Surgical treatment
CIN 3	Surgical excision rather than ablation is favoured		
ACIS	In those who wish to conserve fertility: Cone biopsy and endocervical curettage Repeat cone if margins positive or CIN or ACIS in endocervical sample Re-evaluate in 6 months with colposcopy, cytology, endocervical curettage Long term follow up if uterus retained Hysterectomy recommended in those who have finished child-bearing		

Special consideration needs to be given to those with any kind of glandular abnormality. While the prevalence of AGC or ACIS cytology in adolescence is low, it may be associated with CIN and adenocarcinomas of the genital tract [114]. All adolescents with any category of glandular abnormality should be referred for colposcopy and endocervical sampling. Endometrial sampling would not be a routine procedure in a young woman unless they are at high risk of endometrial cancer [31, 78, 103]. These lesions are hard to diagnose on colposcopy, as changes can be minimal, they may extend into canal, and can be multifocal. Cone biopsy with histological assessment is the gold standard diagnostic procedure, although negative margins does not always mean complete excision, and hysterectomy is the treatment of choice in those who have completed childbearing. In young women cone biopsy, and endocervical curettage, with careful attention to margins and histology has failure rates of 8%, and is accepted treatment. Long term follow up is required for those who undergo conservative treatment [31, 103, 115, 116].

The HPV Vaccines

Efficacy

The fact that the major capsid L1 proteins when propagated into eukaryotic cells self-assemble into virus-like particles (VLPs) resembling HPV has underpinned the development of successful prophylactic HPV vaccines. These VLPs do not contain viral genetic material; hence are non-infectious. Currently there are two prophylactic vaccines available: Gardasil™ (Merck) is a 3 dose quadrivalent HPV (Types 6,11,16,18) L1 vaccine given intramuscularly in the deltoid at 0, 2 and 6 months and Cervarix™ (Glaxo Smith Kline) a bivalent HPV (Type 16,18) L1 vaccine, also intramuscularly in the deltoid, 0, 1 and six month schedules. While both vaccines are estimated to prevent 70% of cervical cancer, around 50% of high-grade dysplasias, the quadrivalent vaccine has also been shown be effective in preventing HPV 6 and 11 related genital warts of which these two viruses contribute to 90% of cases [35]. Vaccine efficacy has been assessed in placebo controlled double blind randomised studies (Table 5). Both vaccines to date show high efficacy against infection and disease from vaccine targeted HPV types, high immunogenicity and high safety. Combined results of the quadrivalent vaccine administered to 20, 583 women show almost 99% protection against preinvasive disease of the cervix, vagina and vulva to the vaccine genotypes, in those who are naïve to those specific HPV types [11]. Although immunity is largely type specific, there is some added benefit in protection for infection as well as CIN for phylogenetically related A7 and A9 genotypes [117]. Studies on the bivalent vaccine demonstrated some added protection of around 10 to 15% for infection from viral types that are phylogenetically related to the vaccine types [34, 118, 119].

Table 5. Prophylactic efficacy of HPV vaccine in those without previous exposure to the targeted HPV types within the vaccine [34, 35, 37, 118-122]#

Author	Mao et al 2006	Villa et al 2005 & Villa et al 2006	Garland et al 2007	Future II Study Group 2007	Harper et al 2004 & Harper 2006 et al	Paavonen et al 2007
Phase	IIa	IIb	III	III	II	III
HPV L1 VLP vaccine type	HPV 16	6,11,16,18	6,11,16,18	6,11,16,18	16,18 (bivalent)	16,18 (bivalent)
Number enrolled	2409	552	5455	12,167	1113	18,644
Age of subjects (years)	16-23	16-23	16-23	15-26	15-25	15-25
Number of sexual partners	0-5	0-4	0-4	0-4	0-6	0-6
Prior Pap abnormalities	Not allowed, but those with current infection or disease were included					
Average length of post dose 3 follow-up	3.5 years	2.5 years for protocol 007, then subset of 241 subjects followed for 5 years	3.0 years	3.0 years	2.25 years for initial randomisation, then subset of 756 subjects followed for 4.5 years	14.8 months
Prevention of HPV 16 or 18 related CIN 2/3 or AIS in Per protocol susceptible* Or intention to treat+	100%*	100%*	100%*	98%*	93.5% * protection against ASCUS, LSIL & HSIL at 2.25 years and 100% protection at 4.5 years	90.4% +
Prevention of HPV 6,11,16,18 related CIN (1-3) and AIS		100%	90%			
Prevention of HPV 6,11, 16 or 18 related genital warts		100%	98.3%			
Prevention of HPV 16 or 18 related VIN or VAIN			100%			

note primary efficacy endpoints vary between trials, as does inclusion criteria for per protocol and intention-to-treat analyses, as does case counting.

Combined general population analyses after administration of the quadrivalent vaccine (including subjects who may have had prior HPV infection or HPV related disease prior to vaccination) has demonstrated a 44% reduction of CIN 2/3 or AIS lesions for vaccine types, a 12 % reduction of these lesions for vaccine and any non-vaccine types, 16.5% reduction in cervical surgery, and 26.5% reduction in surgery to the external genital tract for all HPV related diseases, compared to placebo. These figures are consistent with the fact that vaccine is not therapeutic and does not protect from prevalent HPV-type disease or infection, but does protect against clinical disease against other vaccine serotypes not found at baseline [34, 37, 118, 119, 123].

Administration

Ideally the vaccine should be administered before sexual exposure. Highest immunogenicity of the vaccine is seen if it is administered before 15 years of age. It should be noted however that given the very high efficacy in the clinical trials, that to date we do not have an immune correlate of protection. In June 2006 the Food and Drug administration approved the use of the HPV vaccine for use in 9-26 year olds, and the Centers for Disease Control and Prevention recommended the vaccine be routinely administered in 11-12 year olds, and 13-26 year olds who had not received the vaccine, with 9-10 year olds being vaccinated at the discretion of the parent and provider [124]. It is administered in 3 doses at baseline, 2 and 6 months. Worldwide access to immunization is not uniform, and therefore uptake is around 20% where the vaccine is licensed. Australia is the first country that has adopted a federally funded policy of school-based quadrivalent HPV vaccination for young girls (year 7) 12-13 years, rolled out as of April 2007, with a catch up program to age 26 years (for a 2 year period only). To date vaccine uptake is high in the school-based program and at around 80%. There has also been recent licensure of bivalent vaccine for 10 to 45-year-old females in some European countries as well as Australia. In the USA, parental consent and parental insurance coverage is required for teenagers prior to any vaccination. Vaccination of young girls against a sexually transmitted infection is a sensitive issue, and endorsement by health professionals play a major role in vaccine acceptance. Subsidization of the vaccine for developing nations is also a priority.

The vaccine will not prevent against 20-30% of cervical cancer caused by HPV types other than HPV 16 and 18; therefore continued cervical screening is an imperative and must be articulated to be vaccinated populations. Optimal protocols post-vaccination are not yet known, but while continued research is being done in this area, cervical screening according to national protocols is advised. Complementary health messages such as delayed sexual debut and use of condoms are important. In developing countries, specific programs aimed at educating, empowering, improving the health and financial status of women will also contribute to a reduction in cervical cancer risk. Education is an important factor for delayed first sexual activity, pregnancy, marriage and child bearing. Furthermore learning about sexual and reproductive health, STD prevention, contraception and AIDS, and how to seek health care allows negotiation of safer sex practices [125].

Cervical Cancer: Invasive Disease in Adolescents

Burden of Disease in Adolescents

Cervical cancer is the second most common cancer in women, and current estimates indicate that almost half a million women are diagnosed with cervical cancer each year of whom just over one quarter of a million die from disease[126]. The introduction of cervical screening programs has seen a dramatic decline in the incidence of cervical cancer in developed nations. Recent introduction of the human papillomavirus vaccine is a major breakthrough in the fight against this disease, estimated to prevent 70% of cervical cancer, however worldwide uptake is currently low. Therefore cervical cancer will continue to be a problem for decades to come. Cervical cancer is increasingly becoming a disease of younger premenopausal women. Around 61% of cervical cancer occurs in the age group between 15 and 49 years [127]. However, in adolescents, while pre-invasive disease is common, cervical carcinoma is uncommon, due to the natural history disease.

The vast burden of invasive disease (more than 80%) occurs in resource poor countries and is associated with disproportionately high mortality. The age standardized incidence in Mali, Africa is 24.4 per 100 000 [60].

In the USA, cervical carcinoma is the most common malignancy of the female genital tract in young women over 15 -25 or 15-29 years, whereas ovarian tumours are the most common when those under 15 are included [48, 97, 98]. There is a sharp increase in incidence of invasive cervical disease in late adolescence after 20 years of age. In the year 2000, the incidence per million per year in the USA was 0, 2.2, 14.8, and 66 for those aged <15, 15-19, 20-24 and 25-29 years respectively. This equates to 159 women aged 24 or less being diagnosed with cervical cancer in that year, 22 of whom were under 20 years. The incidence was higher in white females than in other races. Overall incidence of cervical carcinoma in 15-24 year olds between 1975 and 2000 was 26.5 per million, and decreased to 17 per million in 2000. The reduction was only seen in 20-24 year olds, highlighting that there has been no decrease in cervical cancer incidence in 15-19 year olds in the USA since 1975 [48].

Similar low trends have been seen in Australia. However, the incidence rate of cervical cancer for 20-24 years olds has decreased from 0.9 per 100 000 /year to 0.5 per 100 000 /year between 1983 and 2001. For 15-19 year olds, the incidence rate was 0.2 per 100 0000/year and has been stable since 1983, similar to the USA [128].

Cell Types

Squamous cell carcinoma accounts for around 80-90% of cervical cancers in women under 35 years, and adenocarcinoma round 15-25%. In a study of 15-25 year olds, the proportion of those diagnosed with SCC was only 52% [97, 129-131]. Unusual variants include clear cell, neuroendocrine and adenosquamous, the former two are not HPV-related.

The decrease in cancer incidence in women aged 20-24 since the mid seventies, is due to a reduction in squamous cell carcinoma, whereas adenocarcinoma increased during this time. Between 1973 and 1996 SEER data identified a 9 fold increase in the combined incidence of ACIS and adenocarcinoma, from 0.2 to 1.8 per 100 000 women per year, mainly to women born after 1945[132]. This is consistent with other international studies from the West, which reported an increase in incidence of cervical carcinoma in young women from the mid 1970's, particularly adenocarcinoma [130,133-139]. This trend was not seen in a large study of nearly 4000 women with cervical cancer from Taiwan; however younger age was significantly associated with an increased risk of adenocarcinoma rather than older age[131].

Tumour grade, depth and width of invasion, and lymphovascular space invasion (LVSI) are prognostic factors. LVSI does not alter FIGO stage but may be an important factor when deciding on treatment, as in early stage tumours LVSI on cone biopsy specimens are associated with over a 5 fold risk of lymph node metastases at radical hysterectomy[140]. Of 45 cervical cancers reported in women aged 35 years or less in Gateshead, only 3 were microinvasive, 3 were adenocarcinoma, and 37 were squamous cell carcinomas of which 9 were anaplastic and 25 were poorly differentiated with tumour differentiation being a prognostic factor [141].

Clinical Presentation

Early disease is usually asymptomatic and first detected on cervical screening alone. Other symptoms depend on the stage and spread of the tumour, and may include abnormal vaginal bleeding (including intermenstrual and postcoital bleeding), vaginal discharge, backache and pain [142]. Studies from the 1980's of women with cervical cancer under 35 years of age reported a delay in diagnosis of around 4-5 months due to low suspicion of cancer despite symptoms [129, 130]. Around 25-34% of women were asymptomatic and detected on routine smear, and 6-13% had an asymptomatic lesion found on examination and in one study (from Queensland, Australia), 57% of subjects had intermenstrual bleeding. In the same study of those who had a Pap smear within the last 2 years (43%), 77% had normal results, suggesting that young women may have more rapid onset of cancers [129, 130, 134, 141]. The youngest reported case of cervical cancer is in a 9 year old with endometrioid adenocarcinoma, who presented with a brown vaginal discharge. She was treated with radical surgery, followed by chemoradiotherapy after recurrence at 2 months [143].

Diagnosis

Cervical cancer is definitively diagnosed on histology after colposcopically directed punch biopsy of the cervix. A cone biopsy of the cervix may sometimes be required before definitive diagnosis, in situations where the punch biopsy cannot exclude frank invasion, or if the upper limit of lesion is not seen on colposcopy. Histology of the cone biopsy will assess morphology, and may provide information for staging of the tumour (depth of invasion and size of the tumour).

Staging

Prior to any treatment, cervical cancers are staged according to the International Federation of Obstetrics and Gynecology (FIGO) staging system (Table 6.)

Table 6. FIGO staging for cervical carcinoma (Montreal 1995) [144]

Stage 0	***Carcinoma in situ***
Stage 1	*Confined to the uterus*
	IA : Diagnosed on microscopy only
	Stromal invasion ≤ 3mm in depth, and horizontal spread ≤7 mm
IA1	Stromal invasion > 3mm & ≤ 5mm in depth, horizontal spread ≤ 7 mm
IA2	
	1B : Preclinical tumours larger than stage 1A or clinically visible tumours confined to the cervix
IB1	Clinically visible lesion ≤ 4 cm in greatest dimension
IB2	Clinically visible lesion > 4 cm in greatest dimension
Stage II	*Invades beyond the uterus , but not to pelvic side wall or lower 1/3 vagina*
IIA	No obvious parametrial involvement
IIB	Obvious parametrial involvement
Stage III	*Extension to pelvic side wall or lower 1/3 vagina*
IIIA	Extension to lower 1/3 vagina, but not to pelvic sidewall Extension to pelvic side wall or
IIIB	causing hydronephrosis or non- functioning kidney
Stage IV	*Extension beyond true pelvis, or involving mucosa or bladder or rectum*
IVA	Extension to adjacent organs
IVB	Distant metastases

Staging guides treatment and prognosis, and is traditionally performed using information obtained from physical examination, colposcopy, histopathology, chest x-ray, IVP, examination under anaesthesia, cystoscopy and sigmoidoscopy. Newer imaging techniques may more accurately assess true extent of disease but as they are not universally available, particularly in developing countries, they are not currently incorporated into FIGO staging [142, 145]. Computerized axial tomography (CT), magnetic resonance imaging (MRI) and positron emission tomography (PET) have been used to assess presence or absence of pelvic lymphadenopathy, although normal size nodal metastases may be missed. MRI may assess depth of invasion of the primary tumour, and degree of bladder or rectal invasion, and may play a particularly useful role in the selection of subject who wish to undergo fertility sparing surgery [146]. Sentinel node mapping by lymphangiography is also used but may have lower sensitivity for lymph node involvement in early stage tumours [147]. Sentinel lymph node biopsy may identify lymphatic drainage, and guide treatment away from radical surgery towards radio-chemotherapy in the event of a positive result on frozen section. Surgical staging using pelvic and para-aortic lymphadenectomy improves accuracy of diagnosis of tumours ≥ stage 1B. Such surgery may be performed transperitoneally, laparoscopically or extraperitoneally [142, 148].

Many studies have demonstrated that younger patients have a more favourable stage distribution than older women [97]. Data from the Automated Central Tumour Registry from the Department of Defence in the USA between 1990 to 2002, demonstrated that around 70% of women under 25 years of age with cervical carcinoma have localised disease, with 5-year survival being high (around 90%) accordingly. Those with regional disease have 5 year survival of around 45% [97]. Other studies of young women including those up to their mid-thirties have demonstrated stage 1 tumours present 66 to 86% of the time. This may be due to more frequent screening and earlier presentation of disease [129-131, 134].

Treatment of Cervical Cancer in Adolescents

In recent years there has been increasing introduction of uterus sparing surgery for early stage cervical carcinoma, giving young women the possibility of future fertility or at least preservation of ovarian function.

Cone Biopsy

Nodal involvement occurs in < 1% of stage IA tumours, with a mortality rate of 1%. Therefore cold knife cone biopsy with clear margins of excision is therapeutic for stage IA1 squamous cell carcinomas, although they may also be treated by simple hysterectomy without pelvic node dissection if fertility is not desired. In the presence of positive LVSI, many would favour treatment with radical surgery or radiotherapy due to the risk of nodal metastases. Stage IA2 tumours have a 7.8% incidence of nodal metastases [149] and only select IA2 squamous cancers may be treated by cone biopsy alone. Adenocarcinoma involving the endocervical canal may sometimes be treated by a long thin cone biopsy removing the entire endocervical canal if fertility is to be spared [150].

Radical Trachelectomy

Radical trachelectomy is a new procedure, which appears to offer fertility preservation with survival comparable to radical hysterectomy in selected women [151]. Dargent first described outcome of pregnancies after radical trachelectomy in 1994 [152]. The procedure involves resection of the cervix up to the isthmus, and resection of parametrial tissue and a vaginal cuff of at least 2cm with conservation of the uterine body, followed by an isthmic-vaginal anastomosis [150]. A permanent isthmic cerclage suture is often tied around a temporary cervical catheter in an attempt to maintain patency for menstruation and reproductive function, while attempting to give strength to the lower uterine segment and reduce the risk of future miscarriage. There is no consensus as to the advantage of this, with some advocating delayed cerclage during pregnancy to reduce the risk of cervical stenosis [153]. Trachelectomy can be done vaginally, abdominally or laparoscopically. While there is less experience with the abdominal approach, it may be more feasible in very young patients who may have narrow vaginal anatomy, and has actually been described in two paediatric patients aged 6 and 8 years with clear cell carcinoma of the cervix [154]. Radical trachelectomy is performed after pelvic lymphadenectomy, which can be performed laparoscopically, or in an open procedure, or extraperitoneally.

It is estimated that around 50% of women with cervical cancer less than 40 years of age may be eligible for the procedure [155]. Careful patient selection is important, and eligibility criteria generally include women younger than 40 years, a strong desire to preserve fertility, no clinical evidence of impaired fertility, lesion size <2 cm, FIGO stage Ia-IB1 lesions, with no involvement of the upper endocervical canal, and negative regional lymph nodes [156]. Therefore, those with positive LVSI or depth of invasion >4 mm on preliminary cone or punch biopsy may require more extensive lymph node evaluation prior to trachelectomy [140]. Those with Stage Ib1 tumours have 16-18% risk of lymph node spread [149], and careful MRI assessment and histology review pre and post surgery is important. In the event of positive lymph nodes, positive surgical margins, or extensive LVSI with a poorly differentiated tumour, further treatment may be required such as chemoradiation or radical hysterectomy.

Postoperatively it is recommended that contraception be used for 6 months. Follow up is recommended every 3 months for the first year and every 4 months for the second year, involving clinical examination and isthmic and vaginal vault smears. There is a 2% false positive rate of isthmic and vault smears due to high numbers of endometrial cells. Smears with squamous cells alone are considered to be unsatisfactory in the first 2 years, and then negative thereafter [157]. Further investigations include colposcopy at 6 and 12 months, and sometimes MRI. After 2 years, checkups may occur every 6 months up to 5 years then yearly until 10 years, before discharge back to the local provider for routine screening, although many continue to have yearly cervical screening [150].

It is important to diagnose pregnancy early, and book into an institution with high level obstetric and perinatal care. Recent reviews of fertility outcome after radical trachelectomy (involving around 400 cases worldwide) have demonstrated that less than half of women after the procedure have tried to conceive. Around 171 pregnancies have resulted in 109 births. If pregnant: do early pregnancy test, book in to institution with high-level obstetric and perinatal care. First and second trimester loss rates are around 21% and 8% respectively. It is unclear if regular ultrasound scans to check the lower uterine segment is useful. Miscarriage may require evacuation of retained product of conception, involving removal of the stitch or hysterotomy. Reinsertion of the cerclage generally requires an abdominal procedure due to minimal or absent cervical tissue being present vaginally. There is an increased risk of chorioamnionitis due to absence of the cervix and cervical mucus plug, with associated risk of preterm rupture of membranes and preterm delivery. Preterm delivery prior to 36 weeks occurs in 21% (compared to 10-15% in the general population). Elective delivery by classical caesarean section is recommended at 37-38 weeks. The lower uterine body mimics the funnel shape of a short cervix during pregnancy, and a lower segment incision cannot be performed safely due to risk of extension into uterine vessels [150, 153].

Radical trachelectomy is thought to be associated with less physical and sexual morbidity than radical hysterectomy, although no randomised controlled trials have been performed. Complications may be immediate and related to surgery and include bladder perforation, uterine perforation, laceration of vaginal fornix, external iliac arteriotomy, rectus sheath haematoma, lymphoedema, genitofemoral or ilioinguinal nerve neuropraxia or neurotmesis. Delayed complications can include dysmenorrhoea (24%), irregular menstruation (17%), isthmic stenosis and haematometra (10%), prolonged amenorrhoea (7%), and recurrent candidiasis (14%). Isthmic stenosis may require exploration in theatre, and may compromise efficacy of follow up cervical smears [150, 151]. A case of pelvic inflammatory disease due to chlamydia has been reported, and while this is most likely due to sexual behaviour rather than the trachelectomy itself it is unclear if the surgery makes one more susceptible to severe infections [158]. This may be of relevance to young women who have higher rates of partner change.

Recurrence rate of cervical cancer post radical trachelectomy is <5% with an associated mortality rate of 2.5%. Recurrences have been reported as early as 7 months and as late as 7-8 years. They occur predominantly in patients with tumours over 3 cm in size. It is unclear if there is a greater risk of recurrence in those with adenocarcinoma [150, 159].

Radical Hysterectomy and Pelvic Lymphadenectomy

In 1896 the Wertheim radical hysterectomy was performed, which involved removal of the uterus with a wide margin of parametrial and paracervical tissue, upper vagina and bulky and enlarged lymph nodes. FIGO Stage IA2, IB1 and IIA cervical cancers may be treated with radical hysterectomy and pelvic lymphadenectomy. Early stage cervical cancer rarely metastasizes to the ovary, and ovarian preservation may be performed in young patients <45 years with early stage (FIGO IA1-IIa <4 cm) squamous cell cervical carcinoma, with macroscopically normal ovaries, and with preserved peripheral unaffected cervical stroma (which could be assessed preoperatively on MRI) [160]. Patients with similar stage adenocarcinomas have a higher risk of ovarian metastases, and should undergo bilateral oophorectomy. Radiotherapy is equally effective, however does not preserve ovarian function.

Adjuvant Radiotherapy or Chemotherapy

Adjuvant radiotherapy is recommended if there is large tumour size, deep stromal invasion, and LVSI [142]. Adjuvant cisplatin based chemoradiation is recommended in those with positive lymph nodes, parametrial invasion, and positive surgical margins [161].

Chemoradiation as Primary Treatment

Chemoradiation is the treatment of choice for patients with stage IB2 (>4 cm) IIB, III, and IVA cervical cancers [142].

Palliative Chemotherapy

Stage IVB cervical cancers are managed with palliative chemotherapy.

Cervical Cancer in Pregnancy

Routine cervical screening in pregnancy has lead to the detection of early stage cervical carcinomas in pregnancy, and is therefore one of the most frequently encountered malignancies in pregnancy. Management is complex and by a multidisciplinary team, and rests on the patient's wishes, the potential for fetal viability and stage of disease. In the first trimester termination is proposed, and in the third trimester, fetal viability allows surgical therapy. Planned treatment delays are acceptable in those with stage I tumours who are ≥20 weeks gestation, and who desire to continue their pregnancy [162]. Tumour stabilisation or regression with neoadjuvant chemotherapy in the second trimester while waiting for viability has been reported. Chemotherapy must be avoided in the first trimester due to the risk of malformation. Mode of delivery depends on tumour stage. Those with stage IA1 cancers treated by cone biopsy may undergo a normal vaginal delivery. Those with stage IA2-IIA tumours may undergo delivery by classical caesarean section to avoid the risk of bleeding and obstruction of birth canal, followed by radical surgery. Those with Stage IIB tumours and beyond require delivery by classical caesarean section followed by chemoradiation in the puerperium [163].

Recurrent Disease

Follow-up should include rectovaginal and nodal examination, and vault smears, every 3-4 months in the first 3 years, 6 monthly until 5 years, then yearly. Most recurrences occur in first 2 years after primary treatment, and are almost always incurable, with <5% alive at 5 years [142]. Options include salvage Chemoradiation after radical hysterectomy if there has been no previous radiotherapy. Pelvic exenteration may be performed after chemoradiation if there is no evidence of metastatic disease [164].

Survival

Mortality from cervical cancer is low in adolescents, most likely reflects early presentation. In the USA, Crude mortality at 20 years of age from the SEER database is 0.2 per 100 000 [165]. The mortality and 5 year survival data from various countries are shown in Table 7. Highest mortality rates are seen in the developing world.

Age-specific mortality rates for cervical cancer increased in women aged 15 to 35 in from the early 1960's through to the 1980's in England and Wales, and in some Australian reports, likely related to mode of therapy, but have been unchanged over the last 10-15 years [130, 167]. Age of the patient is known to be an important prognostic factor in cervical carcinoma, and younger women are thought to have more aggressive disease and poorer prognosis, when controlling for histological type and stage [134, 168-172]. However a retrospective analysis of 3678 cases of invasive cervical cancer between 1977 and and 1994 in National Taiwan University Hospital revealed that younger age was associated with better survival rate for stage I and II disease, but not for Stage III or IV disease [131]. Other studies have found a strong association between old age and poor prognosis [173]. Probably because younger women more likely to undergo screening, surgical treatment and surveillance [131].

Table 7. Mortality and 5 year survival for cervical cancer in adolescents [48, 166]

Country	Age group (years)	Year	Deaths per 100, 000	5 year survival
USA	15-19	1975-2000	0.01	91%
USA	20-24	1975-2000	0.19	89%
USA	25-29	1975-2000	0.84	87%
Australia	15-19	1997-2004	0.00	
	20-24	1997-2000	0.2	
	20-24	2000-2004	0.1	

Quality of Life in Long-Term Cervical Cancer Survivors

Long-term follow-up studies have shown that younger aged survivors of cervical cancer experience greater survivor specific distress than that of older women. While most women who are disease free experience good physical, social and emotional functioning compared to norms, survivors still experience ongoing concerns about the possibility of recurrent disease, sexual problems (such as vaginal dryness, pain with penetration), and reproductive concerns and sadness about inability to bear children or talk openly about their infertility[174]. Providers should be aware that these concerns may persist long after cure of disease has been achieved.

Vaginal & Vulvar Carcinomas

Most vaginal and vulvar cancers most commonly present in postmenopausal women and are extremely rare in the young, and together account for 4% gynaecological cancers in those aged 25 or less [97]. The commonest cell type is squamous cell.

Vaginal Cancer

Vaginal carcinoma is particularly rare as the vagina does not have a transformation zone vulnerable to HPV infection, although anogenital HPV infection is usually multifocal, commonly involving the vaginal squamous epithelium. Consequently HR-HPV infection, as well as a past history of CIN or cervical cancer is more often associated with vaginal cancer. Non-HPV related risks include previous radiation therapy, chronic irritation, and diethylstilbestrol exposure in utero (the latter causing adenocarcinomas in young women). Routine screening of the general population for vaginal cancer is inappropriate due to the low incidence of disease and also because the malignant potential of vaginal epithelial neoplasia (VAIN) is unknown. Patients with vaginal cancer may present with painless vaginal bleeding. Most carcinomas are located in the upper third of the vagina on the posterior wall. Radiotherapy is the treatment of choice. Overall 5 year survival is 44% [175].

Vulvar Cancer

Squamous cell carcinoma of the vulva occurs as two distinctive clinico-pathological groups, arising from two independent aetiological pathways. That seen in older women in their mid fifties is associated with concurrent vulval dystrophy or lichen sclerosis, not HPV related and histologically are keratinising squamous cell carcinoma. In younger women, vulvar squamous cell cancers are increasing in frequency, the histological type being basaloid or warty and is associated with HR HPV infection, predominantly type16. The precancerous lesion is known as vulva intraepithelial neoplasia grade 2/3 (VIN 2/3). Despite this vulvar cancer it is exceedingly rare in adolescents. VIN is graded according to the depth of involvement of the epidermis, and has low malignant potential. In a study of 60 adolescents undergoing colposcopic evaluation for cervical cytological abnormality, concomitant presence of VIN was 10%, the vast majority being VIN 1, representing the cytopathic effect of viral infection [176]. Recognizing that HPV infection of the vulvar is synonymous with VIN1 (as is CIN 1 in the cervix) the International Society for the Study of Vulvovaginal Disease (ISSVD) nomenclature has now changed, only recognizing the precursor lesions VIN 2/3 [177]. Other risk factors for VIN 2/3 and carcinoma in young women are smoking, condylomas, and HIV positivity.

There are rare case reports of children or adolescents with VIN or vulvar squamous cell carcinoma. Transmission of HPV may be perinatal in these cases, with reactivation of latent infection in the context of immunosuppression [178-180]. Patients may present with itching burning or discomfort, while those with invasive malignancy may present with a solitary vulval lump, or ulceration usually on the labia majora. Diagnosis involves colposcopic examination and biopsy.

The management approach should optimise the chance of cure while minimising disfiguring surgery. Spontaneous resolution of VIN 1 over a couple of years is usual [181]. Topical treatment with imiquimod has been used in women with biopsy confirmed VIN2/3, with response rates of around 77%, although recurrence rates are high (reported to be around 20% at 16 months) [182]. Cryosurgery, electrodessication, and laser are also other treatment possibilities, although surgical excision with rotational skin flaps may be required [183]. Radical local excision is the appropriate treatment in a young person with early invasive disease, with inguinofemoral lymphadenectomy in those with stromal invasion of > 1 mm.

Anal Carcinoma

Anal carcinoma is rare in children and adolescents. Anal squamous cell cancer is preceded by anal intraepithelial neoplasia (AIN) of various grades. HIV positive subjects have high rates of anal HPV infection, independent of anal intercourse although this is the prevalent mode of transmission [184]. Women who are HIV positive with anal HPV are at increased risk of AIN if they smoke, have high risk HPV infection, and have CD4 T cell counts <500 /mm^3 [185]. Screening for anal carcinoma can be done by anal cytology, and is recommended for those at risk. It may be done every 2-3 years in subjects with CD4 counts

>500 cells/mm^3 and yearly in those with lesser counts. There is no consensus regarding screening in adolescents or children [65].

Recurrent Respiratory Papillomatosis (RRP)

RRP is characterized by the development of recurrent warty papillomas in the respiratory tract, predominantly the larynx, but also the trachea and lungs. It is the most common benign tumour of the larynx in children and adolescents, and can cause severe morbidity and distress for patients and their families. It has a bimodal distribution, juvenile onset (JORRP) commonly occurring before the age of 5, with an incidence of 4.3 per 100 0000, and adult onset (AORRP) usually presenting after 20 years of age. RRP in those over 15 years has an incidence of 1.8 per 100 000[186].

JORRP is caused by vertical transmission of HPV and is more severe than AORRP, where mode of transmission is less clear, although sexual transmission is most likely.

Risk factors for JORRP include a history of maternal genital warts, although up to 50% of associated maternal HPV infections may be subclinical. Prolonged labour (therefore increased exposure to HPV) in young primigravid women may increase the risk of transmission, and risk is increased in firstborns. There is insufficient evidence to support routine caesarean section in all women with condylomas and caesarean section is not totally protective.

HPV 6,11 cause the majority of JORRP, and HPV 16 and 18 are also implicated [187]. Those with HPV 11 are likely to have more aggressive disease. Impaired cell mediated immunity in the host may play a role in risk of infection and recurrence. Oncoproteins E6 and E7 may result in uncontrolled cellular proliferation.

Children may clinically present with hoarseness, choking, stridor and airway obstruction, and may be misdiagnosed with asthma or croup. Treatment is required to maintain airway patency and improve voice. Direct laryngoscopy is required for diagnosis and staging. HPV typing may assist prognosis. Biopsy is required for histological confirmation and to rule out malignancy.

Treatment requires recurrent debulking during micro-laryngoscopy, with CO2 laser or microdebrider excision. Recurrence is common with repeated treatments often required, sometimes as often as monthly with average number of lifetime treatments reaching 20. Tracheostomy may be required in around 15% of cases, and is more likely in those with HPV 11. Side effects may include scarring, webbing, airway stenosis, airway fire, airway perforation and haemorrhage. Adjuvant therapy may be required in 10%, and may include the use of alpha interferon, cidofovir or acyclovir, which may slow regrowth but are not curative. Intralesional cidofovir is under study. Spontaneous remission may occur, while in others disease may recur and continue into adulthood. Malignant transformation to squamous cell carcinoma may occur in 3-5%, and is more likely to occur in those with chronic relapsing disease, cigarette smoking, prior radiation therapy, and infection with HPV 11 and 16[188]. There is hope that the HPV vaccine may contribute to elimination of this disease, and trials are awaited.

Conclusion and Key Points

- HPV is the most common sexually transmitted infection and may uncommonly cause a variety of anogenital tract neoplasias, as well as recurrent respiratory papillomatosis which may undergo malignant transformation in young women.
- Anal, vaginal and vulval HPV related disease are all very rare in adolescents.
- Cervical intraepithelial neoplasia is common in adolescents due to high rates of partner change and cervical factors, yet progression to malignancy in that age group is rare due to high rates of regression and viral clearance, plus the natural history of disease.
- Aggressive treatment of pre invasive is associated with concomitant long term obstetric risks and providers should become familiar with new guidelines recommending later onset of cervical screening in young women, and more conservative management of low grade changes.
- Fertility sparing options for treatment of cervical carcinoma are a real option for young women.
- It is hoped that with the introduction of prophylactic HPV vaccines on a large scale, these diseases may be largely prevented, but until worldwide uptake of the vaccine increases, they will continue to be a problem for young women and health providers for decades to come.

References

[1] Genital HPV infection- CDC Fact Sheet. Centers for Disease Control and Prevention; 2004.

[2] Munoz, N., Castellsague, X., de Gonzalez, A.B., and Gissman, L. (2006). Chapter1: HPV in the etiology of human cancer. *Vaccine*, 24 (suppl 3):S1-10.

[3] Parkin, D.M. and Bray, F. (2006). Chapter 2: the burden of HPV related cancers. *Vaccine*, 24 (suppl 3):S11-25.

[4] Schiffman, M., Castle, P.E., Jeronimo, J., Rodriguez, A.C., and Wacholder, S. (2007). Human papillomavirus and cervical cancer. *Lancet*, 370:890-907.

[5] World Health Organisation: Overview of CAH : Adolescent Health and Development. Accessed January 2008.

[6] Dunne, E.F., Unger, E.R., Sternberg, M., McQuillan, G., Swan, D.C., Patel, S.S., and Markowitz, L.E. (2007). Prevalence of HPV infection among females in the United States. *JAMA*, 297:813-819.

[7] Ho, G., Bierman, R., Beardsley, L., Chang, C.J., and Burk, R.D. (1998). Natural history of cervicovaginal papillomavirus infection in young women. *N Engl J Med.* 338:423-428.

[8] Manhart, L.E., Holmes, K.K., Koutsky, L.A., Wood, T.R., Kenney, D.L., Feng, Q., and Kiviat, N.B. (2006). Human papillomavirus infection among sexually active young women in the United States: Implications for developing a vaccination strategy. *Sex Transm Dis.* 33:502-508.

[9] Brown, D., Shew, M., Qadadri, B., Neptune, N., Vargas, M., Tu, W., Juliar, B.E., Breen, T.E., and Fortenberry, J.D. (2005). A longitudinal study of genital human papillomavirus infection in a cohort of closely followed adolescent women. *J Infect Dis.* 191:182-192.

[10] Garland, S., for the WHINURs group (2006). Will vaccination prevent cervical cancer in indigenous and non-indigenous women, abstract. In *Public Health Association of Australia National Immunisation Conference*; *Sydney*.

[11] The Future II Study Group (2007). Effect of prophylactic human papillomavirus L1 virus-like-particle vaccine on risk of cervical intraepithelial neoplasia grade 2, grade 3, and adenocarcinoma in situ: a combined analysis of four trials. *Lancet*, 369:1861-1868.

[12] Ho, L., Chan, S.Y., Burk, R.D., Das, B.C., Fujinaga, K., Icenogle, J.P., Kahn, T., Kiviat, N., Lancaster, W., Mavromara-Nazos, P., et al. (1993). The genetic drift of human papillomavirus type 16 is a means of reconstructing prehistoric viral spread. *J Virol.* 67:6413-6523.

[13] Burd, E.M. (2003). Human papillomavirus and cervical cancer. *Clin Microbiol Rev.* 16:1-17.

[14] de Villiers, E.M., Fauguet, C., Broker, T.R., Bernard, H.U., and zur Hausen, H. (2004). Classification of papillomaviruses. *Virology*, 324:17-24.

[15] Garland, S. (2002). Human papillomavirus update with a particular focus on cervical disease. *Pathology*, 34:213-214.

[16] Smith, J.S., Lindsay, L.J., Hoots, B., Keys, J., Franceschi, S., Winer, R., and Clifford, G.M. (2007). Human papillomavirus type distribution in invasive cervical cancer and high-grade cervical lesions: a meta-analysis update. *Int J Cancer*, 121:621-632.

[17] Stevens, M.P., Tabrizi, S.N., Quinn, M.A., and Garland, S.M. (2006). Human papillomavirus genotype prevalence in cervical biopsies from women diagnosed with cervical intraepithelial or cervical cancer in Melbourne, Australia. *Int J of Gynecol Cancer*, 16:1017-1024.

[18] Madeleine, M.M., Daling, J.R., Schwartz, S.M., Shera, K., McKnight, B., Carter, J.J., Wipf, G.C., Critchlow, C.W., McDougall, J.K., Porter, P., et al. (2001). Human papillomavirus and long-term oral contraceptive use increase the risk of adenocarcinoma in situ of the cervix. *Cancer Epidemiol Biomarkers Prev.* 10:171-177.

[19] Bosch, F.X., Manos, M.M., Sherman, M.E., Jansen, A., Peto, J., Schiffman, M.H., Moreno, V., and Shah, K.V. (1995). Prevalence of HPV DNA in cervical cancer in 22 countries. *J Natl Cancer Inst.* 87:796-802.

[20] Castellsagué, X., Díaz, M., de Sanjosé, S., Muñoz, N., Herrero, R., Franceschi, S., Peeling, R.W., Ashley, R., Smith, J.S., Snijders, P.J.F., et al. (2006). Worldwide human papillomavirus etiology of cervical adenocarcinoma and its cofactors: Implications for screening and prevention. *J Natl Cancer Inst.* 98:303-315.

[21] Monteiro, D.L., Trajano, A.J., da Silva, K.S., and Russomano, F.B. (2006). Pre-invasive cervical disease and uterine cervical cancer in Brazilian adolescents: prevalence and related factors. *Cadernos de Saude Publica.* 22:2539-2548.

[22] Winer, R.L., Lee, S., Hughes, J.P., Adam, D.E., Kiviat, N., and Koutsky, L.A. (2003). Genital human papillomavirus infection: incidence and risk factors in a cohort of female university students. *Am J Epidemiol.* 157:218-226.

[23] Moscicki, A.B., Winkler, B., Irwin, C.E., J.S. (1989). Differences in biological maturation, sexual behaviour, and sexually transmitted disease between adolescents with and withot cervical intraepithelial neoplasia. *J Pediatr.* 115:487-493.

[24] Kahn, J.A., Rosenthal, S.L., Succop, P.A., Ho, G.Y.F., and Burk, R.D. (2002). The interval between menarche and age of first sexual intercourse as a risk factor for subsequent HPV infection in adolescent and young adult women. *J Pediatr.* 141:718-723.

[25] Garland, S.M., Faulkner-Jones, B., Fortune, D.F., and Quinn, M. (1992). Cervical Cancer - what role for human papillomavirus? *MJA*, 156:204-212.

[26] Woodman, C.B., Collins, S., Winter, H., Bailey, A., Ellis, J., Prior, P., Yates, M., Rollason, T.P., and Young, L.S. (2001). Natural history of cervical human papillomavirus infection in young women: a longitudinal cohort study. *Lancet*, 357:1831-1836.

[27] Moscicki, A.B., Hills, N., Shiboski, S., Powell, K., Jay, N., Hanson, E., Miller, S., Clayton, L., Farhat, S., Broering, J., et al. (2001). Risks for incident human papillomavirus infection and low-grade squamous intraepithelial lesion development in young females. *JAMA*, 285:2995-3002.

[28] Villa, L.L. and Schlegel, R. (1991). Differences in transformation activity between HPV 18 and HPV 16 map to the viral LCR-E6-E7 region. *Virology*, 181:374-377.

[29] Solomon, D., Davey, D.D., Kurman, R.J., Moriarty, A., O'Connor, D., Prey, M., Raab, S., Sherman, M., Wilbur, D., Wright, T.J., et al. (2002). The 2001 Bethesda System: terminology for reporting results of cervical cytology. *JAMA*, 287:2116.

[30] Jones, B.A. and Novis, D.A. (2000). Follow-up of abnormal gynecologic cytology: a college of American pathologists Q-probes study of 16132 cases from 306 laboratories. *Arch Pathol Lab Med.* 124:665-671.

[31] National Health and Medical Research Council: Screening to prevent cervical cancer: guidelines for management of asymptomatic women with screen detected abnormalities. June 2005.

[32] Ludicke, F., Stalberg, A., Vassilakos, P., Major, A.L., and Campana, A. (2001). High and intermediate-risk human papillomavirus infection in sexually active adolescent females. *J Pediatr Adolesc Gynecol.* 14:171-174.

[33] Mount, S.L. and Papillo, J.L. (1999). A study of 10296 pediatric and adolescent Papanicolaou diagnoses in northern New England. *Pediatrics*, 103:539-545.

[34] Paavonen, J., Jenkins, D., Bosch, F.X., Naud, P., Salmerón, J., Wheeler, C.M., Chow, S., Apter, D.L., Kitchener, H.C., Castellsague, X., et al. (2007). Efficacy of a prophylactic adjuvanted bivalent L1 virus-like-particle vaccine against infection with human papillomavirus types 16 and 18 in young women: an interim analysis of a phase III double-blind, randomised controlled trial. *Lancet*, 369:2161-2170.

[35] Garland, S.M., Hernandez-Avila, M., Wheeler, C.M., Perez, G., Harper, D.M., Leodolter, S., Tang, G.W.K., Ferris, D.G., Steban, M., Bryan, J., et al. (2007). Quadrivalent HPV6/11/16/18 vaccine to prevent cervical, vulvar and vaginal disease. *N Engl J Med.* 356:1928-1943.

[36] Bjorge, T., Gunborud, A.B., Langmark, F., Skacre, G.B., Thorenson, S.O. (1994). Cervical mass screening in Norway - 510, 000 smears a year. *Cancer Detect Prev.* 18:463-470.

[37] The Future II Study Group (2007). Quadrivalent vaccine against human papillomavirus to prevent high-grade cervical lesions. *New Engl J Med.* 356:1915-1927.

[38] Winer, R.L., Kiviat, N.B., Hughes, J.P., Adam, D.E., Lee, S.K., Kuypers, J.M., and Koutsky, L.A. (2005). Development and duration of human papillomavirus lesions, after initial infection. *J Infect Dis.* 191:731-738.

[39] Moscicki, A.B., Shiboski, S., Hills, N.K., Powell, K.J., Jay, N., Hanson, E.N., Miller, S., Canjura-Clayton, K.L., Farhat, S., Broering, J.M., et al. (2004). Regression of low-grade squamous intra-epithelial lesions in young women. *Lancet,* 364:1678-1683.

[40] Koutsky, L.A., Ault, K.A., Wheeler, C.M., Brown, D.R., Barr, E., Alvarez, F.B., Chiacchierini, L.M., and Jansen, K.U. (2002). Proof of Principle Study Investigators: A controlled trial of a human papillomavirus type 16 vaccine. *N Engl J Med.* 347:1645-1651.

[41] The Atypical Squamous Cells of Undetermined Significance/ Low-grade Squamous Intraepithelial Lesions Triage Study (ALTS) Group: Human papillomavirus testing for triage of women with cytologic evidence of low grade squamous intraepithelial lesions: baseline data from a randomised trial. *J Natl Cancer Inst* 2000, 92:397-402.

[42] The ASCUS-LSIL Triage Study (ALTS) Group: Results of a randomized trial on the management of cytology interpretations of atypical squamous cells of undetermined significance. *Am J Obstet Gynecol* 2003:1383-1392.

[43] The ASCUS-LSIL Triage Study (ALTS) Group: A randomized trial on the management of low-grade squamous intraepithelial lesion cytology interpretations. *Am J Obstet Gynecol* 2003, 188:1393-1400.

[44] Van Oortmarssen, G.J. and Habbema, J.D.F. (1991). Epidemiological evidence for age-dependent regression of pre-invasive cervical cancer. *Br J Cancer,* 64:559-565.

[45] Bos AB, van Ballengooijen M, vanden Akker-van Marle ME, Habbema JDF: Less pap-2 results ('minor abnormalities') in the population screening for cervical cancer since the introduction of new guidelines in 1996. *Ned Tijdschr Geneeskd* 2002, 146:1586-1590.

[46] Campion, M.J. (2005). Preinvasive disease. In *Practical Gynecologic Oncology.* Edited by Berek JS, Hacker NF: Lippincott Williams and Wilkins; 265-336.

[47] Mclndoe, W.A., McLean, M.R., Jones, R.W., and Mullins, P.R. (1984). The invasive potential of carcinoma in situ of the cervix. *Obstet Gynecol.* 64:451-458.

[48] O'Leary, M., Sheaffer, J., Finklestein, J., Olshan, A., and Brown, J. (2006). Chapter 14: Female Genital Tract Cancer. In *Cancer Epidemiology in Older Adolescents and Young Adults 15-29 years of age, Including SEER Incidence and Survival: 1975-2000. National Cancer Institute, NIH Pub. No. 06-5767.* Edited by Bleyer, W.A., O'Leary, M., Barr, R., Ries, L.A.G. (Eds), NIH; 163-173.

[49] Vaccarella, S., Herrero, R., Dai, M., Snijders, P.J., Meijer, C.J., Thomas, J.O., Hoang Anh, P.T., Ferreccio, C., Matos, E., Posso, H., et al. (2006). Reproductive factors, oral contraceptive use, and human papillomavirus infection: pooled analysis of the IARC HPV prevalence surveys. *Cancer Epidemiol Biomarkers Prev.* 15:2148-2153.

[50] Naud, P., Matos, J., Hammes, L., Stuckzynski, J., Brouwers, K., Magno, V., Dias, E., Crusius, P., d'Avila, A., Campos, C., et al. (2006). Factors predicting intermediate endpoints of cervical cancer and exposure to human papillomavirus (HPV) infections in young women screened as potential targets for prophylactic HPV vaccination in south of Brazil. *Eur J Obstet Gynecol Reprod Biol.* 124:110-118.

[51] International Collaboration of Epidemiological Studies of Cervical Cancer (2006). Cervical carcinoma and reproductive factors: collaborative reanalysis of individual data on 16,563 women with cervical carcinoma and 33,542 women without cervical carcinoma from 25 epidemiological studies. *Int J Cancer*, 119:1108-1124.

[52] Winer, R.L., Hughes, J.P., Feng, Q., O'Reilly, S., Kiviat, N.B., Holmes, K.K., and Koutsky, L.A. (2006). Condom use and the risk of genital human papillomavirus infection in young women.[see comment]. *New Engl J Med.* 354:2645-2654.

[53] Manhart, L.E. and Koutsky, L.A. (2002). Do condoms prevent genital HPV infection, external genital warts, or cervical neoplasia? A meta-analysis. *Sex Transm Dis.* 29:725-735.

[54] Anttila, A., Pukkala, E., Söderman, B., Kallio, M., Nieminen, P., and Hakama, M. (1999). Effect of organised screening on cervical cancer incidence and mortality in Finland 1963-1995: Recent increase in cervical cancer incidence. *Int J Cancer*, 83:59-65.

[55] Finnish Cancer Registry: Cancer Statistics, updated on 20.03.2007. http://www.cancerregistry.fi Accessed April 2007.

[56] Grunbaum, J., Kann, L., Kinchen, S., Williams, B., Ross, J.G., Lowry, R., and Kolbe, L. (2002). Youth risk behaviour surveillance - United States 2001. *MMWR Surveill Summ.* 51:1-64.

[57] Rissel, C.E., Richters, J., Grulich, A.E., de Visser, R.O., and Smith, A.M. (2003). Sex in Australia:first experiences of vaginal intercourse and oral sex among a representative sample of adults. *Aust NZ J Public Health*, 27:131-137.

[58] Guido, R. (2004). Guidelines for screening and treatment of cervical disease in the adolescent. *J Pediatr Adolesc Gynecol.* 17:303-311.

[59] Gibbs, N. (1998). Anogenital papillomavirus infections in children. *Curr Opin Pediatr.* 10:393-397.

[60] Bayo, S., Boxch, X., Sanjose, S., Munoz, N., Combita, A., and Meijer, C.J. (2002). Risk factors for invasive cervical cancer in Mali. *Int J Epidemiol.* 31:202-209.

[61] Chaouki, N., Bosch, F.X., Munoz, N., Meijer, C., Gueddari, B., J.W. (1998). The viral origin of cervical cancer in Rabat, Morocco. *Int J Cancer*, 75:546-554.

[62] Mathur, S., Greene, M. and Malhotra, A. (2003). Too young to wed: the lives, rights and health of young married girls. International Center for Research on Women, Washington.

[63] Joint United Nations Programme on HIV and AIDS: World AIDS campaign 2004: women, girls, HIV & AIDS [cited 2006 Aug 31].

[64] Centers for Disease Control: 1993 revised classification system for HIV infection and expanded surveillance case definition for AIDS among adolescents and adults. *MMWR Recomm Rep* 1992, 41:1-19.

[65] Einstein, M.H. and Kadish, A.S. (2004). Anogenital neoplasia in AIDS. *Curr Opin Oncol.* 16:455-462.

[66] Clarke, B. and Chetty, R. (2002). Postmodern cancer: the role of human immunodeficiency virus in uterine cervical cancer. *Mol Pathol.* 55:19-24.

[67] Bower, M., Mazhar, D. and Stebbing, J. (2006). Should cervical cancer be an acquired immunodeficiency syndrome-defining cancer? *J Clin Oncol.* 24:2417-2419.

[68] Frisch, M., Biggar, R.J. and Goedert, J.J. (2000). Human papillomavirus-associated cancers in patients with human immunodeficiency virus infection and acquired immunodeficiency syndrome. *J Natl Cancer Inst.* 92:1500-1510.

[69] Clifford, G.M., Polesel, J., Rickenbach, M., Dal Maso, L., Keiser, O., Kofler, A., Rapiti, E., Levi, F., Jundt, G., Fisch, T., et al. (2005). Cancer risk in the Swiss HIV Cohort Study: Associations with immunodeficiency, smoking, and highly active

[70] antiretroviral therapy. *J Natl Cancer Inst.* 97:425-432.

[71] Bosch, F.X. and de Sanjose, S. (2003). Human papillomavirus and cervical cancer burden and assessment of causality. *J Natl Cancer Inst Mongr.* 31:3-13.

[72] Tate, D.R. and Anderson, R.J. (2002). Recrudescence of cervical dysplasia among women who are infected with the human immunodeficiency virus: a case-control analysis. *Am J Obstet Gynecol.* 186:880-882.

[73] International Collaboration on HIV and Cancer (2000). Highly active antiretroviral therapy and incidence of cancer in human immunodeficiency virus-infected adults. *J Natl Cancer Inst.* 92:1823-1830.

[74] Mueller, B.U. and Pizzo, P.A. (1996). Malignancies in pediatric AIDS. *Curr Opin Pediatr.* 8:45-49.

[75] Moscicki, A.B., Ellenberg, J.H., Vermund, S.H., Holland, C.A., Darragh, T., Crowley-Nowick, P.A., Levin, L., and Wilson, C.M. (2000). Prevalence of and risks for cervical human papillomavirus infection and squamous intraepithelial lesions in adolescent girls: impact of infection with human immunodeficiency virus. *Arch Pediatr Adol Med.*, 154:127-134.

[76] American Cancer Society: Can cervical cancer be prevented? 2006. http://www.cancer.org/docroot/CRI/content/CRI_2_4_Accessed Jan 2008

[77] USPHS: USPHS/ISDA Guidelines for the Prevention of Opportunistic Infections in Persons Infected with Human Immunodeficiency Virus 1997. Report No.46 (No-RR-12)

[78] Massad, L.S., Schneider, M.F., Watts, D.H., Strickler, H.D., Melnick, S., Palefsky, J., Anastos, K., Levine, A.M., and Minkoff, H. (2004). HPV testing for triage of HIV-infected women with Papanicolau smears read as atypical squamous cells of uncertain significance. *J Womens Healh (Larchmt)* 13:147-153.

[79] Wright, T.C., Jr., Massad, L.S., Dunton, C.J., Spitzer, M., Wilkinson, E.J., Solomon, D., American Society for C, Cervical Pathology-sponsored Consensus C. (2007). 2006 consensus guidelines for the management of women with abnormal cervical cancer screening tests. *Am J Obstet Gynecol.* 197:346-355.

[80] Petry, K.U., Scheffel, D., Bode, U., Gabrysiak, T., Kochel, H., Kupsch, E., Glaubitz, M., Niesert, S., Kuhnle, H., and Schedel, I. (1994). Cellular immunodeficiency enhances the progression of human papillomavirus-associated cervical lesions. *Int J Cancer*, 57:836-840.

[81] Ho, G.Y.F., Studentsov, Y., Hall, C.B., Bierman, R., Beardsley, L., Lempa, M., et al. (2002). Risk factors for subsequent cervicovaginal human papillomavirus infection and the protective role of antibodies to HPV-16 virus-like particles. *J Infect Dis.* 186:737-742.

[82] Thomas, D.B. and Ray, R.M. (1996). Oral contraceptive use and invasive adenocarcinomas and adenosquamous carcinoma of the uterine cervix. The World Health Organization Collaborative Study of Neoplasia and Steroid Contraceptives. *Am J Epidemiol.* 144:281-289.

[83] Cox, J.T. (1995). Epidemiology of cervical intraepithelial neoplasia: the role of human papillomavirus. *Baillieres Clin Obstet Gynaecol.* 9:1-37.

[84] Frisch, M., Smith, E., Grulich, A., and Johansen, C. (2003). Cancer in a population-based cohort of men and women in registered homosexual partnerships. *Am J Epidemiol.* 157:966-972.

[85] Marrazzo, J.M., Koutsky, L.A., Stine, K.L., Kuypers, J.M., Grubert, T.A., Galloway, D.A., Kiviat, N.B., and Handsfield, H.H. (1998). Genital human papillomavirus infection in women who have sex with women. *J Infect Dis.* 178:1604-1609.

[86] McIntyre-Seltman, K., Castle, P.E., Guido, R., Schiffman, M., Wheeler, C., for the ALTS Group (2005). Smoking is a risk factor for cervical intraepithelial neoplasia grade 3 among oncogenic human papillomavirus DNA-positive women with equivocal or mildly abnormal cytology. *Cancer Epidemiol Biomarkers Prev.* 14:1164-1170.

[87] Critchlow, C.W., Wolner-Hanssen, P., Escherbach, D.A., Kiviat, N.B., Koutsky, L.A., Stevens, C.E., and Holmes, K.K. (1995). Determinants of cervical ectopia and of cervicitis: age, oral contraception specific cervical infection, smoking and douching. *Am J Obstet Gynecol.* 173:534-543.

[88] Oliveira, L., Rosa, M., Pereira, C., Vasconcel, G., Silva, R., Barrese, T., Carvalho, M., Abibab, G., Rodrigues, E., and Cavalcanti, S. (2006). Human papillomavirus status and cervical abnormalitites in women from public and private health care in Rio de Janeiro State, Brazil. *Rev Inst Med trop S. Paulo,* 48:279-285.

[89] Khan, M.J., Partridge, E.E., Wang, S.S., and Schiffman, M. (2005). Socioeconomic status and the risk of cervical intraepithelial neoplasia grade 3 among oncogenic human papillomavirus DNA-positive women with equivocal or mildly abnormal cytology. *Cancer*, 104:61-70.

[90] Vaccarella, S., Franceschi, S., Herrero, R., Munoz, N., Snijders, P.J.F., Clifford, G.M., Smith, J.S., Lazcano-Ponce, E., Sukvirach, S., Shin, H., et al. (2006). Sexual Behavior, Condom Use, and Human Papillomavirus: Pooled Analysis of the IARC Human Papillomavirus Prevalence Surveys. *Cancer Epidemiol Biomarkers Prev.* 15:326-333.

[91] Sykes, P., Harker, D. and Peddie, D. (2005). Findings and outcome of teenage women referred for colposcopy at Christchurch Women's Hospital, New Zealand. *New Zealand Med J.* 118:U1350-1356.

[92] Case, A.S., Rocconi, R.P., Straughn, J.M., Jr., Wang, W., Roark, K., Waltman, E.E., and Huh, W.K. (2006). Cervical intraepithelial neoplasia in adolescent women: incidence and treatment outcomes. *Obstet Gynecol.* 108:1369-1374.

[93] Sadler, L., A.S, Wang, W., Exeter, M., Whittaker, J., and McCowan, L. (2004). Treatment for cervical intraepithelial neoplasia and risk of preterm delivery. *JAMA*, 291:2100-2106.

[94] Kyrgiou, M., Koliopoulos, G., Martin-Hirsch, P., Arbyn, M., Prendiville, W., and Paraskevaidis, E. (2006). Obstetric outcomes after conservative treatment for intraepithelial or early invasive cervical lesions: systematic review and meta-analysis. *Lancet*, 367:489-498.

[95] Canfell, K., Barnabas, R.V., Patnick, J., and Beral, V. (2004). The predicted effect of changes in cervical screening practice in the UK: results from a modelling study. *Br J Cancer*, 91:530-536.

[96] Sasieni, P., Adams, J. and Cuzick, J. (2003). Benefit of cervical screening at different ages:evidence from the UK audit of screening histories. *Br J Cancer*, 89:88-93.

[97] Rieck, G.C., Tristram, A., Hauke, A., Fielder, H., and Fiander, A.N. (2006). Cervical screening in 20-24 year olds. *J Med Screen*, 13:64-71.

[98] You, W., Dainty, L.A., Rose, G.S., Krivak, T., McHale, M.T., Olsen, C.H., and Elkas, J.C. (2005). Gynecologic malignancies in women aged less than 25 years. *Obstetrics & Gynecology*, 105:1405-1409.

[99] Bleyer, A., Viny, A. and Barr, R. (2006). Cancer in 15 to 29 year- olds by primary site. *Oncologist*, 11:590-601.

[100] Toivonen, T., Nieminen, P., Tarkkanen, J., Timonens, T., Krogerus, L., and Klemi, P. (2005). Cytopathology in Finland. *Cytopathology*, 16:210-214.

[101] National Health Service: NHS Cervical Screening Program. Edited by; Accessed April 2007.

[102] Medical Practitioners Board of Victoria: *Consent for treatment and confidentiality in young people*. Melbourne, Victoria; September 2004.

[103] English, A. and Kenney, K.E. (2003). State minor consent laws: a summary. (2nd Ed.), Edited by. Chapel Hill (NC): Center for Adolescent Health and the Law.

[104] ACOG Committee Opinion: Evaluation and management of abnormal cervical cytology and histology in the adolescent. Number 330, April 2006. *Obstet Gynecol* 2006, 107:963-968.

[105] Williams, A.R. (2006). Liquid-based cytology and conventional smears compared over two 12-month periods. *Cytopathology*, 17:82-85.

[106] Denton, K.J. (2007). Liquid based cytology in cervical cancer screening. *BMJ*, 335:1-2.

[107] Ronco, G., Cuzick, J., Pierotti, P., Cariaggi, M.P., Dalla Palma, P., Naldoni, C., Ghiringhello, B., Giorgi-Rossi, P., Minucci, D., Parisio, F., et al. (2007). Accuracy of liquid based versus conventional cytology: overall results of new technologies for cervical cancer screening: randomised controlled trial. *BMJ*, 335:28.

[108] Davey, E., d'Assuncao, J., Irwig, L., Macaskill, P., Chan, S.F., Richards, A., and Farnsworth, A. (2007). Accuracy of reading liquid based cytology slides using the ThinPrep Imager compared with conventional cytology: prospective study. *BMJ*, 335:31.

[109] Moss, S.M., Gray, A., Marteau, T., Legood, R., Henstock, E., and Maissi, E. (2004). Evaluation of HPV/LBC cervical screening pilot studies. Report to the Department of Health, October. www.cancerscreening.nhs.uk/cervical/evaluation-hpv-2006feb.pdf.

[110] Petignat, P., Faltin, D., Goffin, F., Billieux, M.H., Stucki, D., Sporri, S., Vassilakos, P. (2005). Age-related performance of human papillomavirus testing used as an adjunct to cytology for cervical carcinoma screening in a population with a low incidence of cervical carcinoma. *Cancer*, 105:126-132.

[111] Boardman, L.A., Stanko, C., Weitzen, S., and Sung, C.J. (2005). Atypical squamous cells of undetermined significance: human papillomavirus testing in adolescents. *Obstet Gynecol.* 105:741-746.

[112] Garland, S.M., S. T. (2006). HPV DNA testing potential clinical applications. *Int J Health Prom Edu.* 44:107-112.

[113] Kyrgiou, M., Tsoumpou, I., Vrekoussis, T., et al. (2006). The up-to-date evidence on colposcopy practice and treatment of cervical intraepithelial neoplasia: the Cochrane colposcopy and cervical cytopathology collaborative group (C5 group) approach. *Cancer Treat Rev.* 32:516-523.

[114] Pearson, S.E., Whittaker, J., Ireland, D., and Monaghan, J.M. (1989). Invasive cancer of the cervix after laser treatment. *BJOG*, 96:486-488.

[115] Kashimura, M., Shinohara, M., Oikawa, K., Hamasaki, K., and Sato, H. (1990). An adenocarcinoma in situ of the uterine cervix that developed into invasive adenocarcinoma after 5 years. *Gynecol Oncol.* 36:128-133.

[116] Soutter, W.P., Haidopoulos, D., Gornall, R.J., et al. (2001). Is conservative treatment for adenocarcinoma in situ of the cervix safe? *BJOG*, 108:1184-1189.

[117] Wright, T.C., Jr., Massad, L.S., Dunton, C.J., Spitzer, M., Wilkinson, E.J., Solomon, D., American Society for Colposcopy Cervical Pathology-sponsored Consensus Conference (2007). 2006 Consensus guidelines for the management of women with cervical intraepithelial neoplasia or adenocarcinoma in situ. *Am J Obstet Gynecol.* 197:340-345.

[118] Brown, D., for the FUTURE Study Group: HPV type 6//11/16/18 vaccine: First analysis of cross-protection against persistent infection, cervical intraepithelial neoplasia (CIN), and adenocarcinoma in situ (AIS) caused by oncogenic HPV types in addition to 16/18. In *47th Annual International Conference on Antimicrobial Agents and Chemotherapy September 17-20*; *Chicago, Illinois*: 2007.

[119] Harper, D.M., Franco, E.L., Wheeler, C., Ferris, D.G., Jenkins, D., Schuind, A., Zahaf, T., Innis, B., Naud, P., De Carvalho, N.S., et al. (2004). Efficacy of a bivalent L1 virus-like particle vaccine in prevention of infection with human papillomavirus types 16 and 18 in young women: a randomised controlled trial. *Lancet*, 364:1757-1765.

[120] Harper, D.M., Franco, E.L., Wheeler, C.M., Moscicki, A.B., Romanowski, B., Roteli-Martins, C.M., Jenkins, D., Schuind, A., Costa Clemens, S., Dubin, G., et al. (2006). Sustained efficacy up to 4·5 years of a bivalent L1 virus-like particle vaccine against human papillomavirus types 16 and 18: follow-up from a randomised control trial. *Lancet*:1247-1255.

[121] Mao, C., Koutsky, L.A., Ault, K.A., Wheeler, C.M., Brown, D.R., Wiley, D.J., Alvarez, F.B., Bautista, O.M., Jansen, K.U., and Barr, E. (2006). Efficacy of human papillomavirus-16 vaccine to prevent cervical intraepithelial neoplasia: a randomized controlled trial. *Obstet Gynecol.* 107:18-27.

[122] Villa, L.L., Costa, R.L., Petta, C.A., Andrade, R.P., Ault, K.A., Giuliano, A.R., Wheeler, C.M., Koutsky, L.A., Malm, C., Lehtinen, M., et al. (2005). Prophylactic quadrivalent human papillomavirus (types 6, 11, 16, and 18) L1 virus-like particle vaccine in young women: a randomised double-blind placebo-controlled multicentre phase II efficacy trial. *Lancet Oncol.* 6:271-278.

[123] Villa, L.L., Costa, R.L., Petta, C.A., Andrade, R.P., Paavonen, J., Iversen, O.E., Olsson, S.E., Hoye, J., Steinwall, M., Riis-Johannessen, G., et al. (2006). High sustained efficacy of a prophylactic quadrivalent human papillomavirus types 6/11/16/18 L1 virus-like particle vaccine through 5 years of follow-up. *British Journal of Cancer*, 95:1459-1466.

[124] Merck & Co. I: *Gardasil [Quadrivalent Human Papillomavirus (Types 6,11,16,18) Recombinant Vaccine. Annotated Prescribing Information.* Whitehouse Station, NJ, 08889, USA; 2006.

[125] Markowitz, L.E., Dunne, E.F., Saraiya, M., Lawson, H.W., Chesson, H., and Unger, E.R. (2007). Centers for Disease Control Prevention Advisory Committee on Immunization Practices: Quadrivalent Human Papillomavirus Vaccine: Recommendations of the Advisory Committee on Immunization Practices (ACIP). *MMWR Recomm Rep.* 56:1-24.

[126] Nour, N.M. (2006). Health consequences of child marriage in Africa. *Emerg Infect Dis.* 12:1644-1649.

[127] Castellsague, X., de Sanjose, S., Aguado, T., Louie, K.S., Bruni, L., Munoz, J., Diaz, M., Irwin, K., Gacic, M., Beauvais, O., et al. (2007). *HPV and Cervical Cancer in the World: 2007 Report.*: WHO/ICO Information Centre on HPV and Cervical Cancer (HPV Information Centre); 2007.

[128] Benedet, J.L., Odicino, F., Maisonneuve, P., Beller, U., Creasman, W.T., Heintz, A.P., Ngan, H.Y., and Pecorelli, S. (2003). Carcinoma of the cervix uteri. 25th volume of the FIGO Annual Report on the results of treatment of gynaecological cancer. *Int J Gynaecol Obstet.* 83 (Suppl 1):41-78.

[129] National Cancer Statistics Clearing House: In *AIHW - AACR 2003a;2003b.* Australian Institute of Health and Welfare; April 2006.

[130] Bouma, J. and Crane-Elders, A.B.F. (1983). Cervical carcinoma in younger patients. *Lancet,* 1:248.

[131] Webb, M.J. and Sheehan, T.M. (1989). Invasive carcinoma of the cervix in young women. *ANZJOG*, 29:47-51.

[132] Chen, R.J, Lin, Y.H., Chen, C.A., Huang, S.C., Chow, S.N., and Hsieh, C.Y. (1999). Influence of Histologic Type and Age on Survival Rates for Invasive Cervical Carcinoma in Taiwan. *Gynecol Oncol.* 73:184-190.

[133] Surveillance, Epidemiology and End Results (SEER) Program Public Use CD-ROM (1973-1996). National Cancer Institute, DCPC, Surveillance Program, Cancer Statisitcs Branch, released April 1999, based on the August 1998 submission.

[134] Roberts, A. (1987). Cervical carcinoma:prognosis in younger patients. *BMJ*, 295:670.

[135] Pinion, S. (1987). Cervical carcinoma: prognosis in younger women (letter). *BMJ*, 295:670.

[136] Chilvers, C., Mant, D. and Pike, M.C. (1987). Cervical adenocarcinoma and oral contraceptives. *BMJ*, 295:1446-1447.

[137] Eide, T.J. (1987). Cancer of the uterine cervix in Norway by histologic type, 1970-1984. *J Natl Cancer Inst.* 79:199-205.

[138] Peters, R.K., Chao, A., Mack, T.M., Thomas, D., Bernstein, L., and Henderson, B.E. (1986). Increased frequency of adenocarcinoma of the uterine cervix in young women in Los Angeles County. *J Natl Cancer Inst.* 76:423-428.

[139] Schwartz, S. and Weiss, N. (1986). Increased incidence of adenocarcinoma of the cervix in young women in the United States. *Am J Epidemiol* 1986, 124:1045-1047.

[140] Smith, H.O., Tiffany, M.F., Qualls, C.R., and Key, C.R. (2007). The rising incidence of adenocarcinoma relative to squamous cell carcinoma of the uterine cervix in the United States - a 24 year population-base study. *Gynecol Oncol.* 78:97-105.

[141] Milam, M.R. Frumovitz, M., dos Reis, R., Broaddus, R.R., Bassett, R.L., Jr., and Ramirez, P.T. (2007). Preoperative lymph-vascular space invasion is associated with nodal metastases in women with early-stage cervical cancer. *Gynecol Oncol.* 106:12-15.

[142] Hall, S.W. and Monaghan, J.M. (1983). Invasive carcinoma of the cervix in younger women. *Lancet*, 2:731.

[143] Petignat, P. and Roy, M. (2007). Diagnosis and management of cervical cancer. *BMJ*, 335:765-768.

[144] Palit, A., McDowell, H.H.C., Rintala, R., and Kokai, G. (1998). Endometrioid adenocarcinoma of the cervix in a 9-year-old girl. *Br J Radiol.* 71:1093-1095.

[145] Creasman, W.T. (1995). New gynecologic cancer staging. *Gynecol Oncol.* 58:157-158.

[146] Hricak, H., Gatsonis, C., Chi, D.S., Amendola, M.A., Brandt, K., Schwartz, L.H., Koelliker, S., Siegelman, E.S., Brown, J.J., McGhee, R.B., Jr., et al. (2005). Role of imaging in pretreatment evaluation of early invasive cervical cancer: results of the intergroup study American College of Radiology Imaging Network 6651-Gynecologic Oncology Group 183. *J Clin Oncol.* 23:9329-9337.

[147] Peppercorn, D.P., Jeyarajah, A.R., Woolas, R., Shepherd, J.H., Oram, D.H., Jacobs, I.J., P.A, Lowe, D., and Reznek, R.H. (1999). Role of MR imaging in the selection of patients with early cervical carcinoma for fertility-preserving surgery: initial experience. *Radiology*, 212:395-399.

[148] Chou, H.H., Chang, T.C., Yen, T.C., Ng, K.K., Hsueh, S., Ma, Y., Chang, C.J., Huang, H.J., Chao, A., Wu, T.I., et al. (2006). Low value of [18F]-fluoro-2-deoxy-D-glucose positron emission tomography in primary staging of early stage cervical cancer. *J Clin Oncol.* 24:123-128.

[149] Plante, M., Renaud, M.C., Tetu, B., Harel, F., and Roy, M. (2003). Laparoscopic sentinel lymph node mapping in early-stage cervical cancer. *Gynecol Oncol.* 91:494-503.

[150] Sevin, B.U., Nadji, M., Averette, H.E., Hilsenbeck, S., Smith, D., and Lampe, B. (1992). Microinvasive carcinoma of the cervix. *Cancer*, 70:2121-2128.

[151] Shepherd, J.H. (2005). Uterus-conserving surgery for invasive cervical cancer. *Best Pract Res Clin Obstet Gynaecol.* 19:577-590.

[152] Grant, P. (2006). Radical trachelectomy. *ANZJOG*, 46:372-374.

[153] Dargent, D., Brun, J.L. and Remy, L. (1994). Pregnancies following radical trachelectomy for invasive cervical cancer. *Gynecol Oncol.* 52:104.

[154] Ungar, L., Smith, J.R., Palfalvi, L., and Del Priore, G. (2006). Abdominal radical trachelectomy during pregnancy to preserve pregnancy and fertility. *Obstet Gynecol.* 108:811-814.

[155] Abu-Rustum, N.R., Su, W., Levine, D., Boyd, J., Sonoda, Y., and LaQuaglia, M.P. (2005). Pediatric radical abdominal trachelectomy for cervical clear cell carcinoma: a novel surgical approach. *Gynecol Oncol.* 97:296-300.

[156] Sonoda, Y., Abu-Rustum, N.R., Gemignani, M.L., Chi, D.S., Brown, C.L., Poynor, E.A., and Barakat, R.R. (2004). A fertility-sparing alternative to radical hysterectomy: how many patients may be eligible? *Gynecol Oncol.* 95:534-538.

[157] Roy, M. and Plante, M. (1998). Pregnancies after radical vaginal trachelectomy for early-stage cervical cancer. *Am J Obstet Gynecol.* 179:1491-1496.

[158] Singh, N., Titmuss, E., Chin Aleong J., Sheaff, M.T., Curran, G., Jacobs, I.J., and Shepherd, J.H. (2004), A review of post-trachelectomy isthmic and vaginal smear cytology. *Cytopathology,* 15:97-103.

[159] Del Priore, G., Ungar, L. and Smith, R. (2005). Complications after fertility-preserving radiacal trachelectomy. *Fertil Steril.* 85:227.e225-227.

[160] Plante, M. and Roy, M. (2006). Fertility-preserving options for cervical cancer. *Oncology*, 20:479-488.

[161] Landoni, F., Maneo, A., Colombo, A., Placa, F., Milani, R., Perego, P., Favini, G., Ferri, L., and Mangioni, C. (1997). Randomised study of radical surgery versus radiotherapy for stage Ib-IIa cervical cancer. *Lancet*, 350:535-540.

[162] Peters, W.A., Liu, P.Y., Barrett, R.J., Stock, R.J., Monk, B.J., Berek, J.S., et al. (2000). Concurrent chemotherapy and pelvic radiation therapy compared with pelvic radiation therapy alone as adjuvant therapy after radical surgery in high-risk early-stage cancer of the cervix. *J Clin Oncol.* 2000:1606-1613.

[163] Goff, B.A., Paley, P.J., Koh, W., et al. (2000). Cancer in the pregnant patient. In *Principles and practice of gynecologic oncology*, edn 3rd. Edited by Hoskins WJ, Perez CA, Young RC: Lippincott Wiliams & Wilkins; 501-528.

[164] Caluwaerts, S., Van Calsteren, K., Mertens, L., Lagae, L., Moermans, P., Hansenss, M., Wuyts, K., Vergote, I., and Amant, F. (2006). Neoadjuvant chemotherapy followed by radical hysterectomy for invasive cervical cancer diagnosed during pregnancy: report of a case and review of the literature. *Int J Gynecol Cancer*, 16:884-943.

[165] Dreyer, G., Snyman, L.C., Mouton, A., and Lindeque, B.G. (2005). Management of recurrent cervical cancer. *Best Pract Res Clin Obstet and Gynaecol.* 19:621-644.

[166] Surveillance,Epidemiology and End Results (SEER) Program. SEER* Stat Database: Incidence - SEER 9 Regs Public Use, Nov 2003 Sub (1973-2001). Surveillance Research Program, Cancer Statistics Branch, released April 2004, based on the November 2003 submission. Available at http://seer.cancer.gov/.Retrieved Mar 23, 2005., edn based on the November 2003 submission. 166. Australian Institute of Health and Welfare (AIHW): Cervical Screening in Australia 2003–2004. In *Cancer Series no. 33*. Canberra2006.

[167] Roberts, A. (1982). Cervical cytology in England and Wales 1965-80. *Health Trends*, 14:41-43.

[168] Flores-Luna, L., Salazar-Martinez, E., Rios, E.D., Gonzalez-Lira, G., Zamora-Munoz, S., and Lazcano-Ponce, E. (2001). Prognostic factors related to cervical cancer survival in Mexican women. *Int J Gynecol Obstet.* 75:33-42.

[169] Gajalakshmi, V., Rajaraman, S. and Shanta, V. (2000). A survival study of cervical cancer in Chenni, India. *Ind J Cancer*, 37:158-164.

[170] Grigsby, P.W. (2001). Cervical cancer: combined modality therapy. *Cancer.* 7 (Suppl):S47-S50.

[171] Rutledge, F.N., Mitchell, M.F., Munsell, M., Bass, S., McGuffee, V., and Atkinson, E.N. (1992). Youth as a prognostic factor in carcinoma of the cervix: a matched analysis. *Gynecol Oncol.* 44:123-130.

[172] Serur, E., Fruchter, R.G., Maiman, M., McGuire, J., Arrastia, C.D., and Gibbon, D. (1995). Age, substance abuse, and survival of patients with cervical carcinoma. *Cancer*, 72:2530-2538.

[173] Adami, H.O., Ponten, J., Sparen, P., Bergstrom, R., Gustafsson, L., and Friberg, L.G. (1994). Survival trend after invasive cervical cancer diagnosis in Sweden before and after cytologic screening. 1960-1984. *Cancer*, 73:140-147.

[174] Wenzel, L., DeAlba, I., Habbal, R., Kluhsman, B.C., Fairclough, D., Krebs, L.U., Anton-Culver, H., Berkowitz, R., and Aziz, N. (2005). Quality of life in long-term cervical cancer survivors. *Gynecol Oncol.* 97:310-317.

[175] Hacker, N.F. (2005). Vaginal Cancer. In *Practical Gynecologic Oncology*. Edited by Berek JS, Hacker NF: Lippincott Williams and Wilkins; 585-596.

[176] Lara-Torre, E. and Perlman, S.E. (2004). Vulvar intraepithelial neoplasia in adolescents with abnormal Pap smear results: a series report. *J Pediatr Adolesc Gynecol.* 17:45-48.

[177] Sideri, M., Jones, R.W., Wilkinson, E.J., Preti, M., Heller, D.S., Scurry, J., Haefner, H., and Neill, S. (2005). Squamous vulvar intraepithelial neoplasia: 2004 Modified Terminology, ISVVD vulvar Oncology Subcommittee. *J Reprod Med.* 50:807-810.

[178] Hampl, M., Ramp, U., Bender, H.G., and Kueppers, V. (2006). A case of a pT3, HPV 52-positive vulvar carcinoma in an 18-year-old woman. *Gynecol Oncol.* 101:530-533.

[179] Godfrey, J.C., Vaughan, M.C. and Williams, J.V. (2003). Successful treatment of bowenoid papulosis in a 9-year-old girl with vertically acquired human immunodeficiency virus. *Pediatrics*, 112:e73-e76.

[180] Giaquinto, C., Del Mistro, A., De Rossi, A., Bertorelle, R., Giacomet, V., Ruga, E., and Minucci, D. (2000). Vulvar Carcinoma in a 12-Year-Old Girl With Vertically Acquired Human Immunodeficiency Virus Infection. *Pediatrics,* 106:e 57.

[181] Stafford, E.M., Greenberg, H. and Miles, P.A. Cervical intraepithelial neoplasia III in an adolescent with bowenoid papulosis. *J Adolesc Health Care,* 11:523-526.

[182] Le, T., Menarda, C., Hicks-Bouchera, W., Hopkinsa, L., Weberpalsa, J., and Fung-Kee-Funga, M. (2007). Final results of a phase 2 study using continuous 5% Imiquimod cream application in the primary treatment of high-grade vulva intraepithelial neoplasia. *Gynecol Oncol.* 106:579-584.

[183] Weitzner, J.M., Fields, K.W. and Robinson, M.J. (1989). Pediatric bowenoid papulosis: risks and management. *Pediatr Dermatol*, 6:303-305.

[184] Piketty, C., Darragh, T.M., Da Costa, M., Bruneval, P., Heard, I., Kazatchkine, M.D., Palefsky, J.M. (2003). High prevalence of anal human papillomavirus infection and anal cancer precursors among HIV infected persons in the absence of anal intercourse. *Ann Intern Med.* 138:453-459.

[185] Durante, A.J., Williams, A.B., Da Costa, M., et al. (2003). Incidence of anal cytological abnormalities in a cohort of human immunodeficiency virus-infected women. *Cancer Epidemiol Biomarkers Prev.* 12:638-642.

[186] Reeves, W.C., Ruparelia, S.S., Swanson, K.I., Derkay, C.S., Marcus, A., and Unger, E.R. (2003). National registry for juvenile onset recurrent respiratory papillomatosis. *Arch Otolaryngol Head Neck Surg.* 129:976-982.

[187] Somers, G.R., Tabrizi, S.N., Borg, A.J., Garland, S.M., and Chow, CW. (1997). Juvenile laryngeal papillomatosis in a paediatric population: a clinicopathologic study. *Pediatr Path Lab Med.*, 17:53-64.

[188] Stamataki, S., Nikolopoulos, T., Korres, S., Felekis, D., Tzangaroulakis, A., and Ferekidis, E. (2007). Juvenile recurrent respiratory papillomatosis: still a mystery disease with difficult management. *Head Neck*, 29:155-162.

In: Cancer in Female Adolescents
Editor: Margarite T. Moorland

ISBN: 978-1-60456-421-1

Chapter III

Fertility Preservation in Female Adolescents with Malignancies

Elad Feigin,[*1, 2] ***Enrique Freud***[1, 2] ***Benjamin Fisch,***[2, 3]
Raoul Orvieto,[4, 5] ***Dragan Kravarusic,***[1, 2] ***Galia Avrahami,***[2, 6]
Avi Ben-Haroush,[2, 3] ***and Ronit Abir,***[2, 3]

[1] Department of Pediatric Surgery, Schneider Children's Medical Center of Israel, Rabin Medical Center-Beilinson Campus, Petach Tikvah, Israel
[2] Sackler School of Medicine, Tel Aviv University, Tel Aviv, Israel
[3] Infertility and IVF Unit, Helen Schneider Hospital for Women, Rabin Medical Center-Beilinson Campus, Petach Tikvah, Israel
[4] Infertility and IVF Unit, Brazilai Medical Center, Ashkelon, Israel
[5] Ben Gurion University, School of Medicine, Beer Sheva, Israel
[6] Institute of Pediatric Oncology, Schneider Children's Medical Center of Israel, Petach Tikvah, Israel

Abstract

With the improvements in anticancer treatment, the survival rate of adolescent cancer victims is increasing. As a consequence of this therapy, many female adolescents suffer from ovarian failure and premature ovarian failure. The level of infertility varies by patient age (the younger the patient, the lesser the likehood of severe ovarian failure) as well as by drug dose, treatment duration, type of treatment (alkylating agents cause severe ovarian damage), and number of agents used. The highest risk is associated with high-dose chemotherapy combined with total body irradiation before bone marrow transplantation. Ovarian damage caused by irradiation is also correlated to the anatomical location of the ovaries in relation to the radiation field in the abdomen.

[*] Corresponding Author: Elad Feigin, MD; Department of Pediatric Surgery; Schneider Children's Medical Center of Israel; 14 Kaplan Street; Petach Tikvah 49 202, Israel; Email: eladf@clalit.org.il, Fax: 972 3 9253930

Unfortunately, cancer patients have limited options for fertility preservation. Most survivors require oocyte donation. However, there is a shortage of donated oocytes in Western countries on the one hand, and most women prefer fertility restoration with self-oocytes on the other. Of the feasible possibilities for fertility preservation from self-oocytes, embryo cryopreservation after in vitro fertilization (IVF) as well as cryopreservation of mature human oocytes are in most cases unsuitable for minors. Therefore, cryopreservation of ovarian tissue containing small immature ovarian follicles remains almost the only practical option. So far, the autologous transplantation of cryopreserved-thawed ovarian tissue in women has resulted in four pregnancies, including two live births. Attempts to establish an *in vitro* maturation system are still in their infancy. This technology followed by routine IVF would eliminate the risks of reseeding malignant cells by ovarian grafts, and could possibly be offered in the future to infertile survivors of adolescent cancer, particularly of hematological malignancies. Obtaining ovarian tissue for cryopreservation requires a surgical procedure, usually laparoscopy, under general anesthesia, which may harbor risks that need to be discussed with the patient and her guardians. Other issues, such as the optimal surgical technique and the amount of tissue that needs to be removed for successful cryopreservation, have yet to be resolved. Although fertility-restoration techniques are still in the experimental stage, ovarian tissue removed from prepubertal and adolescent cancer patients is being frozen-stored in some medical centers worldwide. Sustaining the option of parenthood for young female patients may convey a message of hope, with a positive psychological effect.

Introduction

Relevant Aspects of Human Oogenesis, Folliculogenesis and Early Pregnancy

In this section, the *in vivo* development of germ cells and follicles from fetal to adult life and the early stages of pregnancy will be discussed briefly, focusing on topics essential for the understanding of later sections [Speroff *et al.*, 1994; Abir *et al.*, 2006].

The female is born with a complete pool of germ cells (oocytes). Their number declines gradually from birth (about one million) to menopause (average age of 51), mostly by atresia but also by ovulations [Faddy and Gosden, 1996].

Human primordial germ cells (PGC) arrive from the yolk sac to the gonad from day 26 of pregnancy, and are then termed oogonia [Gosden, 1995; Abir *et al.*, 2006]. Thereafter, three events induce the development of the female fetal germ cells in the gonad (ovary): mitotic division cycles of the oogonia; meiotic division; and follicular assembly. The number of female germ cells in the fetal ovary peaks at about seven million in mid-pregnancy, and then drops dramatically during the third trimester. Meiotic division usually commences gradually in the third month of gestation, and the diplothen stage is achieved within weeks of its initiation. At this point, the oogonia increase in size and acquire more intracellular organelles and the nucleus becomes round and large: *germinal vesicle (GV).* These germ cells are now termed oocytes. Just before birth, the oocytes are arrested at the diplothen stage of the prophase of the first meiotic division. They have completed genetic recombination and do not undergo any additional nuclear maturation until puberty when menstrual cycles are initiated.

Follicular formation in humans begins during the fourth month of gestation. During follicular assembly, there is a rapid proliferation of the nearby cells, and the oocytes become surrounded by a single layer of flattened somatic cells, termed granulosa cells (GC) [Gougeon, 1996; Abir *et al.*, 2006]. These cellular complexes, called *primordial follicles*, measure 30-50 μm in diameter, and can be identified in humans from around 22 gestational weeks. Most of the follicles in human fetal as well as in adult ovaries remain in the quiescent primordial form. Their growth regulation is not hormonal, and the exact factors that stimulate their development are unknown [Abir *et al.*, 2006]. Primordial follicles are activated when their GC become cuboidal, and they are then termed *primary follicles* (50-80 μm in diameter).

Primary follicles develop to *secondary follicles* (80 μm -0.2 mm in diameter) with an increased proliferation rate of the GC and consequent formation of a multilaminar layer. In humans, a definitive *theca layer* is created from the stroma cells surrounding the secondary follicle. Steroid hormones are synthesized through complex interactions between the GC and theca cells. During the secondary follicular stage, the oocyte starts to grow, and a glycoprotein coat, the *zona pellucida (ZP)*, forms between the oocyte and the innermost layer of the GC. The final follicular stage consists of development of *antral follicles* (early antral follicle: 0.2-0.4 mm in diameter) containing a fluid-filled cavity within several layers of cuboidal GC; the innermost layers surrounding the oocytes are termed *cumulus cells*.

At puberty, the hypothalamic gonadotrophin releasing hormone (GnRH) is secreted in pulsatile discharges and stimulates the normal production of the pituitary gonadotrophins: follicle stimulating hormone (FSH) and lutenizing hormone (LH) [Speroff *et al.*, 1994]. FSH levels rise in the first half of the menstrual cycle before ovulation, inducing follicular development and growth from secondary stages (the *follicular phase*) [Speroff *et al.*, 1994; Abir *et al.*, 2006]. A primordial follicle reaches the ovulatory antral size (18-20 mm in diameter) within six to nine months [Gougeon, 1996]. Ovulation occurs at the mid menstrual cycle and is stimulated by a drastic increase in baseline LH levels (*LH surge*) [Speroff *et al.*, 1994]. During ovulation, the first meiotic division is completed, with the extrusion of the first polar body enclosed between the oocyte and the ZP, forming a mature oocyte. The ovarian site from which ovulation occurs, develops into a progesterone-secreting gland, the *corpus luteum*. The remaining days until the end of the cycle are termed the *luteal phase*.

The ovarian phases are directly associated with changes in the uterine endometrium. The increased estrogen secretion during the follicular phase stimulates endometrial proliferation until a final preovulatory thickness of over 8 mm is achieved. After ovulation, endometrial development is affected by fluctuations in progesterone and estrogen levels, and is characterized by the appearance of glandular cells, coiling of spiral blood vessels, and expression of sex steroid receptors on the endometrial blood vessels. Implantation occurs on days 21-22 of the cycle, followed by the formation and proliferation of the decidual cells from the endometrium on day 23, under the influence of progesterone. The decidual layer is essential for the invasiveness of the embryonic trophoblast required for normal implantation.

Recently, studies have reported the presence proliferating PGC in ovaries of adult mice [Johnson *et al.*, 2004; 2005]. Although PGC have also been identified in the bone marrow (BM) of mice [Johnson *et al.*, 2005], ovarian function in humans has not been restored after BM transplantation (BMT) for cancer therapy (see next section). The presence of these cells in human adult ovaries is not only controversial but also highly unlikely, taking menopause into account [Faddy and Gosden, 1996; Gougeon, 1996]. Moreover, although some authors observed that PGC developed in cultures of human surface ovarian cells [Bukovski *et al.*, 2004; 2005], others failed to identify them in ovaries from women aged 28-53 years [Liu *et al.*, 2007].

Fertility in Survivors of Childhood or Adolescent Cancer

General Aspects of Childhood and Adolescent Malignancies

Childhood cancer is relatively rare with an annual incidence of around 110 to 130 cases per one million children [Stiller, 2004]; and 1 in every 600 children will develop cancer in the first 15 years of life [Bath *et al.*, 2002]. The estimated relative frequencies of pediatric cancers are as follows: leukemias, 34% (acute lymphoblastic leukemia-ALL ~one third; acute myeloid leukemia-AML ~20%) [Leung *et al.*, 2000; Brougham and Wallace, 2005]; brain/spinal cancer, 24% (central nervous system-CNS tumors are the second most common solid cancers in childhood) [Wallace *et al.*, 2005a]; embryonic cancer, 15%; lymphomas, 11% (Hodgkin lymphoma-HL is the most common solid tumor in adolescents); soft tissue cancer, 6%; bone cancer, 5%; and others, 5% [Leung *et al.*, 2000; Brougham and Wallace, 2005; Wallace *et al.*, 2005a]. Breast cancer is rare in adolescence, with an incidence of <0.1 per 100000 individuals <20 years of age, accounting for <1% of all childhood cancers. Its most common form, secretory cancer, occurs more frequently in children than in adults [Shannon and Smith, 2003].

Major advances in anticancer treatment in recent decades, particularly the use of multi-agent chemotherapeutic regiments, have resulted in a significant increase in the survival rates of children and adolescents to 70%-80% [Linet *et al.,* 1999; Mertens *et al.*, 2001; Brougham and Wallace, 2005; Sklar *et al.*, 2006]. The current survival rate for various forms of leukemia is at least 70% [Hann *et al.*, 2000; Bath *et al.*, 2002]. Today 1 in every 100 adults in their third decade is a survivor of childhood cancer, and by 2010, an estimated 1 in every 715 adults in the general population will be a survivor of childhood or adolescent cancer [Bath *et al.*, 2002]. With the rise in the number of survivors, some long-term side effects of anticancer treatment have become apparent, and their potential effect on quality of life. One of these is fertility problems which in most cases are detected only later in life [Bath *et al.*, 2002; Brougham and Wallace, 2005; Wallace *et al.,* 2005a].

General Aspects of Subfertility after Anticancer Treatment

The potential adverse effects of anticancer treatment on reproductive function in female survivors may be mediated through the ovary [Bath *et al.*, 2002], the uterus [Bath *et al.*, 1999; 2002], or the hypothalamus-pituitary-ovarian axis [Bath *et al.*, 2001; 2002]. Specifically, systemic chemotherapy or spinal, abdominal, or pelvic radiotherapy can accelerate oocyte depletion and lead to various degrees of ovarian failure [Meirow and Nugent, 2001; Brougham and Wallace, 2005].

Chemotherapeutic agents affect dividing cells, and therefore, the mechanism by which they damage the quiescent primordial follicles is unknown [Meirow, 2000; Meirow and Nugent, 2001]. Although the common assumption is that they do so by initiating apoptosis [Tilly, 1996], limited evidence has been provided so far by only two *in vitro* studies [Perez *et al.,* 1997; Meirow, 2000; Meirow and Nugent, 2001]. Indeed, investigations initiated in our laboratory did not identify any traces of apoptosis in postchemotherapy ovarian follicles of patients aged 6-39 (mean: 17±10 years) (Figure 1).

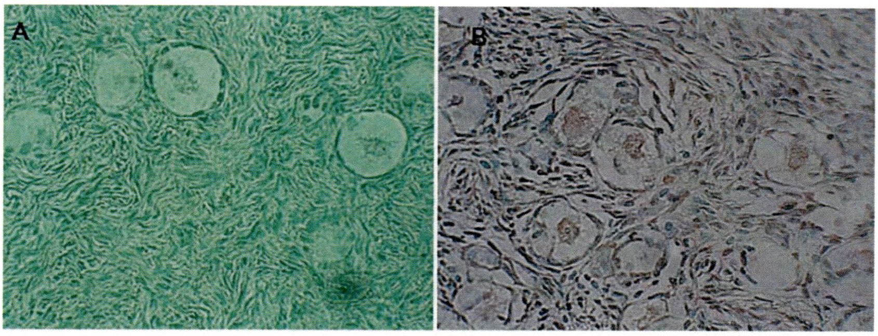

Figure 1. Photographs showing outcome of staining to detect apoptosis. (A) Ovarian section from a 15-year-old patient with HL after chemotherapy that included cyclophosphamide. Note the primordial (arrowheads) and primary follicles (arrows), the exclusively methyl green staining, with lack of brown staining for apoptosis. Original magnification, X400. (B) Positive control of an ovarian section treated with DNase from a 17-year-old patient with HL after chemotherapy that included cyclophosphamide. Note the primary follicle (arrow), and the brown staining indicating apoptosis, in addition to the background methyl green staining. Original magnification, X400.

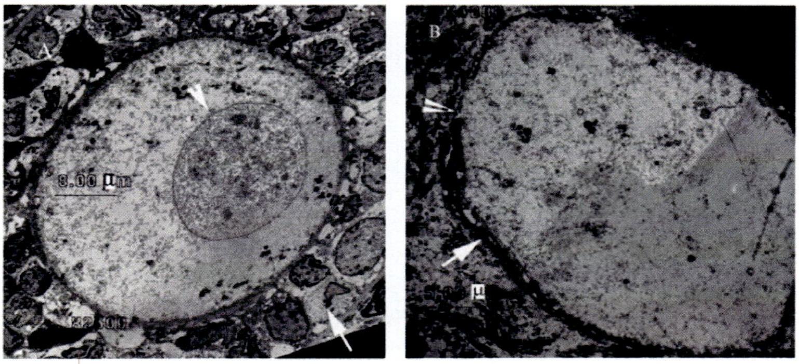

Figure 2. Photographs from transmission electron microscopy sections (TEM). A. TEM ovarian section from a 13-year-old patient before anticancer treatment. Note the normal secondary follicle with its GV (arrowhead) and normal GC layer (arrow). Original magnification, X2500. (B) TEM ovarian section from the same patient as in figure 1 (B). Note the primordial follicle with its damaged GC layer and nuclei (arrow) and basement membrane (arrowhead). Original magnification, X4000.

This was also true at 4 days after treatment onset in a 14-year-old patient [Abir *et al.*, 2008]. However, we did find a significant decrease in follicular quality, as indicated by the reduction in normal GC nuclei and concomitant increase in oocyte vacuolization (Figure 2). Given that follicles cannot remain viable without normal interactions between the oocytes and the GC [Gougeon, 1996], the follicular destruction after chemotherapy could occur in response to changes in the GC. Although large numbers of follicles were identified in ovaries of girls ≤20 years old after therapy, it is possible that a portion of them will eventually deteriorate because of poor quality, especially of the GC [Abir *et al.*, 2008].

The level of ovarian damage varies by patient age at the time of treatment and the chemotherapy agents used [Meirow and Nugent, 2001; Abir *et al.*, 2008]. Regarding age, young girls, especially at prepubertal ages, appear to be relatively protected against chemotherapy-induced ovarian damage, probably because of their larger reserve of surviving primordial follicles [Meirow and Nugent, 2001; Brougham and Wallace, 2005; Abir *et al.*, 2007]. Some studies also attributed this finding to the premenarcheal hormonal status [Marcello *et al.*, 1990; Abir *et al.*, 1998], although our results do not confirm this association [Abir *et al.*, 2008].

Regarding the treatment protocol, the integrity of the ovaries is affected by the type of chemotherapeutic agents, the cumulative dose, the total dose, and the duration of the treatment [Abir *et al.*, 1998]. The risks of ovarian damage associated with the various preparations are summarized in Table 1 [Grundy *et al.*, 2001; Meirow and Nugent, 2001; Wallace *et al.*, 2005a; Lee *et al.*, 2006]. In general, alkylating agents pose the highest risk of infertility, although the risk is equally high for certain nonalkylating agents such as porcarbazine [Meirow and Nugent, 2001; Wallace *et al.*, 2005a]. It rises even further when alkylating agents are combined with high levels of abdominal-pelvic radiation [Wallace *et al.*, 2005a]. The pre-BMT conditioning protocol of busulfan and cyclophosphamide leads to high sterilization rates, whereas high-dose melfalan seems safer [Meirow and Nugent, 2001; Wallace *et al.*, 2005a]. Nevertheless, when a pre-BMT conditioning regimen that included cyclophosphamide was used in children, only 5% had ovarian failure, emphasizing the importance of young age as an ovarian protector [Bath *et al.*, 2002]. Pre-BMT total body irradiation (TBI), and high doses of chemotherapeutic agents were found to create a high risk of severe ovarian dysfunction [Abir *et al.*, 1998; Meirow, 2000; Meirow and Nugent, 2001; Wallace *et al.*, 2005a].

Table 1. Risk levels for infertility promoted by various chemotherapeutic agents

Risk level	Agents
High	Alkylating agents: cyclophosphamide, ifosfamide, chlormethine, busulfan, melphalan, chlorambucil, carmustine, lomustine, mechlorethamine; procarbazide
Medium	Cisplatin, carboplatin, doxorubicin
Low	Vincristine, methotrexate, dactinomycin, bleomycin, mercaptopurine, vinca alkaloids (vinblastine), fluorouracil
Risk exists-unknown level	Nitrosources & antimetabolites: cytosine arabinoside
Unknown risk	Taxanes, oxaliplatin, monoclonal antibodies (trastuzumab, bevacizumab, cetuximab), tyrosine kinase inhibitors (eriotinib, imatinib)

Modified from Grundy *et al.*, 2001; Wallace *et al.*, 2005a; Lee *et al.*, 2006.

Effects of Radiation Therapy on the Ovary

TBI before BMT, and abdominal or pelvic radiation can by itself also result in ovarian damage. The degree of impairment depends on the radiation dose, location of the ovaries relative to the radiation field, fractionation schedule, and age at treatment [Abir *et al.,* 1998; Brougham and Wallace, 2005]. Even scattered radiation may cause ovarian damage [Abir *et al.,* 1998]. The extent of oocyte depletion after radiotherapy depends on the size of the existing oocyte pool. Therefore, the younger the irradiated patient, the later the onset of premature ovarian failure (POF) [Brougham and Wallace, 2005].

The human oocyte is very sensitive to radiation and the lethal dose required for the destruction of 50% of the oocytes is ~<2 Grey (Gy) [Wallace *et al.*, 2003; Brougham and Wallace, 2005]. Childhood TBI at 10-15.75 Gy can result in 90% POF of various degrees [Bath *et al.*, 1999; Brougham and Wallace, 2005; Wallace *et al.,* 2005b; Edgar and Wallace, 2007], while 20-30 Gy can lead to 97% ovarian failure [Edgar and Wallace, 2007]. However, one study reported that 56% of girls treated prepubertally with TBI had spontaneous puberty [Sarafogolu *et al.*, 1997], and those in whom ovarian failure developed were older at the time of radiotherapy (8.6 vs 6.1 years). Pregnancies have also been reported in patients who were treated with TBI in childhood/adolescence [Sanders *et al.*, 1996; Bath *et al*, 2002].

Effects of Radiation Therapy on the Uterus

TBI and abdominal or pelvic radiation at doses of 14-30 Gy in children and adolescents can often disrupt uterine anatomy and function (receptivity and maintenance of pregnancy) [Sanders *et al.*, 1996; Bath *et al.*, 1999; 2002; Brougham and Wallace, 2005; Edgar and Wallace, 2007]. This might be a result of diminished radiotherapy-induced elasticity of the uterine musculature, uterine fibrosis, and vascular damage, possibly associated with cervical incompetence as well. Uterine growth at puberty is stimulated by ovarian estrogen production. Therefore, the final uterine volume after radiotherapy depends on the age and pubertal status of the patient at the time of treatment [Critchley and Wallace, 2005; Signorello *et al.,* 2006; Edgar and Wallace, 2007]. The risk of uterine damage is probably greater in girls treated before menarche. Uterine irradiation was found to reduce uterine volume in 100 survivors of childhood cancer [Larsen *et al.*, 2004; Edgar and Wallace, 2007].

Unfortunately, current medical technologies are limited and uterine changes can be only partially assessed before pregnancy, and mostly only after puberty [Bath *et al.,* 2002]. Ultrasound scanning is a reliable means for evaluating uterine size, shape, blood supply, and endometrial thickness. Normal uterine sizes and volume have been well documented for prepubertal, pubertal, and menopausal patients. In addition, the uterine shape changes throughout puberty and is therefore an indicator of the pubertal stage. Using Doppler scanning clinicians can identify uterine artery blood flow and quantify it by the degree of resistance to the flow. In addition, endometrial biopsies can be easily obtained and prepared for histologic study and assays of the relevant immunohistochemical markers.

Studies of pregnancy outcome after uterine irradiation in childhood/adolescence have reported an increased incidence of nulliparity, premature birth and/or low birth weight, intrauterine growth retardation, stillbirth, and possibly, spontaneous miscarriages [Chiarelli *et al.*, 2000; Green *et al.*, 2002a; 2002b; Brougham and Wallace, 2005; Edgar and Wallace, 2007]. The recent Childhood Cancer Survivor Study (CCSS) investigated the long-term outcome of a cohort of 5-year survivors of childhood/adolescent cancer who were diagnosed before age 21 years, between 1970 and 1986 [Edgar and Wallace, 2007]. A total of 2201 singleton infants were born to 1264 survivors exposed to uterine irradiation [Signorello *et al.*, 2006; Edgar and Wallace, 2007]. There were significant risks of preterm birth (<37 weeks), low birth weight (<2500gr), and small for gestational age (SGA: <10th centile) babies; all of which were significantly correlated with maternal receipt of high cumulative dose of uterine radiotherapy (>50 Gy) before menarche [Edgar and Wallace, 2007].

Cranial Irradiation

Cranial or cranio-spinal radiation treatment may have adverse effects on reproductive function, mediated by the hypothalamic-pituitary-ovarian axis [Bath *et al.*, 2001; 2002]. Studies have reported disruptions in the hypothalamic–pituitary-gonadal axis in patients treated with high dose cranial or craniospinal irradiation (>23 Gy) for brain tumors, with a 60% risk of gonadotrophin deficiency by 4 years from treatment [Hall *et al.*, 1994; Bath *et al.*, 2001; 2002]. Delayed puberty, pubertal arrest, and primary amenorrhea were often documented (see next two chapters on treatment) [Bath *et al.,* 2001; Brougham and Wallace, 2005; Edgar and Wallace, 2007]. Abnormal gonadotrophin levels and delayed puberty were less common following exclusive CNS radiation [Brougham and Wallace, 2005; Chow *et al.*, 2007; Edgar and Wallace, 2007]. In contrast, elevated gonadotrophin levels associated with ovarian dysfunction were noted in many children treated with craniospinal radiation, probably as a result of the damaging effects of the chemotherapy on the ovary [Hamre *et al.*, 1987].

Given the high survival rates of childhood and adolescent ALL, more attention should be directed to the effects of low-dose cranial irradiation (18-24 Gy) often administrated to patients with CNS involved ALL or recurrent ALL [Bath *et al.*, 2001; Edgar and Wallace, 2007]. Irregularities in menarche are often reported after such treatment, although the findings are conflicting [Bath *et al.*, 2001]. One study investigated 188 survivors, all diagnosed at a mean age of 7 years, most of whom received cranial radiotherapy, but only 14% were exposed to alkylating agents [Mills *et al.*, 1997]. Significantly higher irregularities in onset of menarche were detected in the survivors treated with cranio/spinal radiation at a dose of 24 Gy or with lower doses (~18 Gy) before the age of 8. The CCSS evaluated 72 survivors of ALL, all of whom were diagnosed prior to menarche and exposed to cranio/spinal radiotherapy (15-29 Gy directed to the brain+10-24 Gy to the spine in 90%), as well as chemotherapy with alkylating agents [Chow *et al.*, 2007]. They found that cranio/spinal radiotherapy was associated with delayed menarche, and cranial radiotherapy with earlier menarche, regardless of radiation level (<20 or $\geq$20 Gy), compared with the patients' siblings. The risk of early menarche was positively correlated with younger age at diagnosis (<5) and radiation doses of >18 Gy. These risks for menarche irregularities were absent in patients treated with chemotherapy only.

Cranial irradiation for ALL during childhood or adolescence may also be associated with lower first-birth rate, as identified in 23 survivors of ALL who delivered 41 children [Nygaard *et al.*, 1991]. A study of gonadotrophin secretion in 12 survivors of ALL with regular menses who were treated prepubertally with cranial irradiation (10-14 Gy) as well as chemotherapy, documented lower than normal estrone secretion throughout the cycle, in addition to lower early follicular phase plasma estradiol and LH levels, particularly during the LH surge, with a shorter luteal phase (≤11 days) [Bath *et al.*, 2001]. Ovarian size, however, was normal as were FSH levels.

Cranial irradiation for treatment of ALL might also indirectly affect fertility by reducing levels of growth hormone (GH) [Bath *et al.*, 2001; 2002], leading to insufficient production of insulin like growth factor 1, to reduction in the effects of gonadotrophins on the ovary, and to inhibition in uterine receptivity [Homburg and Farhi, 1995].

POF and Acute Ovarian Failure (AOF)

A study of 1067 women treated for adolescent cancer (diagnosis before the age of 20 years) with radiotherapy and chemotherapy (including also alkylating agents), yielded a 42% rate of POF by age 31 years, representing a four fall greater risk than in other women in their early twenties [Byrne *et al.*, 1992; Bath *et al.*, 2002; Brougham and Wallace, 2005]. Moreover, the CCSS reported that in 2819 survivors of childhood cancer the risk for developing POF was 13-fold higher than that of their siblings, with a cumulative incidence of 8% by age 40 [Sklar *et al.*, 2006]. Ovarian radiation was identified as the greatest risk factor for POF. The increased risk was directly correlated with exposure to high doses of ovarian irradiation (≥10 Gy), although even low scattered doses (<1 Gy) induced POF. Alkylating agents were also implicated with a direct correlation of risk with the dose received. The cumulative risk approached 30% in patients after treatment with alkylating agents as well as abdominopelvic radiation. Attained age also affected POF, although it was unclear if the elevated risk was related to older childhood/adolescent age at diagnosis [Byrne *et al.*, 1992; Sklar *et al.*, 2006]. Therapy for HL was also identified as a risk factor for POF, but this finding is because the patients had been treated with the older, gonadotoxic protocols (see also next section) [Sklar *et al.*, 2006]. Moreover, in nearly 50% of the survivors, POF was surgically induced by hysterectomy [Chiarelli *et al.*, 1999; Sklar *et al.*, 2006].

Survivors of childhood and adolescent cancer are considered to have AOF if they never menstruated, ceased having menses within 5 years of their cancer diagnosis, or experienced a complete loss of ovarian function within 5 years of diagnosis [Chemaitilly *et al.*, 2006]. AOF has been reported only in 6.3%-12% of survivors of pediatric and adolescent cancer [Stillman *et al.*, 1981; Larsen *et al.*, 2003; Chemaitilly *et al.*, 2006]. Ovarian irradiation is its most significant risk factor [Stillman *et al.*, 1981; Chemaitilly *et al.*, 2006], and the risk is directly correlated with increased doses [Chemaitilly *et al.*, 2006]. In the earliest study of this issue [Stillman *et al.*, 1981], a 12% rate of AOF was reflected in 182 childhood cancer survivors, of whom 29% had Wilms tumor. The next study, performed more than 20 years later [Larsen *et al.*, 2003], reported an 8% AOF rate in 100 survivors diagnosed before age 15 years. The CCSS reported only a 6.3% rate of AOF in 3390 survivors, and highlighted additional risk factors [Chemaitilly *et al.*, 2006]: exposure to chemotherapeutic drugs, specifically alkylating agents such as cyclophosphamide in patients diagnosed at an older age (13-20 years), or to procarbazine in patients diagnosed at any age (mostly treated by older HL protocols; see next section), older age at diagnosis (especially above 12 years), and cancer diagnosis of lymphoma, Wilms tumor, or soft tissue sarcoma.

Effects of Current Cancer Treatments for Certain Malignancies on Fertility

The recent trend in ALL treatment is to increase the intensity of chemotherapy [Bath *et al.*, 2001], while reducing the dose of gonadotoxic agents, particularly cyclophosphamide [Brougham and Wallace, 2005]. Indeed, one outcome study of this protocol in 40 survivors of childhood ALL reported normal puberty in all cases, 37 had regular menses, and 9 gave birth to 14 live offspring [Wallace *et al*, 1993; Bath et al., 2002]. More intensive treatment regimens in prepubertal and pubertal girls resulted in higher FSH levels after GnRH administration, although the time of puberty onset was normal, as was estrogen production [Quigley *et al.*, 1989]. Furthermore, intrathecal chemotherapy has in many centers replaced cranial radiation for the prevention of ALL with CNS disease, but its possible effect on the hypothalamic-pituitary-ovarian pathway is still unknown [Bath *et al.*, 2002].

Regarding AML, the treatment today is more intensive, over a shorter time. It is based predominantly on anthracycline agents and cytarabine, which may affect fertility [Bath *et al.*, 2002]. At the same time the use of BMT for AML has decreased in the last decade, such that in many patients, fertility is preserved naturally [Leung *et al.,* 2000; Bath *et al.*, 2002; Brougham and Wallace, 2005]. It contrast, however, one long-term follow up study of AML survivors who received radiotherapy, confirmed the high rates of infertility.

In the last decade one of the important modifications for the treatment of HL is the replacement of gonadotoxic chemotherapeutic agents, such as procarbazine, and of alkylating agents such as chlorambucil, mustine and cyclophosphamide, with the less gonadotoxic, anthracycline drugs [Bath *et al.,* 2002; Brougham and Wallace, 2005]. The safest treatment protocol for the ovary consists of adriamycin, bleomycin, vinblastine and decarbazine (ABVD) [Brougham and Wallace, 2005]. The older protocols, such as mechlorethamine, vincristine, procarbazine and prednisolone (MOPP) [Edgar and Wallace, 2007], or procarbazine without radiotherapy, induced POF with elevated gonadotrophin levels in over 50% of survivors of childhood or adolescence HL [Mackie *et al.*, 1996; Edgar and Wallace, 2007]. There are, however, reports of normal ovarian function, including pregnancies, in some patients treated with the old protocols [Mackie *et al.*, 1996; Bath *et al.*, 2002].

Be that as it may, girls exposed to mediastinal and/or axillary lymph node (mantle) radiotherapy for HL, specifically during the time of growth of the mammary tissue (age 10-16 years), are at a 75-fold higher risk of acquiring breast cancer during the reproductive period [Shannon and Smith, 2003]. The higher risk is detectable even 10 years after treatment, and increases progressively 15 years or more later, with a cumulative probability of 35% for breast cancer at age 40 years. Therefore, it is highly recommended that these survivors be mammographically screened at regular intervals, even as soon as 8 years after irradiation. The secondary breast malignancy is often treated with cyclophosphamide, further diminishing fertility potential (see also chapter on "Ethical and Psychological Issues and Counseling").

Because each malignancy is now treated with a specific protocol, it is currently possible to approximate the risk of diminished fertility by type of disease (Table 2) [Bath *et al.*, 2002; Wallace *et al.,* 2005a]. However, it should be stressed that this list is just an estimation, and infertility risk in girls should be assessed on case-by-case basis, with consideration that the same therapy can affect individuals differently.

Table 2. Estimated risk levels for infertility according to specific malignancies

Risk level	Malignancy or treatment
High >80%	TBI, localized pelvic radiotherapy, chemotherapy conditioning for BMT, HL (alkylating agent based therapy), metastatic sarcoma (similar to risks of pre-BMT conditioning protocols)
Medium	AML, hepatoblastoma, osteosarcoma, Ewing sarcoma, soft tissue sarcoma, neuroblastoma, NHL, HL (with ABVD therapy), brain tumor (with craoniospinal irradiation), cranial irradiation >24 Gy
Low <20%	ALL, Wilms tumor, soft tissue sarcoma stage I, germ cell tumors (with gonadal preservation and no radiotherapy), retinoblastoma, brain tumors (with surgery and cranial irradiation of 24 Gy)

Modified from Bath *et al.*, 2002; Wallace *et al.,* 2005a.

Hormonal Replacement Therapy (HRT) for Delayed Puberty and Development

Delayed puberty or lack of resumption of the normal pubertal course after anticancer treatment in adolescent survivors can be a result of the effects of the treatment on the ovary (follicular depletion), the uterus (radiation induced abnormalities that interfere with normal endocrine function), or the hypothalamic–pituitary-gonadal axis (hyopgonadotrophic hypogonadism) [Speroff *et al.*, 1994; Bath *et al.*, 1999, 2001; Brougham and Wallace, 2005; Chemaitilly *et al.,* 2006; Edgar and Wallace, 2007]. The first priority in these cancer survivors is to evaluate the cause and source of the delay, and to initiate appropriate therapy. The medical evaluation for delayed puberty usually includes X-rays for bone age, measurement of serum gonadotrophins, prolactin, GH and adrenal and gonadal steroids, assessment of thyroid function, ultrasound ovarian scanning with emphasis on volume and number of antral follicles and skull imaging (in hypogonadotrophic hypogonadism) [Speroff *et al.*, 1994; Bath *et al.*, 2002, 2001].

In patients with POF (hypogonadism), hormonal therapy is essential not only to initiate and sustain the maturation and function of the secondary sexual characteristics developed at adolescence, but also to promote the full height potential, including the increase in bone density [Speroff *et al.,* 1994]. Treatment consists of very small daily doses of unopposed estrogen, either conjugated estrogen or estradiol, for 6-12 months. After onset of breast development and uterine growth, treatment should be switched to a sequential program of increased daily maintenance levels of estrogen with the addition of cyclic medroxyprogesterone acetate during the first 12 days each month in order to induce cyclic vaginal withdrawal bleeding [Speroff *et al.,* 1994; Abir *et al.*, 2001a]. In some girls (excluding those with AOF), HRT triggers the initiation or resumption of puberty, and development continues spontaneously, thereafter, when the bone age reaches 13 years [Speroff *et al.,* 1994].

Delayed puberty due to cranial radiation-induced hyopgonadotrophic hypogonadism may be accompanied by growth failure as a result of GH deficiency [Bath *et al.,* 2002, 2001]. In these cases, the adolescents should be treated with GH as well, because it stimulates alone or with HRT the growth and maturation of the epiphyseal growth plates [Abir *et al.*, 2001a]. Treatment with GH should be continued until either the final target height is achieved or near-epiphyseal fusion precludes a significant effect. When planning the optimal HRT to induce puberty in girls receiving GH, especially those with AOF, clinicians should consider the biphasic effect of estrogen on growth, namely, stimulatory at low doses and inhibitory at high doses. Furthermore, estrogen should not be used alone for growth promotion, and when used for feminization induction in conjunction with ongoing GH therapy, further growth augmentation may not occur. Therefore, the timing of estrogen administration to induce puberty may have an important impact on growth. In girls receiving GH, estrogen should not be given when bone age is less than 11 or 12 years or until near-final height has been achieved, that is, when only one more year of GH therapy is required. However, although the addition of very low estrogen doses to GH therapy in girls aged 12-15 years might have beneficial effects on final height, poor outcome may be due to late initiation of GH therapy and to early use of estrogen therapy.

Fertility Preservation/Restoration

Fertility Assessment

To preserve or restore fertility in adolescent cancer patients or survivors, the first priority is to assess the direct cause of the possible or putative fertility problem [Speroff *et al.*, 1994; Bath et al., 2001; Bath *et al.*, 1999; Brougham and Wallace, 2005; Chemaitilly *et al.*, 2006; Edgar and Wallace, 2007]. In most cases, the infertility is due to depletion in ovarian follicles [Abir *et al.*, 1998; Meirow, 2000; Meirow and Nugent, 2001]. Assessment of gonadal function includes clinical evaluation of pubertal progression, biochemical analysis of plasma gonadotrophins and sex steroids, menstrual history, and ultrasound examination of the uterus and ovaries [Wallace *et al.*, 2005a; Broekmans *et al.*, 2006]. Raised concentrations of FSH will often be detected in the early follicular stage, despite healthy ovulatory cycles.

As the hypothalamic-pituitary-gonadal axis is fairly quiescent before and during puberty, the biochemical assessment of ovarian reserve and function is unreliable [Bath *et al.*, 2002, 2003; Brougham and Wallace, 2005; Broekmans *et al.*, 2006], although anti-Mullerian hormone (AMH, a granulosa cell product which indicates the presence of preantral and early antral follicles) or inhibin B (a glycoprotein secreted from small developing antral follicles), may serve as potential markers, even in prepubertal patients [Brougham and Wallace, 2005]. The follicular reserve can be evaluated by various clinical methods [Bath *et al.*, 2003]. One study investigated 20 survivors of heterogenic childhood/adolescent malignancies aged >16 years at recruitment, with regular menses, of whom 10 were being treated with the combined oral contraceptive pill. FSH, AMH and inhibin B levels were measured in the serum, and ovarian volume and follicular numbers were identified by ultrasound scanning. The results showed elevated levels of FSH, lower levels of AMH, lower ovarian volume, and fewer antral follicles, compared with normal controls. FSH administration to the cancer survivors and controls taking the oral contraceptive pill, resulted in undetectable inhibin B levels, and lower antral follicle counts, compared with controls.

Fertility Restoration Options with Emphasis on Practical Technologies

The options for fertility preservation and restoration in young cancer patients, specifically adolescents, are limited (Figure 3) [Greenberg and Urbach, 2006]. Currently, egg donation with *in vitro* fertilization (IVF) is almost their only chance for pregnancy, especially after ovarian failure [Larsen *et al.*, 2000; Abir *et al.*, 2006]. However, there is a shortage of donated oocytes worldwide. Potential ways to increase the pool of donated oocytes include using immature oocytes from ovaries of aborted human fetuses [Biron-Shental *et al.*, 2004] or developing oocytes from embryonic stem cells [Hubner *et al.*, 2003]. However, not only are these options highly controversial, and forbidden in some countries, but the development of these technologies is still in its infancy [Hubner *et al.*, 2003; Abir *et al.*, 2006]. Moreover, most women prefer to use their own oocytes. Therefore, methods to preserve and restore self-fertility are required.

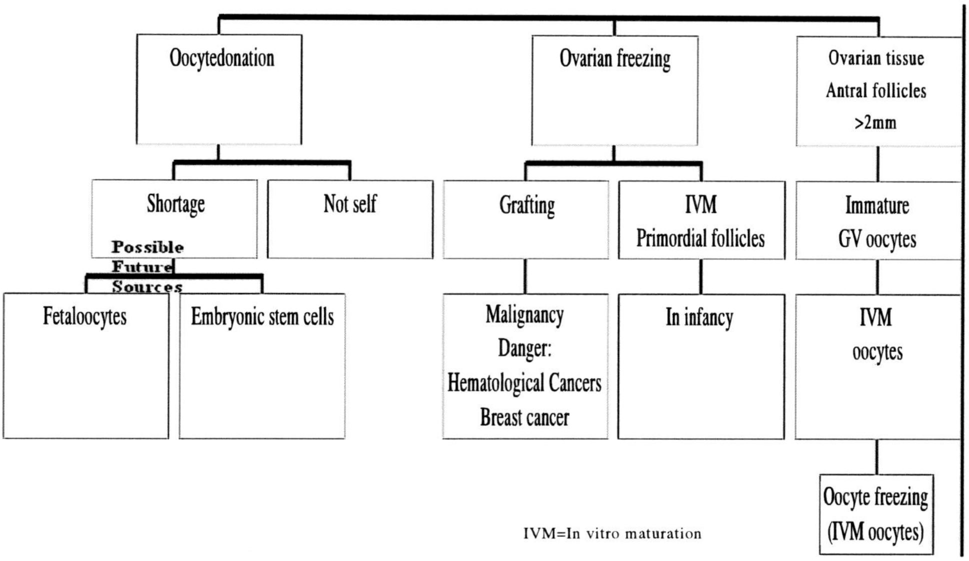

Figure 3. Schematic diagram of fertility preservation options for adolescents with cancer.

A practical option for fertility preservation is IVF treatment followed by cryopreservation of the embryos [Abir *et al.*, 1998]. However, this solution is usually unsuitable and unethical for adolescents, especially prepubertal ones, because IVF requires hormonal treatment for superovulation with unpleasant side effects, and also in the rare cases of estrogen-dependent adolescent breast cancer, such treatment can enhance the malignancy. In addition, the use of donor sperm for IVF in these cases seems unethical. IVF with embryo cryopreservation can be considered in older adolescent minors (~17-18 years old) who are married or in very stable relationships, although occasionally even in these cases, anticancer therapy cannot be postponed to allow 2-4 weeks of IVF treatment [Greenberg and Urbach, 2007].

Technologies for the cryopreservation of mature oocytes have greatly improved in the last decade. Their use to date has resulted in about 120 live births [Jain and Paulson, 2006, Lee *et al.*, 2006; Oktay *et al.*, 2006]. However, as the overall success rates remain lower than those of standard IVF procedures, the method is usually not applied to preserve fertility in cancer patients. Nevertheless, one group recently reported a live birth after intracytoplasmic sperm injection to an oocyte cryopreserved before treatment for HL [Yang *et al.*, 2007]. Like for embryo cryopreservation, this option is usually unsuitable for adolescents, as it requires intense hormonal stimulation.

Ovarian Cryopreservation for Fertility Preservation

Almost the only option for fertility preservation in adolescents is cryopreservation of ovarian tissue containing primordial follicles retrieved by a simple laparoscopic operation (figure 4) [Abir *et al.,* 1998; Meirow, 2000; Meirow and Nugent, 2001]. The cryopreservation of ovarian cortical fragments was recently reported by our group in 23 girls of average age 13.5 years (range 5-17.5 years) [Feigin *et al.*, 2007] (see also chapter on "Our Experience with Ovarian Retrieval from Adolescents"), and by others in 47 girls of average age 5 years (range 10 months to 15 years) [Poirot *et al.*, 2007], with heterogenic malignancies.

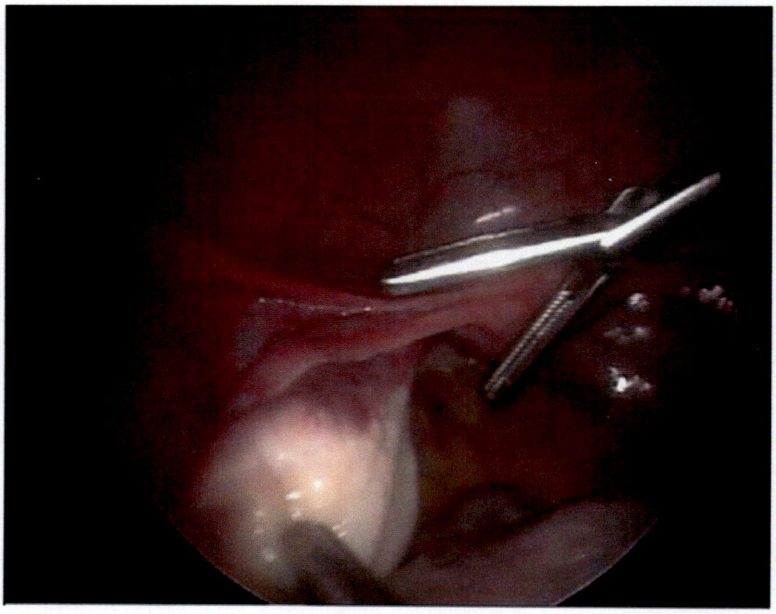

Figure 4. Laparoscopic procedure for retrieval of ovarian tissue. Laparoscopic view of normal ovary during ovarian retrieval for cryopreservation.

Ovarian cryopreservation should preferably be performed before initiation of any form of anticancer therapy, especially BMT [Meirow *et al.*, 2001; Abir *et al.*, 2007]. However, in many patients, cancer treatment cannot be postponed, and in cases of recurrent malignancies, tissue may not have been cryopreserved after the initial diagnosis. Therefore, the justification of preserving ovarian tissue after cancer treatment remains a major dilemma. One live birth has been reported in a 25-year-old cancer survivor who was treated prior to ovarian cryopreservation with high-dose chemotherapy protocols that included cyclophosphamide [Meirow *et al.*, 2005]. A recent study from our laboratory described large numbers of viable (Figure 5) nonapoptotic (Figure 1A) follicles in ovaries of patients ≤20 years old [Abir *et al.*, 2008], suggesting that age is a major determinant for the application of postchemotherapy ovarian cryopreservation. Therefore, in adolescents, ovarian cryopreservation after treatment can indeed be considered.

During surgery for fertility preservation, surgical and anesthetic risks should be kept to a minimum (Figure 4). It seems prudent to perform other necessary procedures that are conducted as part of the standard course of treatment at the same time, such as line insertion or BM harvesting [Poirot *et al.*, 2007; Weintraub *et al.*, 2007]. It is important that the amount of tissue retrieved be sufficient for fertility preservation. Therefore, in young patients with small ovaries an entire ovary is usually removed, whereas in patients with larger ovaries, partial oophorectomy may suffice [Feigin *et al.*, 2007]. Electrocautery is not recommended because it could damage the retrieved tissue during manipulation of the ovary intended for preservation. Laparosopic procedures have been described using two [Poirot *et al.*, 2007] or three trocars according to surgeons' preference.

The most common method of cryopreservation is slow, gradual freezing of thinly sliced ovarian cortical fragments in a medium containing dimethylsulphoxide or ethylene glycol or propandiol combined with sucrose [Hovatta, 2005]. Other techniques are currently being investigated and include vitrification with a high concentration of combinations of cryoprotectants for rapid freezing [Rahimi *et al.*, 2003] and cryopreservation of whole ovaries (see subsection *"Follicular loss due to ischemia and possible preventive methods"*).

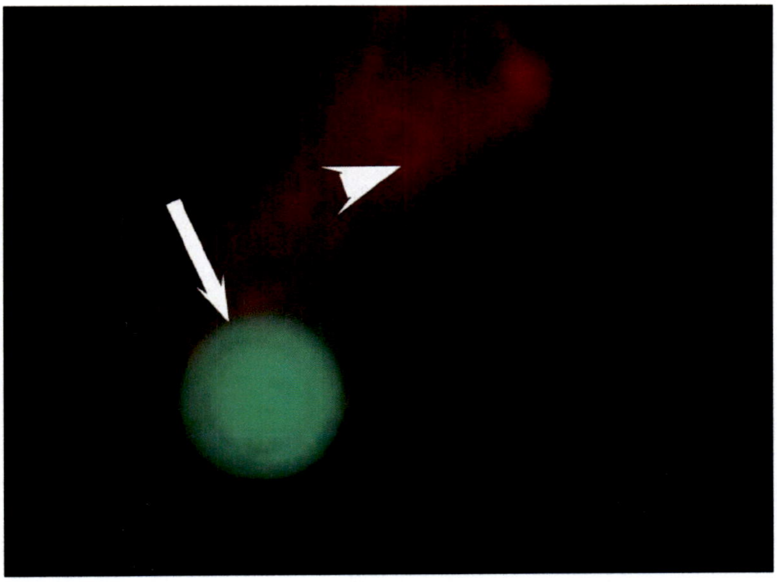

Figure 5. Photograph of fluorescence viability staining. Isolated secondary follicle from a 14-year-old patient with anaplastic ependymoma after chemotherapy that included cyclophosphamide. The follicle itself is stained only with green calcein in the GC layer as well as the oocyte (arrow) (esterase activity in viable cells). The red reflection in the background (arrowhead) is caused by the red ethidium homodimer staining in the dead stroma cells below the follicle (membranes of dead cells become permeable to this stain). Original magnification, X400.

Restoration of Fertility via Frozen-Thawed Ovarian Grafts

There is a trend today to attempt to restore of ovarian function by reimplantation of frozen-thawed ovarian cortical fragments to the ovarian site [Donnez *et al.,* 2004, Meirow *et al.*, 2005, 2007, Schmidt *et al.*, 2005; Demeestere *et al.*, 2006; Rosendahl *et al.*, 2006]. The utilization of this technique in former cancer patients has so far led to 4 pregnancies, including two live births [Donnez *et al.,* 2004, Meirow *et al.*, 2005, 2007]. Similarly, grafting ovarian tissue from fertile monozygotic twins to their infertile twins has led to 6 pregnancies [Silber *et al.,* 2005; Silber and Gosden, 2007], including at least one live birth [Silber *et al.,* 2005]. The advantage of retransplantation to the natural site is that it makes spontaneous conception [Donnez *et al.,* 2004; Demeestere *et al.*, 2006] as well as IVF pregnancy possible [Meirow *et al.*, 2005, 2007; Silber *et al.,* 2005; Rosendahl *et al.*, 2006; Silber and Gosden, 2007]. Better results were obtained by transplanting strips of thawed tissue (1.5 cm X 1.5 cm in diameter, 0.1-0.2 cm in thickness) rather than injecting small fragments into the ovary [Meirow *et al.,* 2005].

However, the scientific disadvantage of reimplantation to the ovarian site is the low probability that pregnancies might originate not from the ovarian graft but from remaining dormant oocytes [Meirow *et al.*, 2005, 2007; Silber *et al.,* 2005; Demeestere *et al.*, 2006; Rosendahl *et al.*, 2006; Silber and Gosden, 2007]. Therefore, the earlier attempts were conducted in other sites, such the pelvis [Oktay and Karlikaya, 2000; Radford *et al.*, 2001; Lee *et al.*, 2006] or subcutaneous areas, namely, the forearm [Oktay *et al.*, 2001; 2003, Lee *et al.*, 2006] and lower abdomen [Oktay *et al.*, 2004; Schmidt *et al.*, 2005; Lee *et al.*, 2006]. Restoration of ovarian endocrine function, menses, and development of antral follicles was documented [Oktay and Karlikaya, 2000; Oktay *et al.*, 2001; 2003, 2004, Radford *et al.*, 2001; Schmidt *et al.*, 2005; Lee *et al.*, 2006]; one group even reported the production of a 4–cell IVF embryo [Oktay *et al.*, 2004]. In forearm and perhaps also in lower abdomen grafting, antral follicles can be detected externally as growing bulges [Oktay *et al.*, 2001; 2003], although these relatively exposed sites might provide insufficient follicular protection and pose a danger of damage from random pressure.

Follicular Loss Due to Ischemia and Possible Prevention Methods

Studies show very little follicular depletion following freezing-thawing of thinly sliced ovarian cortical tissue [Abir *et al.*, 2001a]. Most follicular loss occurs as a result of the ischemia induced by the slow graft revascularization after transplantation. Therefore, methods to improve and hasten graft vascularization are urgently needed. The antioxidant vitamin E was found to improve follicular survival by reducing ischemia in murine hosts [Nugent *et al.*, 1998], whereas in bovine ovarian tissue incubated at 37^0C, the antioxidant ascorbic acid reduced stroma cell but not follicular apoptosis [Kim *et al.*, 2004]. The administration of recombinant LH and FSH to upregulate ovarian angiogenic factors in mouse hosts in which ovarian grafts were placed in the poorly vascularized abdominal wall [Imthurn *et al.*, 2000] successfully increased follicular survival only when the recipients were treated 2 days before and 2 days after grafting. This finding was explained by the necessary presence of effective amounts of angiogenic factors before transplantation to induce neovascularization and prevent ischemia immediately after grafting. Vitamin E treatment [Nugent *et al.*, 1998] as well as gonadotrophin stimulation [Imthurn *et al.*, 2000] before and after grafting can be attempted also in transplantation trials in women.

Systemic treatment with angiogenic factors should probably not be attempted, owing to risk of side effects, such as bleeding or clotting in other body parts. Some methods that increased revasculization of ovarian grafts in rodents are also unsuitable for humans: grafting ovarian tissue to males [Weissman *et al.*, 1999]; host treatment with testosterone [Arrau *et al.*, 1983]; bilateral oophorectomy with transplantation to other sites [Laschke *et al.*, 2002, 2003]; and wound creation in grafting sites a few days before transplantation with implantation into the angiogenic granulation tissue [Israeli *et al.*, 2006]. The latter might cause bleeding complications before the actual transplantation.

Cryopreservation of whole ovaries with their vascular pedicles may reduce revascularization time after ovarian transplantation with vascular surgery and minimize follicular ischemia [Martinez-Madrid *et al.*, 2007]. Our own experience with preparation of human ovarian tissue yielded extreme infiltration difficulties due to the dense tissue structure [Abir *et al.*, 2001b, 2008]. This might also cause insufficient equilibrium of whole ovaries with cryoprotectant solutions and result in inadequate freezing.

The first ovarian grafting trial was performed only in 2000 [Oktay and Karlikaya, 2000], so there are as yet no reports on the transplantation of tissue from survivors of adolescent cancer. It is already clear, however, that ovarian grafts have a limited active endocrine period [Demeestere *et al.*, 2006; Meirow *et al.*, 2007], probably because of the extensive follicular loss immediately after implantation. As ovaries of adolescents, specifically prepubertal girls, contain large numbers of follicles [Marcello *et al.*, 1990; Gougeon, 1996; Abir *et al.*, 2008], it is highly likely that grafts from such patients will function longer than those from older cancer survivors [Oktay and Karlikaya, 2000; Oktay *et al.*, 2001; 2003, 2004; Meirow *et al.*, 2005, 2007; Demeestere *et al.*, 2006; Rosendahl *et al.*, 2006]. An additional advantage in adolescents might be that their oocytes could yield higher fertility and pregnancy rates with fewer chromosomal anomalies than those of older women [Dudzinski, 2004].

Danger of Reseeding Cancer with Ovarian Grafts and Putative Techniques for Its Elimination

In some cancers, such as hematological malignancies (leukemias), certain types of NHL and breast cancer, replantation of ovarian tissue carries a risk of reseeding the cancer [Shaw and Trounson, 1997; Meirow *et al.*, 1998, Abir *et al.*, 2006]. These malignancies also occur in adolescents [Leung *et al.*, 2000; Shannon and Smith, 2003; Brougham and Wallace, 2005; Wallace *et al.*, 2005a], but the ovary is not involved in the adolescence abundant [Leung *et al.*, 2000; Brougham and Wallace, 2005; Wallace *et al.*, 2005a] HL [Meirow *et al.*, 1998; Kim *et al.*, 2001; Seshadri *et al.*, 2006], and probably also not in most NHL [Kim *et al.*, 2001]. The estimated risks for ovarian metastasis of malignancies are summarized in Table 3 [Sonmezer *et al.*, 2005].

Table 3. Estimated risk levels for ovarian metastasis according to specific malignancies

Risk level	Malignancy
High	Squamous cell carcinoma of the cervix, Ewing sarcoma, breast cancer (stage I-III, infiltrative ductal), Wilms tumor, osteosarcoma, non-genital rhadomyosarcoma
Moderate	Breast cancer (stage IV and iniltrative lobular), colon cancer (including tumors of rectum and appendix), adeno/adenosquamous carcinoma of the cervix, upper gastrointestinal system malignancies
Low	Burkitt lymphoma, neuroblastoma and genital rhabdomyosarcoma
None (probably)	HL, most NHL

Modified from Meirow *et al.*, 1998; Kim *et al.*, 2001; Sonmezer *et al.*, 2005; Seshadri *et al.*, 2006.

Eliminating the risk of retransmission of cancer by ovarian grafts could theoretically be achieved by *in vitro* maturation (IVM) of primordial follicles from frozen-thawed ovarian tissue, followed by routine IVF and embryo transfer [Abir *et al.*, 2006]. However, this technique to date has only been achieved in murine models [O'Brien *et al.,* 2003]. Given the complexity of human follicular development and the uncertainty of the signals activating primordial follicles [Gougeon, 1996], the successful *in vitro* culture of primordial follicles from patients in the near future seems impractical. So far, human primordial follicles have only developed in culture to secondary stages [Abir *et al.*, 2001b, 2006]. However, as adolescent patients are very young, this option might be available to them when they are older, and will provide an excellent safe alternative of fertility restoration for the many survivors of leukemia as well as other cancers.

Another possible method of restoring fertility without the danger of retransmitting malignant cells is transplantation of isolated primordial ovarian follicles instead of tissue. However, both the isolation and the handling of the tiny human primordial follicles are extremely difficult [Abir *et al.*, 2001b], and keeping them intact requires embedding them in matrices such as collagen gels [Telfer *et al.*, 1990; Abir *et al.*, 2001b] or plasma clots (hematological glue) before grafting [Gosden, 1990a, 1990b; Carroll *et al.,* 1990; Carroll and Gosden, 1993]. Such grafts have promoted follicular development and survival in rodents [Telfer *et al.*, 1990; Laschke *et al.*, 2002, 2003], and even led to the birth of live pups in mice [Gosden, 1990a, 1990b; Carroll *et al.,* 1990; Carroll and Gosden, 1993]. A very recent study described the transplantation of isolated human follicles embedded in plasma clots to murine hosts for one week [Dolmans *et al.*, 2007]. Although there was evidence of GC proliferation in most of the isolated follicles, stroma cells surrounding the follicles were detected as well. Therefore, before it can be used clinically, the follicle isolation procedure needs to be improved to eliminate the risk of the presence of residual stroma cells, possibly by using collagenase [Abir *et al.*, 2001b] instead of liberase [Dolmans *et al.*, 2007] for isolation, followed by delicate manual dissection [Abir *et al.*, 2001b].

A more feasible fertility preservation strategy combines cryopreservation of ovarian tissue with retrieval of immature cumulus-enclosed GV stage oocytes from small antral follicles ($\geq$2 mm), followed by their *in vitro* maturation [Revel *et al.*, 2004; Huang *et al.*, 2007] and subsequent slow gradual freezing [Revel *et al.*, 2004] or vitrification [Huang *et al.*, 2007]. This technique does not require hormonal stimulation, and is, therefore, suitable also for adolescents with cancer. Moreover, ovaries of postpubertal adolescents usually contain relatively high numbers of small antral follicles resulting from normal cyclic FSH stimulation; occasionally, very low numbers of such follicles can be detected even in ovaries of prepubertal adolescents as a result of basal FSH levels [Speroff *et al.*, 1994]. However, the aspiration of immature oocytes soon after chemotherapy is not recommended, because these oocytes are not quiescent and originate from growing follicles, and therefore, might have been affected by chemotherapy [Meirow *et al.*, 2001].

Other Methods for Fertility Preservation

Young patients who are due to receive pelvic irradiation may have their ovaries shielded or moved as far as possible from the radiation field by oophoropexy, performed by a simple laparoscopic operation, if laparotomy is not needed for removal of the primary tumor (Figure 6) [Leporrier *et al.*, 1987; Williams *et al.*, 1999; Brougham and Wallace, 2005; Lee *et al.*, 2006]. Because of the risk of spontaneous relocation of the ovaries, the procedure should be performed in close proximity to the radiation treatment [Williams *et al.*, 1999; Lee *et al.*, 2006]. The ovary is sutured at a lateral position, usually behind the uterus or into the paracolic gutters [Leporrier *et al.*, 1987; Williams *et al.*, 1999; Brougham and Wallace, 2005]. However, scattering radiation and alterations in ovarian blood supply limit the overall success rate of this ovarian protection strategy to approximately 50% [Damewood *et al.*, 1990; Clough *et al.*, 1996; Zinger et al., 2004; Lee *et al.*, 2006]. There is a possibility that the procedure may complicate future oocyte retrieval and promote some ovarian dysfunction and development of cysts. Nevertheless, spontaneous conception following this procedure has been reported [Lee *et al.*, 2006]. A combined approach of transposition of one ovary with retrieval of tissue for cryopreservation from the second ovary might be considered [Martin *et al.*, 2007].

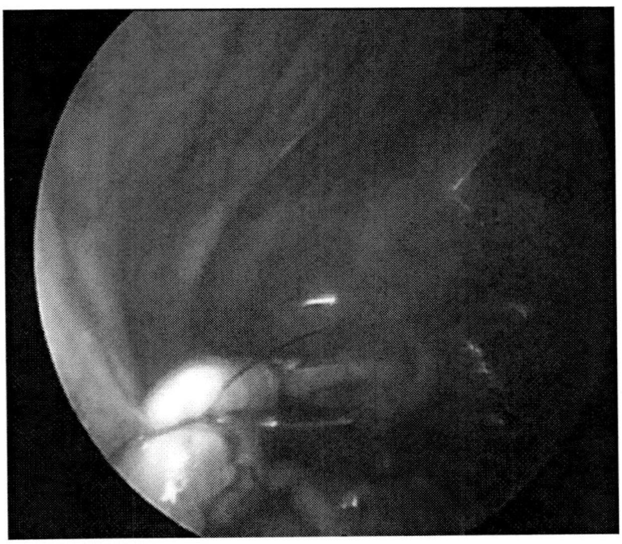

Figure 6. Laparoscopic oophoropexy. Laparoscopic view of an ovary transfixed to the abdominal wall.

A controversial strategy with unclear benefits for ovarian protection is suppression ovarian activity by GnRH analog administration. This inhibits the hypothalamic-pituitary-ovarian axis and, thereby, gonadotrophin release and follicular development, possibly mimicking the prepubertal situation [Abir *et al.*, 1998; Pereyra Pacheco *et al.*, 2001; Brougham and Wallace, 2005; Lee *et al.*, 2006; Blumenfeld *et al.*, 2007]. However, the mechanism whereby GnRH protects primordial follicles is unknown, as they do not express FSH receptors, and their growth is FSH-independent [Brougham and Wallace, 2005]. It is possible that GnRH analogs interrupt the FSH increase induced by alkylating agents or decrease uterine-ovarian perfusion and, thus, ovarian exposure to chemotherapy; they might also act directly on the ovary or on ovarian anti-apoptotic molecules [Blumenfeld *et al.*, 2007]. This treatment is probably of no benefit to prepubertal girls, nor does it diminish radiation-induced damage.

GnRH analog was administered to 12 postmenarcheal patients (age 14.7 to 20 years) with normal menses before anticancer therapy that included also cyclophosphamide [Pereyra Pacheco *et al.*, 2001]. The patients were followed for 5 years, and their fertility was preserved as indicated by the resumption of normal menses as well as ovulations, even in patients treated with high-dose chemotherapy before BMT. Because of the possible protective effects of GnRH analogs as well as the benefits of conducting anticancer treatment without menstrual withdrawal bleeding, in various medical centers including our own, this treatment is usually offered to postmenarcheal adolescents before or during cancer therapy.

Fertility Problems as a Result of Uterine and Cranial Irradiation

Attempts to correct radiation induced uterine abnormalities and improve function by medical means have failed [Edgar and Wallace, 2007]. The administration of sex steroid replacement therapy to survivors of adolescent and childhood cancer, previously exposed to TBI or abdominal and/or pelvic radiation, failed to improve uterine blood flow, endometrial thickness, or uterine volume [Bath *et al.*, 1999; Larsen *et al.*, 2004; Edgar and Wallace, 2007]. Findings were discouraging even when high-dose estrogen was used, suggesting that the uterine damage might be irreversible (see also: "Pregnancy Complications in Survivors of Childhood or Adolescent Cancer").

The mechanism underlying cranial irradiation-related infertility and amenorrhea may involve the suppression of pulsatile GnRH secretion, leading to hyopgonadotrophic hypogonadism and oligoamenorrhea [Speroff *et al.*, 1994; Bath *et al.*, 2001]. This condition is usually diagnosed before adulthood on the basis of findings of abnormal growth and puberty development (see previous chapter). The defect is confirmed by measuring lower levels of the serum gonadotrophins FSH as well as LH [Speroff *et al.*, 1994; Bath *et al.*, 2001]. Sometimes, however, ammenoreic hypoestrogenic patients (with negative progestational withdrawal) will frequently have normal (immunoactive but not bioactive) circulating levels of FSH and LH. In hyopgonadotrophic patients, replacement therapy with exogenous GnRH or, more practically, with gonadotrophin preparations containing FSH and LH may induce folliculogenesis and lead to adequate steroid production (usually with human menopausal gonadotrophin) [Ben Rafael and Orvieto, 1998]. However, because this treatment is expensive and emotionally stressful owing to the need for frequent serum determinations and ultrasonography, it is advisable that the clinicians conduct the entire fertility investigation (including serum gonadotrophin and semen analysis) before considering administration of gonadotrophins.

The Gonadotrophin preparation is usually injected intramuscularly on day 3 to day 5 of menstruation or withdrawal bleeding. If withdrawal bleeding cannot be induced, an arbitrary day is chosen, provided that pregnancy has already been ruled out. The patient returns 3 to 4 days later for measurement of serum 17 β estradiol (E2) and progesterone levels and ovarian utrasonography. The gonadotrophin injections are administered daily until the serum E2 levels findings reach appropriate value and adequate follicular growth is verified. When a mature follicle (>16 mm) is identified, human chorionic gonadotrophin is usually injected to trigger ovulation, mimicking the LH surge. If pregnancy does not occur, treatment is continued for at least 3 ovulatory cycles. Thereafter, it can be combined with intrauterine insemination for 3 more cycles, even with a normal semen analysis, before resorting to more aggressive methods (such as IVF).

Pregnancy rates in women with hypothalamic hypogonadotrophic amenorrhea, unassociated with anticancer therapy, are high (20-30% per treatment cycle, ~80% after 6 cycles and 93% after 12 cycles) [Speroff *et al.*, 1994; Mausner *et al.*, 2006], but there are as yet no reported statistics on survivors of adolescent cancer. As many of these survivors were treated also with therapy affecting the ovary/uterus, their pregnancy rates might be lower.

Our Experience with Ovarian Retrieval from Adolescents for Fertility Preservation

Between 1998 and 2006, we operated on 27 female adolescents aged 10-18 years (median 15 years) with various malignancies (Table 4) to harvest ovarian tissue. Twelve girls were scheduled for anticancer treatment (Table 4, patients 2, 4, 7, 8, 10, 13, 14, 18, 19, 22, 24, 26) and 15 had already undergone some form of chemotherapy (Table 4, patients 1, 3, 5, 6, 9, 11, 12, 15-17, 20, 21, 23, 25, 27). Only five of the patients were premenarcheal (Table 4, patients 1, 2, 5, 7, 9).

The surgery was performed laparoscopically under general anesthesia using one 10-mm port positioned at the umbilicus and two 5-mm ports, one at the left lower quadrant and one at the right. Partial or complete, unilateral oophorectomy was performed according to the consensus decision of the pediatric oncologist, the surgeon, and the medical staff of the IVF unit, based on ovarian size and the anticancer treatment protocol. The ovaries were completely removed in 12 patients (Table 4, patients 1, 8, 9, 11, 12, 14, 15, 16, 18, 19, 24, 27), and partially in 15 (Table 4, patients 2-7, 10, 13, 17, 20-23, 25, 26).

Appropriate instruments were used, at the surgeon's preference, to reduce as much as possible tissue damage, and especially to avoid electrocautery. The harvested tissue was placed in a plastic bag, and immediately transferred to the laboratory for cryopreservation preparation. All patients but one (Table 4, patient 24) had a benign postoperative course; most released on the first postoperative day. The patient with a complicated course had a vascular injury that was identified intraopertively; its immediate correction required conversion from a laparoscopic to an open procedure, followed by five days of hospitalization. In no case did the ovarian retrieval process delay the initiation of anticancer treatment. One patient (Table 4, patient 14) underwent transposition of the remaining ovary prior to pelvic irradiation one year after ovarian harvesting, with no difficulty.

Table 4: Characteristics of adolescents who underwent ovarian cryopreservation

Patient	Age	Illness	Treatment	Pubertal status
1	10	Meduloblastoma	After	Premenarcheal
2	13	Osteosarcoma	Before	Premenarcheal
3		HL	After	Pubertal
4		CML	Before	Pubertal
5		Osteosarcoma	After	Premenarcheal
6		Ewing sarcoma	After	Pubertal
7		CML	Before	Premenarcheal
8	14	Ewing sarcoma	Before	Pubertal
9		Ewing sarcoma	After	Premenarcheal
10		Ewing sarcoma	Before	Pubertal
11		Anaplastic ependymoma	After	Pubertal
12		HL	After	Pubertal
13	15	Rhabdomyosarcoma	Before	Pubertal
14		Rhabdomyosarcoma	Before	Pubertal
15		HL	After	Pubertal
16		HL	After	Pubertal
17	16	Ewing sarcoma	After	Pubertal
18		HL	Before	Pubertal
19		HL	Before	Pubertal
20		Primitive neuroectodermal tumor	After	Pubertal
21	17	HL	After	Pubertal
22		Ewing sarcoma	Before	Pubertal
23		HL	After	Pubertal
24	18	HL	Before	Pubertal
25		AML	After	Pubertal
26		HL	Before	Pubertal
27		NHL	After	Pubertal

Note: Patients are arranged in every age group chronologically: the youngest patient is first and the oldest last.

Treatment=before thearpy/after any form of anticancer therapy.

CML=chronic myeloid leukemia.

Pregnancy Complications in Survivors of Childhood or Adolescent Cancer

Uterine Complications

Women who received uterine irradiation during childhood or adolescence, especially before the onset of menarche, should be carefully monitored during pregnancy and considered at high risk of pregnancy complications [Edgar and Wallace, 2007]. Good communication between the patient and the obstetrician is essential (see also next chapter). Uterine defects in the patient population with normal gonadotrophin levels, is often followed by preterm deliveries or recurrent pregnancy losses (see also Introduction: Fertility in survivors of childhood or adolescent cancer). In cases of early recurrent pregnancy losses, progesterone supplementation can be attempted; however, miscarriages due to uterine abnormalities usually occur during the second trimester, when progesterone support is not beneficial [Ornoy and Abir, 1994]. In cases of recurrent premature deliveries, complete rest, especially during the third trimester, with steroid therapy to accelerate fetal lung maturation from 24 gestational weeks, can be attempted [Gojnic and Pervulov, 2005]. In cases of consistent recurrent abortions or preterm deliveries with offsprings that do not survive, IVF treatment with gestational surrogacy may be considered [Brinsden, 2003]. This option allows survivors to have their own genetic children.

Cardiac Complications

Cardiac decompensation during pregnancy is a concern in patients who received significant doses of anthracycline therapy [Edgar and Wallace, 2007]. However, in a study of 53 women who had been treated for childhood cancer with a protocol that included anthracycline (mean cumulative dose 267 mg/m^2) clinical heart failure during pregnancy was not identified [Sorensen *et al.*, 2003; Edgar and Wallace, 2007], indicating a low risk of this complication in survivors of childhood or adolescent cancer. In the rare cases of adolescent breast cancer survivors, the contribution of radiation therapy in addition to anthracylines and taxanes on cardiac toxicity is still unknown [Shannon and Smith, 2003]. Be that as it may, clinicians should be aware of these women's medical history, and carefully monitor them for cardiac complications [Shannon and Smith, 2003; Sorensen *et al.*, 2003; Edgar and Wallace, 2007].

Ethical and Psycological Issues and Counseling

General Aspects Regarding Fertility Preservation

Most patients wish to have their own biological offspring instead of adoption or egg donation. Moreover, in some instances, patients choose to receive less effective anticancer treatment if it is less gonadotoxic than the optimal therapy [Partridge *et al.*, 2004]. Anticancer therapy, by itself, has unpleasant immediate side effects, and is very difficult to endure, often causing distress and even depression [Wallace *et al.,* 2005a]. This problem is complicated in adolescence, which is a period of emotional and psychological instability, during which issues of sexuality are of particular importance, and the potential prospect of infertility due to anticancer treatment can be devastating. Our group and others [Saito *et al.*, 2005] have observed a positive psychological effect in patients in whom the option of parenthood is preserved, even if never ultimately used. Many patients and their families regard open discussions on future fertility and actions for its preservation as sources of hope and reassurance of the curative aim of the anticancer treatment that will result in a normal life, including parenthood.

Surgical Consideration and Risks

Although the laparoscopy procedure employed to harvest tissue for ovarian preservation is usually simple and safe, it can cause unexpected complications, such as injuries to major blood vessels [Kravarusic *et al.*, 2005; Schmidt *et al.*, 2007]. These risks must be clearly presented to the patient and her parents/guardians. They will have to consider that the anticancer therapy itself is extremely stressful and difficult, and to decide if it is worthwhile to undergo an additional operation that will probably cause some extra physical pain, and might be associated with complications, although the risk is very low. Some concern has been expressed regarding the hazard of disseminating disease during surgical procedures such as on the pelvis. However, there is only one case report in the literature of abdominal trocar site metastases in an adult, and we are unaware of such cases in minors [Picone *et al.*, 2003].

Risks after Fertility Restoration

Patients and their parents should also be made aware of the risks of reseeding malignant cells with future ovarian grafting, mostly in cases of hematological cancers. They may be assured that the ovary is not involved in HL and probably not in most NHL [Abir *et al.*, 2006]. They should be warned that ovarian tissue will probably not be implanted if risk of retransmission of malignant cells is high. The young age of the patients should be emphasized, as it is possible that by the time they become adults, safer technologies for fertility restoration, such as *in vitro* maturation of primordial follicles, might be developed. Furthermore, with improvements in genetic/molecular biology and other screening methods, it might eventually be possible to precisely evaluate in which malignancies the ovary is involved, or even conduct individual patient testing [Ohali *et al.*, 2004].

Given that primordial follicles contain quiescent oocytes [Gougeon, 1996], and that oocytes should not be aspirated from antral follicles shortly after initiation of anticancer treatment [Meirow *et al.,* 2001], patients should be assured that they are at almost no risk for chemo/radiotherapy-induced congenital anomalies or even neoplastic disease in offspring conceived either from the cryostored gametes or naturally. Moreover, various epidemiological studies showed no increase in congenital malformations in cancer survivors who underwent chemotherapy [Arnon *et al.*, 2001].

Informed Consent Session

As most of the reported cases of fertility preservation dealt with adults [Meirow and Nugent, 2001], and work with minors is at a relatively early, experimental stage, the issue of informed consent in minors is still unresolved. Informed consent should be obtained only by protocols approved by institutional review boards [Lee *et al.*, 2006]. It has been suggested that these patients and their guardians be approached by the clinical professionals in charge of the therapy or by a multidisciplinary team who will explain the risks for subfertility resulting from the anticancer therapy and the purpose and the potential of cryopreservation of ovarian tissue [Wallace *et al.*, 2005a; Lee *et al.*, 2006; Weintraub *et al.*, 2007]. These clinicians should be involved in all stages of the procedure, and jointly deal with the medical, surgical, scientific, and ethical issues [Wallace *et al.*, 2005a; Weintraub *et al.*, 2007]. All pertinent, available, updated information should be presented as plainly and clearly as possible, and the expectations should be carefully defined to avoid unrealistic hope. The medical staff should emphasize that they are offering an experimental technique of fertility preservation, with possible early and late consequences, some of which are as yet unknown. At the same time, they need to point out that if the parent or guardian opts out of fertility preservation, the opportunity to have biological children might be missed.

We expect that in most cases, parents will represent their children. The advantage of parents over other guardians is that they are usually emotionally close to their offspring and come from the same background and culture, so they can more practically foresee the patient's future. Adolescents should be allowed to take an active part in the consent process, according to their wishes and capabilities. In some centers, like ours, not only the guardians but also the minors themselves (above 7 years of age) sign the informed consent form. Besides the question of the legal rights of minors, active signing may add a positive psychological effect, ensuring the patient that she is involved in the planning of her future. Nevertheless it is the adult parent/guardian who makes the final decision to cryostore gametes. The decision of how to use the gametes is made by the cancer survivor herself in adulthood.

Guidelines and Recommendation for Fertility Preservation in Minors

There are as yet no definitive recommendations regarding fertility preservation in minors. Guidelines for ovarian cryopreservation should be formed on the basis of available information, and modified when new findings come to light [Brougham and Wallace, 2005; Wallace *et al.*, 2005a]. Guidelines for cryopreservation of gonadal tissue have been formulated by the Royal College of Obstetrics and Gynecology [Grundy *et al.*, 2001]. In addition, the world's largest pediatric oncology collaboration, the Children's Oncology Group (COG), have published long-term follow-up guidelines for survivors of childhood and adolescent cancers, including a comprehensive review of the risk factors for infertility (http://www.childrensoncologygroup.org) [Heath and Stern, 2006]. These reports [Grundy *et al.*, 2001, Heath and Stern, 2006] are important initial steps in establishing standard protocols. However, the COG recommendations for fertility preservation focus on minors likely to receive a cumulative dose equivalent to 7.5 g/m^2 cyclophosphamide, 6-10 Gy abdominal/pelvic irradiation, or 24 Gy spinal irradiation. As various levels of ovarian damage can be induced also by lesser intensities of these anticancer therapies or by other protocols, many centers have lower thresholds for offering fertility preservation [Weintraub *et al.*, 2007].

Legal Issues

Uniform laws regarding fertility preservation in minors have not yet been created. Therefore, we may eventually expect, law suits claiming damage due to side effects of ovarian retrieval procedures or unsuccessful fertility restoration, and also claims related to the failure of health care givers to disclose the hazardous effects of anticancer therapy on fertility and the available options for fertility preservation [Crockin, 2005]. It is also possible that some survivors of adolescent cancer will claim damages from their guardians for deciding not to opt for fertility preservation procedures, further emphasizing the importance of the minor's participation in the informed consent session.

Delayed Puberty

In cases of delayed puberty due to anticancer treatment, appropriate hormonal therapy should be started early, not only for the development of normal female sexual characteristics and bone density, but also to minimize psychological stress [Speroff *et al.*, 1994; Abir *et al.*, 2001a]. Monthly menstruation is an important experience for adolescent girls and reinforces their femininity. Specifically in cancer patients, its presence may minimize their fear of being different, especially if the disease and its treatment prevented normal activities of adolescence/childhood [Speroff *et al.*, 1994].

Psycholgical-Gynecological Counseling in Adulthood

Psycholgical-Gynecolgical counseling should also be offered to adult survivors of childhood and adolescent cancer. The women with regular menstrual cycles should be told that because of their increased risk for POF their fertility might diminish with time, and therefore, pregnancy should not be postponed too long [Edgar and Wallace, 2007].

Women who received uterine irradiation in childhood or early adolescence should also be made aware of the pregnancy risks (miscarriages and early deliveries) due to possible irreversible uterine damage. Survivors of adolescent HL treated with mantel radiation should be informed of their higher risk of breast cancer [Shannon and Smith, 2003], which might also further diminish their fertility prospects-an additional consideration for not delaying pregnancy too long. Moreover, patients with infertility due to childhood/adolescence cranial irradiation may find their good prospects for fertility restoration with appropriate hormonal treatment an important source of hope [Ben Rafael and Orvieto, 1998].

Conclusion

Fertility preservation in female adolescents undergoing gonadotoxic chemotherapeutic and irradiation therapy for cancer, is an exciting and promising prospect, but it harbors many riddles and uncertainties. The size of the target population has been steadily increasing over the last decades with improvements in cancer treatment. Some of these patients may need to be treated already in adolescence for delayed puberty resulting from the anticancer treatment.

The motivation for preserving fertility for future biological reproduction is natural and high, as patients usually prefer to have their own biological offspring rather than adopting or using egg donation. Ovarian tissue can be retrieved for long term cryobanking by a relatively simple and uncomplicated surgical procedure under general anesthesia, with minimal or no delay in the initiation of anticancer treatment. The decision not to undergo ovarian cryostorage before anticancer treatment might be irreversible in terms of fertility preservation.

Although methods for fertility restoration using frozen-thawed ovarian tissue are not optimal as yet, the technique for freezing-thawing ovarian tissue seems to be successful, and it is reasonable to exercise some scientific optimism. However, at present, gamete cryostorage may be done only as a part of a study protocol under institutional review board guidelines, with adherence to local laws and ethics. It is noteworthy that a minority of the survivors of adolescent cancer may suffer from fertility problems due to uterine or cranial irradiation. These patients should be treated mostly in adulthood, when the inability to produce offspring becomes apparent.

Clinicians as well as scientists dealing with fertility preservation and restoration must be aware that the benefits-risk ratio is unknown. Like any other experimental treatment, further information will be gathered with time. For adolescent cancer patients, ovarian cryostorge, despite its experimental nature, is almost their only chance for fertility preservation. Therefore, the scientific and medical community should be kept abreast of progress in the field, and should openly and constantly inform patients and their guardians of new knowledge and advances. Fertility preservation for adolescents is not a direct part of treating cancer, nor does it change cancer statistics. It is about the future of cancer survivors and their desire to lead a normal productive and reproductive life.

Acknowledgment

Our original studies were partially sponsored by research grants from the Israel Cancer Association and Tel Aviv University. We are greatly indebted to Gloria Ganzach of the Editorial Board of Rabin Medical Center for the English editing.

References

Abir, R, Fisch, B, Raz, Ah, Nitke, S and Ben Rafael, Z. (1998) Preservation of fertility in women undergoing chemotherapy-current approach and future prospects. *J. Assist. Reprod. Genet., 15*, 469-77.

Abir, R, Fisch, B, Nahum, R, Orvieto, R, Nitke, S and Ben Rafael Z. (2001a) Turner's syndrome and fertility: current status and possible future prospects, *Hum. Reprod. Update., 7,* 603-10.

Abir, R, Fisch, B, Nitke, S, Okon, E, Raz, Ah and Ben-Rafael Z. (2001b) Morphological study of fully and partially isolated early human follicles. *Fertil Steril., 75*, 141-6.

Abir, R, Nitke, S, Ben-Haroush, A and Fisch, B. (2006) In vitro maturation of human primordial ovarian follicles-Clinical significance, progress and methods for growth evaluation, *Histol. Histopathol., 21*, 887-98.

Abir, R, Ben-Haroush, A, Felz, C, Okon, E, Raanani, H, Orvieto, R, Nitke, S and Fisch B. (2007) Selection of patients before and after anticancer treatment for ovarian cryopreservation. *Hum. Reprod.,* electronic publication before press, 2008.

Arnon, J., Meirow, D, Lewis-Roness, H and Ornoy A. (2001) Genetic and teratogenic effects of cancer treatments on gametes and embryos. *Hum. Reprod. Update., 7,* 394-403.

Arrau, J, Roblero, L, Curry, L and Gonzalez R. (1983) Effect of exogenous sex steroids upon the number of germ cells and the growth of foetal ovaries grafted under the kidney capsule of adult ovariectomised hamsters. *J. Embryol. Exp. Morphol., 78*, 33-42.

Bath, LE, Critchley, HO, Chambers, SE, Anderson, RA, Kelnar, CJ and Wallace WH. (1999) Ovarian and uterine characteristics after total body irradiation in childhood and adolescence: response to sex steroid replacement. *Br. J. Obstet. Gynaecol, 106*, 1265-72.

Bath, LE, Anderson, RA, Critchley, HO, Kelnar, CJH and Wallace, WHB. (2001) Hypothalamic-pituitary-ovarian dysfunction after prepubertal chemotherapy and cranial irradiation for acute leukaemia. *Hum. Reprod, 16*, 1838-44.

Bath, LE, Wallace, WH and Critchley, HO. (2002) Late effects of the treatment of childhood cancer on female reproductive system and the potential for fertility preservation. *BJOG., 109*, 107-14.

Bath, LE, Wallace, WHB, Shaw, MP and Anderson RA. (2003) Depletion of ovarian reserve in young women after treatment for cancer in childhood: detection by anti-Mullerian hormone, inhibin B and ovarian ultrasound. *Hum. Reprod, 18*, 2368-74.

Ben-Rafael, Z and Orvieto, R. (1998) Infertility due to defective ovulation. In: Rodriguez-Armas O, Hedon B, eds. *Clinical Infertility and Contraception*. UK: The Parthenon Publishing Ltd, 22-36.

Biron-Shental, T, Fisch, B, Van Den Hurk, R, Felz, C, Feldberg, D and Abir, R. (2004) Survival of frozen-thawed human ovarian fetal follicles in long-term organ culture. *Fertil. Steril., 81,* 716-9.

Blumenfeld, Z, Avivi, L, Eckman, A, Epelbaum, R, Rowe, JM and Dann, EJ. (2007) Gonadotropin-releasing hormone agonist decreases chemotherapy-induced gonadotoxicity and premature ovarian failure in young female patients with Hodgkin lymphoma. *Fertil. Steril.*, electronic publication ahead of print.

Brinsden, PR. (2003) Gestational surrogacy. *Hum. Reprod. Update., 9*, 483-91.

Broekmans, FJ, Kwee, J, Hendriks, DJ, Mol, BW and Lambalk, CB. (2006) A systematic review of tests predicting ovarian reserve and IVF outcome. *Hum. Reprod. Update.*, 12, 685-718.

Brougham, MFH and Wallace, WHB. (2005) Subfertility in children and young people treated for solid and haematological malignancies. *Br. J. Haemtol., 131*, 143-55.

Bukovsky, A, Caudle, MR, Svetlikova, M and Upadhyaya, NB. (2004) Origin of germ cells and formation of new primary follicles in adult human ovaries. *Reprod. Biol. Endocrinol., 2*, 20.

Bukovsky, A, Svetlikova, M and Caudle, MR. (2005) Oogenesis in cultures derived from adult human ovaries. *Reprod. Biol. Endocrinol., 3*, 17.

Byrne, J, Fears, TR, Gail, MH, Pee, D, Connely, RR, Austin, DF, Holmes, GF, Holmes, FF, Latourette, HB and Meigs, JW. (1992) Early menopause in long-term survivors of cancer during adolescence. *Am. J. of Obstet. Gynecol., 166*, 788-93.

Carroll, J and Gosden, R. (1993) Transplantation of frozen-thawed mouse primordial follicles. *Hum. Reprod., 8*, 1163-7.

Carroll, J, Whittingham, DG, Wood, MJ, Telfer, E and Gosden, RG. (1990) Extraovarian production of mature viable mouse oocytes from frozen primary follicles. *J. Reprod. Fertil., 90*, 321-7.

Chemaitilly, W, Mertens, AC, Mitby, P, Whitton, J, Stovall, M, Yasui, Y, Robison, LL and Sklar, CA. (2006) Acute ovarian failure in the childhood cancer survivor study. *J. Clin. Endocrinol. Metab., 91*, 1723-8.

Chiarelli, AM, Marrett, LD and Darlington, GA. (1999) Early menopause and infertility in females after treatment for childhood cancer diagnosed in 1964 to 1988 in Ontario, Canada. *Am. J. Epidemiol., 150*, 245-54.

Chiarelli, AM, Marrett, LD and Darlington, GA. (2000) Pregnancy outcomes in females after treatment for childhood cancer. *Epidmiology, 11,* 161-6.

Chow, EJ, Friedman, DL, Yasui, Y, Whitton, JA, Stovall, M, Robinson, LL and Sklar, CA. (2007) Timing of menarche among survivors of childhood leukemia: a report from the childhood cancer survivor study. *Pediatr. Blood Cancer.,* Electronic publication ahead of print.

Clough, KB, Goffinet, F, Labib, A, Renolleau, C, Campana, F, de la Rochefordiere, A and Durand, JC. (1996) Laparoscopic unilateral ovarian transposition prior to irradiation: Prospective study of 20 cases. *Cancer., 77*, 2638-45.

Critchley, HO and Wallace, WH. (2005) Impact of cancer treatment on uterine function. *J. Natl. Cancer Inst. Mongr., 34*, 64-8.

Crockin, SL. (2005) Legal issues related to parenthood after cancer. *J. Natl. Cancer Inst. Monogr.,* 34, 111-3.

Damewood, MD, Hesla, HS, Lowen, M and Schultz, MJ. (1990) Induction of ovulation and pregnancy following lateral oophoropexy for Hodgkin's disease. *Int. J. Gynaecol. Obstet., 33*, 369-71.

Demeestere, I, Simon, P, Buxant, F, Robin, V, Fernandez, SA, Centner, J, Delbaere, A, Englert, Y. (2006) Ovarian function and spontaneous pregnancy after combined heterotopic and orthotopic cryopreserved ovarian tissue transplantation in a patient previously treated with bone marrow transplantation: a case report. *Hum. Reprod, 21,* 2010-14.

Dolmans, M-M, Martinez-Madrid, B, Gadisseux, E, Guiot, Y, Yuan, Yuan Yuan, W, Torre, A, Camboni, A, Van Langendonckt, A and Donnez, J. (2007) Short-term transplantation of isolated human ovarian follicles and cortical tissue into nude mice. *Reproduction.*, *134*, 253-62.

Donnez, J, Dolmans, MM, Demylle, D, Jadoul, P, Picard, C, Squifflet, J, Martinez-Madrid, B and Van Langendonckt, A. (2004) Livebirth after orthotopic transplantation of cryopreserved ovarian tissue. *Lancet, 364*, 1405-10.

Dudzinski, DM. (2004) Ethical issues in fertility preservation for adolescent cancer survivors: oocyte and ovarian tissue cryopreservation. *J. Pediatr. Adolesc. Gynecol., 17*, 97-102.

Edgar, AB and Wallace WHM. (2007) Pregnancy in women who had cancer in childhood. *European Journal of Cancer, 43*, 1890-4.

Faddy, MJ and Gosden RG. (1996) A model confirming the decline in follicle numbers to the age of menopause in women. *Hum. Reprod., 11*, 1484-6.

Feigin, E, Abir, R, Fisch, B, Kravarusic D, Steinberg R, Nitke S, Avrahami G, Ben-Haroush A and Freud E. (2007) Laparoscopic ovarian tissue preservation in young patients at risk of ovarian failure as a result of chemotherapy/irradiation for primary malignancy. *J. Pediatr. Surg., 42*, 862-4.

Gojnic, M and Pervulov, M. (2005) Artificial fetal lung maturation-prevention of antenatal complications in premature deliveries. *Clin. Exp. Obstet. Gynecol., 32*, 61-4.

Gosden, RG. (1990a) Restitution of fertility in sterilized mice by transferring primordial ovarian follicles. *Hum. Reprod., 5*, 117-22.

Gosden, RG. (1990b) Restitution of fertility in sterilized mice by transferring primordial ovarian follicles. *Hum. Reprod., 5*, 499-504.

Gosden RG (1995) Oocyte development throughout life. In: Grudzinshes JG, Yovici JL, eds. *Gametes-The Oocyte*. Cambridge, UK: Cambridge University Press, 119-149.

Gougeon, A. (1996) Regulations of ovarian follicular development in primates: facts and hypotheses. *Endocrinol. Rev.*, 17, 121-54.

Green, DM, Whitton, JA, Stovall, M, Mertens, AC, Donaldson, SS, Ruymann, FB, Pendergrass, TW and Robison, LL. (2002a) Pregnancy outcome of female survivors of childhood cancer: a report from the Childhood Cancer Survivor Study. *Am. J. Obstet Gyncecol., 1887*, 1070-80.

Green, DM, Peabody EM, Nan, B, Peterson, S, Kalapurakal, JA and Breslo, NE. (2002b) Pregnancy outcome after treatment for Wilms tumor: a report from the National Wilms Study Group. *J. Clin. Oncol., 20*, 2506-13.

Greenberg, ML and Urbach, SL. (2006) Preserving the fertility of children with cancer. *MJA., 185*, 532-3.

Grundy, R, Gosden, RG, Hewitt, M, Larcher, V, Leiper A, Spoudeas, HA, Walker D and Wallace, WHB. (2001) Fertility preservation for children treated for cancer (1): Scientific advances and research dilemmas. *Arch. Dis. Child., 84*, 355-9.

Hall, JE, Martin, KA, Whitney, HA, Landy, H and Crowley, WF Jr. (1994) Potential for fertility with replacement of hypothalamic gonadotrophin-releasing hormone in long term female survivors of cranial tumors. *J. Clin. Endocrionol. Metab., 79,* 1166-72.

Hamre, MR, Robison, LL, Nesbit, ME, Sather, MN, Meadows, AT, Ortega, JA, D'Angio, GJ and Hammond, GD. (1987) Effect of radiation on ovarian function in long-term survivors of childhood acute lymphoblastic leukemia: A report from the Children Cancer Study Group. *J. Clin. Oncol., 5,* 1759-65.

Hann, I, Vora, A, Richards, S, Hill, F, Gibson, B, Lilleyman, J, Kinsley, S, Mitchell, C and Eben, OB. (2000) Benefit of intensified treatment for all children with acute lymphoblastic leukaemia: results from MRC UK acute lymphoblastic leukaemia XI and MRC acute lymphoblastic leukaemia 97 trials. UK Medical Research Council's Working Party on Childhood Leukemia. *Leukemia., 14,* 356-63.

Heath, JA and Stern, CJ. (2006) Fertility preservation in children newly diagnosed with cancer: existing standards of practice in Australia and New Zealand. *MJA., 185,* 538-41.

Homburg, R and Farhi, J. (1995) Growth hormone and reproduction. *Curr. Opin. Obstet. Gynecol., 7,* 220-3.

Hovatta, O. (2005) Methods for cryopreservation of human ovarian tissue. *Reprod. BioMedicine Online., 10,* 729-34.

Huang, JY, Tulandi, T, Holzer, H, Tan, SL and Chian, RC. (2007) Combining ovarian tissue cryobanking with retrieval of immature oocytes followed by in vitro maturation and vitrification: an additional strategy of fertility preservation. *Fertil. Steril.,* Electronic publication ahead of print.

Hubner, K, Fuhrmann, G, Christenson, LK, Kehler, J, Reinbold, R, De La Fuente, R., Wood, J., Strauss, III JF, Boiani, M and Scholer, HR. (2003) Derivation of oocytes from mouse embryonic stem cells. *Science, 300,* 1251-6.

Imthurn, B, Cox, SL, Jenkin, G, Trounson, AO and Shaw, JM. (2000) Gonadotrophin administration can benefit ovarian tissue grafted to the body wall: Implications for human ovarian grafting. *Mol. Cell Endocrinol., 163,* 141-6.

Israeli, T, Nevo, N, Harmelin, A, Neeman, M and Tsafriri, A. (2006) Reducing ischaemic damage in rodent ovarian xenografts transplanted into granulation tissue. *Hum. Reprod., 21,* 1368-79.

Jain, JK and Paulson, RJ. (2006) Oocyte cryopreservation. *Fertil. Steril., 86* (supplement 4), 1037-46.

Johnson, J, Canning, J, Kaneko T, Pru JK and Tilly JL. (2004) Germline stem cells and follicular renewal in the postnatal mammalian ovary. *Nature., 428,* 145-50.

Johnson, J, Bagley, I, Skznik-Wikiel, M, Lee, HJ, Adams, GB, Niikura, Y, Tschudy, KS, Tilly, JC, Cortes, ML, Forkert, R, Spitzer, T, Iacomini, I, Scadden, DT and Tilly, JL. (2005) Oocyte generation in adult mammalian ovaries by putative germ cells in bone marrow and peripheral blood. *Cell., 122,* 303-15.

Kim, SS, Radford, J, Harris, M, Varley, J, Rutherford, AJ, Lieberman, B, Shalet, S and Gosden, R. (2001) Ovarian tissue harvested from lymphoma patients to preserve fertility may be safe for autotransplantation. *Hum. Reprod., 16,* 2056-60.

Kim, SS, Yang, HW, Kang, HG, Lee, HH, Ko, DS and Gosden, RG. (2004) Quantitative assessment of ischemic tissue damage in ovarian cortical tissue with or without antioxidant (ascorbic acid) treatment. *Fertil. Steril., 82*, 679-85.

Kravarusic, D, Dlugy, E, Steinberg, R, Paloi, B, Baazov, A, Fegin, E and Freud, E. (2005) Two year experience with minimal access surgery at Schneider Children's Medical Center of Israel. *Isr. Med. Assoc. J.*, 7, 564-7.

Larsen, EC, Loft, A, Holm, K, Muller, J, Brocks, V and Andersen, AN. (2000) Oocyte donation in women cured of cancer with bone marrow transplantation including total body irradiation in adolescence. *Hum. Reprod., 15*, 1505-8.

Larsen, EC, Muller, J, Schmieglow, K, Rechnitzer, C and Andersen, A. (2003) Reduced ovarian function in long-term survivors of radiation-and chemotherapy treated childhood cancer. *J. Clin. Endocrinol. Metab., 88*, 5307-14.

Larsen, EC, Schmieglow, K, Rechnitzer, C, Loft, A, Muller, J and Andersen, A. (2004) Radiotherapy at a young age reduces uterine volume of childhood cancer survivors. *Acta Obstet. Gynecol. Scand, 83*, 96-102.

Laschke, MW, Menger, MD and Vollmar, B. (2002) Ovariectomy improves neovascularization and microcirculation of freely transplanted ovarian follicles. *J. Endocrinol., 172,* 535-44.

Laschke, MW, Menger, MD and Vollmar, B. (2003) Cryopreservation does not affect neovascularization of freely transplanted ovarian follicles. *Fertil. Steril., 79*, 1458-60.

Lee, SJ, Schover, LR, Partridge, AH, Patrizio, P, Wallace, WH, Hagerty, K, Beck, LN, Brennan, LV and Oktay, K. (2006) American society of clinical oncology recommendations on fertility preservation in cancer patients. *J. Clin. Oncol., 24*, 2917-31.

Leporrier, M, von Theobald, P, Roffe, JL and Muller, G. (1987) A new technique to protect ovarian function before pelvic irradiation. Heterotopic ovarian autotransplantation. *Cancer., 60*, 2201-4.

Leung, W, Hudson, MM, Strickland, DK, Phipps, S, Srivastava, DK, Ribeiro, RC, Rubnitz, JE, Sandlund, JT, Kun, LE, Bowman, LC, Razzouk, BL, Mathew, P, Shearer, P, Evans, WE and Pui, CH. (2000) Late effects of treatment in cancer survivors of childhood acute myeloid leukemia. *Journal Clin. Oncol., 18*, 3273-9.

Linet, M, Ries, LAG, Smith, MA, Tarone, RE and Devesa, SS. (1999) Cancer surveillance series: Recent trends in childhood cancer incidence and mortality in the United States. *J. Natl. Cancer Inst., 91*, 1051-8.

Liu, Y, Wu, C, Qifeng, L, Yang, D, Albertini, DF, Keefe, DL and Liu, L. (2007) Germline stem cells and neo-oogenesis in the adult human ovary. *Dev Biol., 306*, 112-20.

Mackie, EJ, Radford, M and Shalet, SM. (1996) Gonadal function following chemotherapy for childhood Hodgkin's disease. *Med. Paediatr. Oncol., 27*, 74-8.

Marcello, MF, Nuciforo, G, Romeo, R, Di Dino, G, Russo, O, Palumbo, G and Schiliro, G. (1990) Structural and ultrastructural study of the ovary in childhood leukemia after successful treatment. *Cancer., 66*, 2099-104.

Martin, JR, Kodaman, P, Oktay, K and Taylor HS. (2007) Ovarian cryopreservation with transposition of a contralateral ovary: a combined approach for fertility preservation in women receiving pelvic radiation. *Fertil. Steril., 87*, 189. e5-7.

Martinez-Madrid, B, Camboni, A, Dolmans, MM, Nottola S, Van Langendonckt, A and Donnez, J. (2007) Apoptosis and ultrastuctural assessment after cryopreservation of whole human ovaries with their vascular pedicle. *Fertil Steril.*, *87*, 1153-65.

Mausner, SJ, Abdallah, RT and Hubayter, Z. (2006) Optimal stimulation protocols for in vitro fertilization. *Fertil. Steril.*, *86*, 267-73.

Meirow, D. (2000) Reproduction post-chemotherapy in young cancer patients. *Mol. Cell. Endocrinol.*, *169*, 123-31.

Meirow, D and Nugent D. (2001) The effects of radiotherapy and chemotherapy on female reproduction. *Hum. Reprod. Update.*, *7*, 535-43.

Meirow, D, Ben Yehuda, D, Prus, D, Poliack, A, Schenker, JG, Rachmilewitz, EA and Lewin, A. (1998) Ovarian tissue banking in patients with Hodgkin's disease: Is it safe? *Fertil. Steril.*, *69*, 996-8.

Meirow, D, Epstein, M, Lewis, H, Nugent, D and Gosden, RG. (2001) Administration of cyclophosphamide at different stages of follicular maturation in mice: effects on reproductive performance and fetal malformations. *Hum. Reprod.*, *16*, 632-7.

Meirow, D, Levron, J, Eldar-Geva, T, Hardan, I, Fridman, E, Zalel, Y, Schiff, E and Dor, J. (2005) Pregnancy after transplantation of cryopreserved ovarian tissue in a patient with ovarian failure after chemotherapy. *N. Engl. J. Med.*, *353*, 318-21.

Meirow, D, Levron, J, Eldar-Geva, T, Hardan, I, Fridman, E, Yemini, Z and Dor, J. (2007) Monitoring the ovaries after autotransplantation of cryopreserved ovarian tissue: endocrine studies, in vitro fertilization cycles, and live birth. *Fertil. Steril.*, *87*, 418.e7-418.e15.

Mertens, AC, Yasui, Y, Neglia, JP, Potters, JD, Nesbit, Jr ME, Ruccione, K, Smithson, WA and Robison, LL. (2001) Late mortality experience in five-year survivors of childhood and adolescent cancer: the Childhood cancer Survivor Study. *J. Clin. Oncol.*, *19*, 3163-72.

Mills, JL, Fears, TR, Robison, LL, Nicholson, HS, Sklar C and Byrne, J. (1997) Menarche in a cohort of 188 long-term survivors of acute lymphoblastic leukemia. *J. Pediatr.*, *131*, 598-602.

Nugent, D, Newton, H, Gallivan, L and Gosden, RG. (1998) Protective effect of vitamin E on ischaemia-reperfusion injury in ovarian grafts. *J. Reprod. Fertil.*, *114*, 341-6.

Nygaard, R, Clausen, N, Siimes, MA, Marky, I, Skejeldestad, FE, Kristinsson, JR, Vuoristo, A, Wegelius, R and Moe, PJ. (1991) Reproduction following treatment of childhood leukemia: a population-based prospective cohort study of fertility and offspring. *Med. Pediatr. Oncol.*, *19*, 459-66.

O'Brien, MJ, Pendola, JK and Eppig, JJ. (2003) A revised protocol for in vitro development of mouse oocytes from primordial follicles dramatically improves their development competence. *Biol. Reprod.*, *68*, 1682-6.

Ohali, A, Avigad, S, Zaizov, R, Ophir, R, Horn-Saban, S, Cohen, IJ, Meller, I, Kollender, Y, Issakov, J and Yaniv, I. (2004) Prediction of high risk Ewing's sarcoma by gene expression profiling. *Oncogene.*, *23*, 8997-9006.

Oktay K and Karlikaya, G. (2000) Ovarian function after transplantation of frozen, banked autologus ovarian tissue. *N Engl J Med.*, *342*, 1919.

Oktay, K, Economos, K, Kan, M, Rucinski, J, Veeck, L Rosenwaks, Z. (2001) Endocrine function and oocyte retrieval after autologuous transplantation of ovarian cortical strips to the forearm. *JAMA., 286*, 1490-3.

Oktay, K, Buyuk, E, Rosenwaks, Z and Rucinski, J. (2003) A technique for transplantation of ovarian cortical strips to the forearm. *Fertil. Steril., 80*, 193-8.

Oktay, K, Buyuk, E, Veeck, L, Zaninovic, N, Xu, K, Takeuchi, T, Opsahl, M and Rosenwaks, Z. (2004) Embryo development after heterotopic transplantation of cryopreserved ovarian tissue. *Lancet., 363*, 837-40.

Oktay, K, Buyuk, E, Veeck, L, Zaninovic, N, Xu, K, Takeuchi, T, Opsahl, M and Rosenwaks Z. (2004) Embryo development after heterotopic transplantation of cryopreserved ovarian tissue. *Lancet., 363*, 837-40.

Oktay, K, Cil, AP and Bang H. (2006) Efficiency of oocyte cryopreservation: a meta-analysis. *Fertil. Steril., 86*, 70-80.

Ornoy, A. and Abir, R. (1994) Recurrent (habitual) abortions: incidence, etiology and prevention, *Issues and Reviews in Teratology., 7*, 139-74.

Partridge, AH, Gelber, S, Peppercorn, J, Sampson, E, Knudson, K, Laufer, M, Rosenberg, R, Przpyszny, M, Rem, A and Winer, EP. (2004) Web-based survey of fertility issues in young women with breast cancer. *J. Clin. Oncol.*, 22, 4174-83.

Pereyra Pacheco, B, Mendez Ribas, JM, Milone, G, Fernandez, I, Kvicala, R, Mila, T, Di Noto, A, Contreras Ortiz, O and Pavlovsky, S. (2001) Use of GnRH analogs for functional protection of the ovary and preservation of fertility during cancer treatment in adolescents: a preliminary report. *Gynecol. Oncol., 81*, 391-7.

Perez, GI, Knufdon, CM, Leykin, L, Korsmeyer, SJ and Tilly JL (1997) Apoptosis-associated signaling pathways are required for chemotherapy-mediated female germ cell destruction. *Nature Med, 3*, 1228-32.

Picone, O, Aucouturier, JS, Louboutin, A, Cosacs, Y and Camus, E. (2003) Abdominal wall metastasis of a cervical adenocarcinoma at the laparoscopic trocar insertion site after ovarian transposition: case report and review of the literature. *Gynecol. Oncol.*, 90, 446-9.

Poirot, CJ, Martelli, H, Genestie, C, Golmard, J-L, Valteau-Couanet, D, Helardot, P, Pacquesment, H, Sauvat, F, Tabone, M-D, Phillippe-Chomette, P, Esperou, H, Baruchel, A and Brugieres, L. (2007) Feasibility of ovarian tissue cryopreservation for prepubertal females with cancer. *Pediatr. Blood Cancer., 49*, 74-78.

Quigley, C, Cowell, C, Jimenez, M, Burger, H, Kirk, J, Bergin, M, Stevens, M, Simpson, J and Silink, M.. (1989) Normal and early development of puberty despite gonadal damage in children treated for acute lymphoblastic leukaemia. *N Engl J Med., 321*, 143-51.

Radford, JA, Lieberman, BA, Brison, DR, Smith, AR, Critchlow, JD, Russel, SA, Watson, AJ, Clayton, JA, Harris, M, Gosden, RG and Shalet, SM. (2001) Orthotopic reimplantation of cryopreserved ovarian cortical strips after high-dose chemotherapy for Hodgkin's lymphoma. *Lancet., 357*, 1172-5.

Rahimi, G, Isachenko, E, Sauer, H, Isachenko, V, Wartenberg, M, Hescheler, J, Mallmann, P and Nawroth, F. (2003) Effect of different vitrification protocols for human ovarian tissue on reactive oxygen species and apoptosis. *Reprod. Fertil. Dev., 15*, 343-9.

Revel, A, Safran, A, Benshushan, A, Shushan, A, Laufer, N and Simon, A. (2004) In vitro maturation and fertilization of oocytes from an intact ovary of a surgically treated patient with endometrial carcinoma: case report. *Hum. Reprod., 19,* 1608-11.

Rosendahl, M, Loft, A, Byskov, AG, Ziebe, S, Schmidt, KT, Andersen, AN, Ottosen, C and Andersen CY. (2006) Biochemical pregnancy after fertilization of an oocyte aspirated from a heterotopic autotransplant of cryopreserved ovarian tissue: case report. *Hum. Reprod., 21*, 2006-9.

Saito, K, Suzuki, K, Iwasaki, A, Yumura, Y and Kubota, Y. (2005) Sperm cryopreservation before cancer chemotherapy helps in the emotional battle against cancer. *Cancer.,* 104, 521-4.

Sanders, JE, Hawley, J, Levy, W, Gooley, T, Buckner, CD, Deeg, HJ, Doney, K, Strorb, R, Sullivan, K, Witherspoon, A and Applebaum, FR. (1996) Pregnancies following high dose cyclophosphamide with or without high-dose busulfan or total body irradiation and bone marrow transplantation. *Blood., 87*, 3045-52.

Sarafogolou, K, Bouland, F, Gillio, A and Sklar, C. (1997) Gonadal function after bone marrow transplantation for acute leukaemia during childhood. *J. Pediatr., 130*, 210-6.

Schmidt, AI, Engelmann, C, Till, H, Kellnar, S and Ure BM. (2007) Minimally-invasive pediatric surgery in 2004: a survey including 50 German institutions. *J. Pediatr. Surg.*, 42, 1491-4.

Schmidt, KLT, Andersen Yding, C, Loft, A, Byskov, AG, Ernst, E and Andersen Nyboe, A. (2005) Follow up of ovarian function post-chemotherapy following ovarian cryopreservation and transplantation. *Hum. Reprod., 20*, 3539-46.

Seshadri, T, Gook, D, Lade, S, Spencer, A, Grigg, A, Tiedemann, K, McKendrick, J, Mitchell, P, Stern, C and Seymour, JF. (2006) Lack of evidence of disease contamination in ovarian tissue harvested for cryopreservation from patients with Hodgkin lymphoma and analysis of factors predictive of oocyte yield. *Br. J. Cancer., 94*, 1007-10.

Shannon, C. and Smith, IE. (2003) Breast cancer in adolescents and young women. *Eur. J. Cancer.,* 39, 2632-42.

Shaw, J and Trounson, A. (1997) Oncological implications in the replacement of ovarian tissue. *Hum Reprod., 12*, 403-5.

Signorello, LB, Cohen, SS, Bosetti, C, Stoball, M, Kasper, CE, Weathers, RE, Whitton, JA, Green, DM, Donaldson, SS, Mertens, AC, Robison, LL, Boice, JD Jr. (2006) Female survivors of childhood cancer: preterm birth and low birth weight among their children. *J. Natl. Cancer Inst., 98*, 1453-61.

Silber, SJ and Gosden, RG. (2007) Ovarian transplantation in a series of monozomic twins discordant for ovarian failure. *N. Engl. J. Med., 353*, 1382-4.

Silber, SJ, Lenahan, KM, Levine, DJ, Pineda, JA, Gorman, KS, Friez, MJ, Crawfored, EC and Gosden RG. (2005) Ovarian transplantation between monozomic twins discordant of premature ovarian failure. *N. Engl. J. Med., 353*, 58-63.

Sklar, CA, Mertens, AC, Mitby, P, Whitton, J, Stovall, M, Kasper, C, Mulder, J, Nichologson, S, Yasui, Y and Robison, LL. (2006) Premature menopause in survivors of childhood cancer: a report from the childhood cancer survivor study. *J. National. Cancer Institute., 98*, 890-6.

Sonmezer, M, Shamonki, MI and Oktay, K. (2005) Ovarian tissue cryopreservation: benefits and risks. *Cell Tissue Res., 322*, 125-32.

Sorensen, K, Levitt, GA, Bull, C, Droup, I and Sullivan, ID. (2003) Late anthracycline toxicity after childhood cancer: a prospective longitudinal study. *Cancer., 97,* 1991-8.

Speroff, L, Glass, RH and Kase, NG. (1994) The Ovary-Embryology and Development, The Uterus, Abnormal puberty and growth problems, Amenorrhea, Induction of ovulation. In: Speroff L, Glass RH, Kase NG, eds. *Clinical Gynecologic Endocrinology and Infertility*. Baltimore, Maryland, USA: Wiliams and Wilkins, 93-152, 361-457, 897-931.

Stiller, CA. (2004) Epidemiology and genetics of childhood cancer. *Oncogene., 23*, 6429-44.

Stillman, RJ, Schinfeld, JS, Schiff, I, Gelber, RD, Greenberger, J, Larson, M, Jaffe, N and Li, FP. (1981) Ovarian failure in long term survivors childhood malignancy. *Am. J. Obste.t Gynecol., 139*, 62-6.

Telfer, E., Torrance, C. and Gosden R.G. (1990) Morphological study of cultured preantral ovarian follicles of mice after transplantation under the kidney capsule. *J. Reprod. Fertil.*, 89, 565-571.

Tilly J (1996) Apoptosis and ovarian function. *Rev. Reprod. 1*, 162-72.

Wallace, WHB, Shalet, SM, Tetlow, IJ, Morris-Jones, PH. (1993) Ovarian function following the treatment of childhood acute lymphoblastic leukaemia. *Med. Pediatr. Oncol., 21*, 333-9.

Wallace, WHB, Thomson, AB and Kelsey, TW. (2003) The radiosensitivity of the human oocyte. *Hum. Reprod., 18*, 117-21.

Wallace, WHB, Anderson, RA and Irvine, DS. (2005a) Fertility preservation for young patients with cancer: Who is at risk and what can be offered? *Lancet Oncol.*, 6, 209-18.

Wallace, WHB, Thomson, AB, Saran, F and Kelsey, TW. (2005b) Predicting age at ovarian failure after radiation to a field that includes the ovaries. *Int. J. Radiat. Oncol, Biol, Physics., 62*, 738-44.

Weintraub, M, Gross, E, Kadari, A, Ravitsky, V, Safran, A, Laufer, N and Revel, A. (2007) Should ovarian cryopreservation be offered to girls with cancer? *Pediatr. Blood Cancer., 48*, 4-9.

Weissman, A, Gotlieb, L, Colgan, T, Jurisicova, A, Greenblatt, EM and Casper, RF. (1999) Preliminary experience with subcutaneous human ovarian cortex transplantation in the NOD-SCID mouse. *Biol. Reprod., 60*, 1462-7.

Williams, RS, Littelll, RD and Mendelhall, NP. (1999) Laparoscopic oophoropexy and ovarian function in the treatment of Hodgkin disease. *Cancer., 86*, 2138-42.

Yang, D, Brown, SE, Nguyen, K, Reddy, V, Brubaker, C and Winslow, KL. (2007) Live birth after the transfer of human embryos developed from cryopreserved oocytes harvested before cancer treatment. *Fertil. Steril., 87*, 1469. e1-4.

Zinger, M, Liu, JH, Husseinzadeh, N and Thomas, MA. (2004) Successful surrogate pregnancy after ovarian transposition, pelvic irradiation and hysterectomy. *J. Reprod. Med., 49*, 573-4.

In: Cancer in Female Adolescents
Editor: Margarite T. Moorland

ISBN: 978-1-60456-421-1

Chapter IV

Ovarian Function Preservation after Cancer Treatment

Ana Carolina Japur de Sá Rosa e Silva*, Bruno Ramalho de Carvalho, Julio César Rosa e Silva and Marcos Felipe Silva de Sá

Human Reproduction Sector, Department of Gynecology and Obstetrics.
Faculty of Medicine of Ribeirão Preto, University of São Paulo, Brazil

Abstract

Currently thousands of teen and adult women are submitted to cancer treatment every year and estimative point to the existence of one survivor of malignant disease during childhood for each group of 250 adults. Improvements in medical care became absolutely necessary, demanding the development of new strategies to diminish the toxic consequences of chemotherapy and improve quality of life of treated patients. Ovarian failure is a frequent complication following cancer treatment, due to the cytotoxic effect of radio and chemotherapy. Temporary or permanent absence of endocrine and reproductive ovarian functions depends, mainly, on patients' age at the moment the gonadotoxic treatment was performed and also on the administered doses. The ovarian failure and consequently the installed hypogonadism culminate with several complications as the augmented incidence of cardiovascular diseases, reduced bone mass density and osteoporosis, precocious climacteric symptoms and infertility. Science advances progressively increase the knowledge on ovarian follicular and hypothalamic-pituitary axis dynamics. Furthermore cryobiology development has permitted physicians to plan and offer distinct strategies intending to maintain gonadal function for patients submitted to malignant neoplasm treatment. This chapter aims to discuss the available options in fertility preservation, especially focusing hormonal/pharmacological methods and cryobiology techniques (oocytes, embryos and ovarian cortical tissue cryopreservation).

* Correspondence: Dr. Ana Carolina Japur de Sá Rosa e Silva; Hospital das Clínicas da FMRP-USP / Campus Universitário; Laboratório de Ginecologia e Obstetrícia - 1° andar; Bairro Monte Alegre / Ribeirão Preto – São Paulo / CEP: 14.048-900; E-mail: anasars@convex.com.br

Context

It is estimated that 678,060 women received a diagnosis of cancer in 2007 and that 270,100 of them will die of the disease (Ries *et al*, 2007). Considering the current scenario showing that hundreds of thousands of girls and women with cancer are submitted to chemotherapy (CT) and radiotherapy (RT) procedures (Oktay and Sonmezer, 2004), estimates for the near future indicate the existence of one survivor of the disease during childhood per 250 adult individuals (Blatt, 1999). The overall decline in the mortality rates due to childhood cancer was approximately 40% between 1975 and 1995, with a significant 2.6% reduction per year against an annual increase of 0.8% in the number of new cases (Ries *et al*, 1999). The malignant neoplasias most commonly diagnosed among women younger than 40 years are cancer of the breast, melanoma, cancer of the uterine cervix, non-Hodgkin's lymphomas and leukemia (Jemal *et al*, 2005).

This context requires science to invest in a reduction of the chemo- and radiotherapeutic sequels, ultimately aiming the maintenance of quality of life for cured patients, which includes the preservation of ovarian steroidogenesis. The cytotoxic action of chemotherapeutic agents and of ionizing radiation, currently used for the treatment of neoplasias very frequently, leads to premature ovarian failure (POF), which occurs at varying degrees of intensity and may imply serious long-term consequences such as increased incidence of cardiovascular diseases, reduction of bone mass and osteoporosis, premature climacteric symptoms and infertility (Schüffner *et al*, 2003). The temporary or permanent absence of endocrine and reproductive ovarian function depends on variables such as location of the disease, drug used, doses administered, route of administration and patient age at the time of gonadotoxic treatment (Donnez *et al*, 2004; Kwon and Case, 2004; Lee *et al*, 2006).

The cytotoxic action of certain drugs on the gonads is a real fact, but it is still not known on which cell type it occurs, contributing to greater aggressiveness in the depletion of primordial follicles or in the prevention of follicular maturation. The structural and functional proximity between granulosa cells and oocyte makes it difficult to establish the exact target of these drugs, but it seems obvious that damage to anyone of these structures would lead to impairment and dysfunction of the other (Gradishar and Schilsky, 1989). Alkylating drugs such as cyclophosphamide, mustard L-phenylalanine, chlorambucil, nitrosoureas, melphalan, busulfan and procarbazine, because of their nonspecific action, are likely to reach both cell types (Blumenfeld *et al*, 1999; Lee *et al*, 2006). Thus, they may cause irreversible damage to gonadal tissue as a consequence of chromosome deletions and prevention of the synthesis of essential cellular proteins secondary to chemical interactions with DNA. The injuries may range from a reduction of the number of follicles to gonadal fibrosis, depending not only on the agent in question, but also on its cumulative dose. Other agents such as 5-fluorouracil, methotrexate, vincristin, bleomicyn, dactinomycin, etoposide and doxorubicin also cause damage, but usually not irreversibly (Shamberger *et al*, 1981; Lee *et al*, 2006).

In a study conducted by Bines *et al*, the rates of ovarian failure ranged from 21 to 71% in young patients and from 49 to 100% in older patients (Bines *et al*, 1996). Also Blumenfeld *et al*, studied the occurrence of POF after CT with cyclophosphamide and observed rates of 100%, 50% and 13% among patients older than 30 years, aged 20 to 30 years, and younger than 20 years, respectively. The younger the patients treated, the lower the damage caused to the ovaries (Blumenfeld *et al*, 2000). Chapman *et al*, reported that, among patients treated for Hodgkin's disease, 69% of those aged 29 years or less presented POF, as opposed to 96% of those aged 30 years or more (Chapman *et al*, 1979). Although a less aggressive effect is documented in younger patients, Rosa e Silva *et al*, observed that despite the normal pubertal development presented by young girls submitted to chemotherapy during childhood, they are likely to present higher FSH levels in comparison to healthy girls, although within normal ranges (Rosa e Silva *et al*, 2007).

RT leads to POF in more than 60% of women submitted to doses higher than 300 cGy (Schüffner *et al*, 2003). In addition to ovarian aggression, there may also be injury of uterine vascularization and development among children and adolescents (Holm *et al*, 1999).

Preservation of Ovarian Function

The continuous evolution of assisted reproduction techniques has led to large numbers of studies aiming the preservation of ovarian function. The technique adopted should try to maintain the quality of life of the patient by restoring steroidogenic function and permitting the possibility of biological maternity. Patient age, diagnosis, the existence of a sex partner, the time available and the possible metastatic involvement of the ovaries should be taken into consideration (Roberts and Oktay, 2005) in addition, of course, of parity and of the wish for new pregnancies. Modern techniques of cryopreservation of oocytes and ovarian cortical tissue have now been added to the universally accepted alternatives of hormonal manipulation, ovary transposition and of embryo and semen cryopreservation, with promising results.

1. Hormonal Methods

The use of combined oral contraceptives, progestagens alone and gonadotropin releasing hormone analogues (a-GnRH) has been proposed in order to maintain ovarian rest and thus minimize the damage caused by chemotherapeutic agents to the follicular reserve.

1.1. Combined Oral Contraceptives and Progestagen Alone

The studies conducted on combined oral contraceptives (COC) in general have demonstrated that they are ineffective for the preservation of ovarian function after chemotherapy with alkylating agents (Longhi *et al*, 2003).

The use of medroxyprogesterone has been associated with follicle protection against the immediate toxicity of CT for Hodgkin's disease, but the maintenance of follicular quality was not achieved and a high rate of atresia was observed on a long-term basis (Familiari *et al*, 1993).

The suppressive effect of COC probably is not sufficient to fully block the hypothalamus-pituitary-ovary axis, thus it prevents follicle dominance and ovulation but not follicular recruitment (Killick *et al*, 1987; Fauser and Heusden, 1997). Therefore, COC, although less invasive, have been ruled out as a treatment option.

1.2. Gonadotropin Releasing Hormone Analogues (GnRHa)

The use of GnRHa as a method for the preservation of ovarian function is still controversial and a source of debate (Lee *et al*, 2006), although Blumenfeld *et al* recently published a non-randomized trial that strongly suggested the gonadoprotective effect of the drugs when administered in parallel to CT (Blumenfeld *et al*, 2007). The strategy intends to provoke a state similar to the prepubertal one, based on the prerogative that ovarian suppression may be a means of preserving oocytes (Kwon and Case, 2004). This theory was based on data published by Ortin *et al* (1990) and by Blumenfeld *et al* (1996), who detected the occurrence of gonadal damage in only 13% of girls younger than 15 years treated for Hodgkin's disease, suggesting a low action of the chemotherapeutic agent on prepubertal ovaries, i.e., ovaries in a resting state (Ortin *et al*, 1990; Blumenfeld *et al*, 1996).

The mechanisms by which protection may occur have not been well established since primordial follicles, theoretically, do not depend on the action of gonadotropins. Also, even though some studies have suggested the participation of GnRH in follicular physiology from the primary stage to atresia (Clayton *et al*, 1992; Whitelaw *et al*, 1995) and the expression of their receptors in granulosa-luteal cells is evident (Peng *et al*, 1994), there are no data demonstrating their action on primordial follicles. One of the theories, advanced by Ataya *et al*, proposes a direct action of the analogues on the ovaries in an earlier phase of folliculogenesis, before the chemosensitive one. There are indications that GnRHa may inhibit the follicular mitotic activity (Ataya *et al,* 1988; Ataya *et al,* 1989; Leung *et al*, 2003), conferring ovarian protection since the cytotoxicity of chemotherapeutic agents is more intense on cells in a process of overt division.

Some studies have encouraged the use of GnRHa for ovarian protection against the action of chemotherapeutic agents alone since there is evidence of an absence of protection in patients submitted to irradiation (Jarrell *et al*, 1991). Blumenfeld *et al* detected a reduction from 61% to 6.7% in the incidence of POF in women submitted to CT combined or not with GnRHa, respectively (Blumenfeld *et al,* 1996), and recently confirmed these data in a trial in which 96.9% of the patients taking GnRHa during CT resumed regular menstrual cycles as opposed to only 63% of control patients submitted to CT alone (Blumenfeld et al, 2007). Recchia *et al* also obtained evidence that led them to state the occurrence of protection of ovarian function on a long-term basis after resumption of the menstrual cycles in 86% of the patients who had taken goserelin in combination with CT for breast cancer (Recchia *et al*, 2002).

Even though there are no definitive data conferring a chemoprotective effect to GnRHa, this drug has a second beneficial effect on women submitted to CT. The presence of alterations of menstrual blood flow, especially hypermenorrhea and menorrhagia secondary to the thrombocytopenia produced by the chemotherapeutic agent, is not uncommon in these patients. Suppression of the hypothalamus-pituitary-ovary axis causing temporary chemical castration may prevent these disorders in these patients. Care must be taken regarding the bone mass of these patients in cases of prolonged hypoestrogenic states, with add back therapy possibly being advisable after a six month use.

2. Ovarian Transposition

Surgical ovarian transposition consists of pexis of the gonads close to the lower renal poles and therefore outside the pelvis and the field of irradiation. The application of this procedure is reserved for patients who are candidate for isolated RT as a preventive measure, since, in view of the maintenance of the vascular pedicle, it does not prevent the adverse action of the chemotherapeutic agent through the bloodstream. This means that in cases where both chemo and radiotherapy are required, this technique is useless. The procedure can be performed by laparotomy and laparoscopy and is indicated in cases of localized pelvic RT, in general for cervical tumors in the initial stages and lymphomas (Kwon and Case, 2004; Rosa e Silva, 2006).

The rates of success can reach 100% when low doses of irradiation are applied in patients younger than 40 years (Clough *et al*, 1996), nevertheless in a long term follow up the results are still discouraging, with the incidence of POF reaching more than 80% after 35 months of the procedure (Kwon and Case, 2004). Williams *et al* reported a small series in which laparoscopic oophoropexy performed before pelvic irradiation for Hodgkin's disease was effective in preserving gonadal function when associated with low doses of CT, but not after excessive cumulative doses (Williams *et al*, 1999).

A limitation of the method is the possibility of occurrence of vascular twisting or stretching during transposition, which may cause flow obstructions (Rosa e Silva, 2006).

3. Cryopreservation

There is no doubt that the use of cryotechnology for the preservation of ovarian function in patients at risk for POF generates good perspectives for the future. Many ethical questions still need to be discussed and more advances must be obtained, but the desired benefits are clear.

Freezing protocols should contemplate methods for freezing and thawing of a given tissue that will maintain viability and functionality (Woods *et al*, 2004). Thus, specific methods are required for each cell or tissue type, based on rapid or slow techniques and on the use of cryoprotective agents. These agents could be alcohols, amines, sugars and proteins which, in order to be effective, should have some properties such as high solubility in water (to reduce the freezing point), high permeability (to minimize the osmotic gradient) and low toxicity. The most common cryoprotective solutions consist of the following combinations: (a) dymethyl-sulfoxide and human serum, (b) ethylene glycol and fetal bovine serum, and (c) 1-2-propanediol, sucrose and human serum albumin (Arnon, 2001; Hovatta, 2003; Oehninger, 2005).

The functional cell damage caused by cryopreservation may be irreversible if the temperature falls below ideal levels. In general, very abrupt thermal variations may interfere with water transport through the cell membrane and favor the formation of ice crystals and salt deposits inside the cells (Mazur, 1963), it may also damage the microtubules of cells in overt division (Oktay and Gosden, 1999) and harm the traffic of molecules and organelles during the process of mitosis (Vincent and Johnson, 1992). Also, the differences in osmotic pressure between the intra- and extracellular environments may lead to changes in cell volume with consequent damage to the plasma membrane and the organelles (Oda *et al*, 1992; Hotamisligil *et al*, 1996). The tissue re-expansion phase (thawing) may also be deleterious if the external medium is inadequate (Pegg and Diaper, 1988).

3.1. Embryo Cryopreservation

Embryo cryopreservation probably is the most diffuse and routine method adopted by Human Reproduction services throughout the world after the first pregnancy obtained from a frozen and thawed embryo was recorded in 1983 (Trounson and Mohr, 1983).

The rate of survival for embryos submitted to freezing and thawing is 70 to 80% (Michelman and Nayudu, 2006), with implantation and clinical pregnancy rates of approximately 14% and 10% for each embryo transferred, respectively (Gelbaya *et al*, 2006). The potential for implantation of thawed embryos is directly related to the number of blastomeres; the use of those that remain intact after the process confers chances of success similar to those obtained for fresh embryos. For the habitual loss of blastomeres a 30% reduction in the implantation potential is expected for cryopreserved embryos (Edgar *et al*, 2000).

The major limitation of the process is the need to postpone the beginning of the antineoplastic treatment for 2 to 6 weeks, since exogenous stimulation of follicular growth requires a period of approximately two weeks after menstruation (Lee *et al*, 2006). Techniques of *in vitro* oocyte maturation will probably solve this problem in the near future, but their experimental nature still prevents their use in clinical practice (Buckett *et al*, 2007), especially in patients in which an unsuccessful procedure may seal the reproductive future.

Among other limitations of the method we may cite: (a) the high costs, especially those related to ovarian stimulation drugs; (b) the risk of developing ovarian hyperstimulation syndrome, a potentially serious event; (c) increased steroid production by the stimulated ovaries, an undesirable event for hormone-dependent neoplasias such as some breast cancers; and (d) the need for a partner or a semen donor for fertilization, a fact that contraindicates the method for prepubertal patients and patients without a sex partner who do not accept semen donation (Kwon and Case, 2004; Oehninger, 2005).

For specific cases of hormone-dependent neoplasias, some studies have documented the use of letrozole and tamoxifen as alternatives to traditional hormonal stimulation, without recurrence of cancer on a short-term basis (Oktay *et al*, 2003a; Oktay *et al*, 2003b; Oktay K, 2005). The perspectives are centered on the expected reduction of ovarian estrogen production when the use of letrozole is started before and maintained during stimulation with gonadotropins (Oktay *et al*, 2003b; Azim and Oktay, 2007), but the small series published thus far are not yet sufficient to recommend these hormones for the maintenance of fertility in cancer patients. Similarly, good results have been demonstrated with tamoxifen stimulation, generating positive expectations for breast cancer patients (Oktay *et al*, 2003b). In the case of endometrial neoplasias, protection can be obtained by the use of the intrauterine system with levonorgestrel (Juretzka *et al*, 2005).

3.2. Oocyte Cryopreservation

Even though the first birth from a frozen human oocyte was obtained more than two decades ago (Chen, 1986), followed by several other reports (Borini *et al*, 2004; Levi Setti *et al*, 2005; Oktay *et al*, 2006), oocyte cryopreservation is still considered to be an experimental technology in many countries (Schüffner *et al*, 2003; Lee *et al*, 2006). The importance of the technique is that it provides an option that minimizes the ethical, legal and religious problems involved in embryo freezing. Thus, it is particularly interesting for women without a partner or who do not accept fertilization with donor semen or who are against embryo freezing for personal reasons. In addition, this technique plays an important role among the options for the preservation of fertility in adolescents, since these girls usually have no defined partner with whom they intend to constitute a family.

Again, a crucial point for this procedure is the time available, since this intervention requires postponement of the beginning of treatment until ovarian stimulation is completed and the oocytes are retrieved by guided aspiration. Another limitation of oocyte cryopreservation is the difficulty in guaranteeing their fertilization after thawing, since they are extremely sensitive to the freezing protocols currently used, regardless of the phase of maturation. Osmotic changes, damage to the zona pellucida, to the cell membrane, to the cytoskeleton, microtubules and organelles, rupture of cortical granulations, chromosome and DNA alterations, and the toxicity of available cryoprotective agents continue to represent a challenge, being responsible for high rates of oocyte destruction (Johnson *et al*, 1988; Vincent and Johnson, 1992; White *et al*, 1998; Dudzinski, 2004; Woods *et al*, 2004; Oehninger, 2005).

Over the last few years there has been a marked progress in the technique. Rates of 2 to 4% successful use of frozen and thawed oocytes were reported by Porcu *et al* (1997), but more recent reports have indicated a refinement of the technique. More recent data estimate a 23 to 75% survival rate of immature oocytes after thawing (Chen, 1986; Mandelbaum *et al*, 1988; Tucker *et al*, 1998; Oehninger, 2005), with 27 to 67% rates of *in vitro* maturation (Tucker *et al*, 1998; Oehninger, 2005). Fertilization rates range from 32 to 57% (Mandelbaum *et al*, 1988; Fabbri *et al*, 2001) and cleavage occurs in 60 to 91% of cases (Chen, 1986; Fabbri *et al*, 2001). Even more encouraging results have been recently published by Cobo *et al,* with oocyte survival rates of the order of 96.7% and pregnancy rates of 65% (Cobo *et al*, 2007).

It has been demonstrated that small temperature variations can damage the microtubules that compose the mitotic spindle and lead to chromosome losses and aneuploidies during the end of first meiotic division in the process of oocyte maturation and even in mature gametes, when the division spindles are very sensitive (Oktay and Gosden, 1999). In addition, they may also harm the transit of molecules and organelles during the process of cell division (Vincent and Johnson, 1992). Thus, it appears that the difficulty in disseminating the technique of oocyte freezing may be related to these effects, although, based on the lately results for this technique many of these obstacles seem to be overcame difficulties.

3.3. Cryopreservation of Ovarian Cortical Tissue

The idea of ovarian tissue transplantation is not recent. The first records date back to the 19th century, and in the 1950 decade studies on the transplantation of ovarian tissue after thawing in female rats documented the occurrence of follicular growth, with the production of estrogen and pregnancy (Deanesly, 1957; Shüffner *et al*, 2003). Since then, the freezing of ovarian tissue by cryopreservation techniques has been the subject of numerous studies, with recent data showing complete recovery of gonadal function after autograft transplants in mice, rats, sheep, primates (Oehninger, 2005) and humans (Donnez *et al*, 2004), as well as the birth of healthy offspring. Even so, larger and more detailed studies are needed to elucidate the potential of frozen and thawed ovarian tissue for the maintenance of reproductive capacity by either *in vivo* maturation of isolated oocytes or autotransplant of cryopreserved tissue.

Today the cryopreservation of ovarian tissue is contemplated to serve specific groups of ′patients for whom the other techniques are not recommended, such as: (1) prepubertal patients whose gonads are not yet under the control of the hypothalamus-pituitary axis, (2) women without a partner who do not want embryos fertilized with donor semen, (3) patients with estrogen-dependent neoplasias such as breast cancer, and (4) women with malignant neoplasias that require an immediate approach, for whom the time needed for ovulation induction would postpone the beginning of treatment. Particularly from this perspective, the advantage of the collection of ovarian cortical tissue for cryopreservation is that it can be performed at any time during the menstrual cycle by videolaparoscopy, permitting the acquisition of hundreds of thousands of primordial follicles (Poirot *et al*, 2002), with the advantage that the anti neoplasic therapy can be started two or three days latter, if no surgical complications occur.

The option of freezing the ovarian cortex is based on the principle that primordial follicles are more resistant to cryotoxicity than follicles in the maturation process (Oktay *et al*, 1997; Oktay, 2000). This resistance may be the result of the peculiar characteristics of inactive follicles, such as reduced metabolism, absence of the zona pellucida and greater ease of cryoprotector penetration due to the smaller follicular size (Oktay, 1998).

The use of cryoprotectors reduces cell damage during tissue preservation (Kim *et al*, 2001a), but these agents may also result in some cytotoxicity in cases of prolonged exposure, with a 15 to 90% loss of primordial ovarian follicles depending on the type of protector and the technique used (Newton *et al*, 1996). The protocols most extensively used to freeze ovarian tissue involve technique of slow progressive freezing and direct/rapid freezing (vitrification in liquid nitrogen). Slow freezing and rapid thawing seem to be the most favorable schemes since data on direct freezing are scarce and suggest that these procedures provide results that, at most, are equal to those obtained with slow freezing (Isachenko *et al*, 2003; Hovatta, 2003; Hovatta, 2004).

A major concern of the scientific community regarding ovary freezing is the establishment of criteria for the evaluation of frozen tissue after thawing. The ideal evaluation of thawed ovarian tissue should consider aspects related to the viability and maintenance of function, since viable tissue is not necessarily functional. Parameters such as dehydration time, the cryoprotectors added and their concentrations and the freezing method are considered in terms of their impact not only on cell survival, but also on the morphology of follicles and oocytes, stromal and pre-granulosa cells, organelles, and collagen bonds. Not only morphology should be considered, but mainly the maintenance of the capacity of oocyte fecundation.

The great limitation of the method still is the risk that the reimplanted cryopreserved tissue will contain metastatic neoplastic cells that may lead to recurrence of the disease. This possibility is directly related to the selection of patients for this option of preservation of gonadal function (Rosa e Silva, 2006). Although favorable results have been reported in the literature regarding the low possibility of reimplantation of tissue containing cancer cells (Kim *et al*, 2001b), this possibility must be taken into consideration.

Ethical Aspects

Patient safety is the major ethical question to be considered when a proposal is made to preserve ovarian function after antineoplastic treatment, since it would be futile to try to preserve fertility if the patient does not have the physical well-being necessary for a healthy maternity.

Regarding the preservation of embryos and oocytes, the risks related to ovarian stimulation should be considered. These risks range from the worsening of estrogen-dependent neoplasias to treatment postponement and to the controversial predisposition to the development of ovarian cancer (Sushan *et al*, 1996; Modan *et al*, 1998; Revel *et al*, 2000). The ovarian hyperstimulation syndrome should also be kept in mind and proper care should be taken (Mathur *et al*, 2005) to prevent the systemic consequences of this process from interfering with the general pre-treatment condition of the patient.

The option to cryopreserve ovarian tissue does not involve the ethical dilemmas of delaying the institution of cancer therapy or of the risks of exogenous stimulation and therefore is an option for young women and girls. However, the habitual risks involved in any surgical procedure such as bleeding and infection should be considered (Dudzinski, 2004).

There is no doubt that the greatest benefits when the preservation of fertility is considered are psychoemotional since the impossibility of biological maternity generates anguish with the sensation of reproductive impotence and causes disorders of social interaction (Dudzinski, 2004).

The possibility of being able to conceive a child after a cancer is a factor that improves self-esteem and that can even contribute to a better acceptance of treatment and of its adverse effects. However, the risk of lack of success should be fully explained since current means do not guarantee that gametes and gonads will be protected by hormonal and surgical interventions or will resist cryopreservation techniques.

Within the experimental context, in which uncertainty prevails, it is extremely important to inform the patient or the person legally responsible for her and the relatives involved in the process, and also to document the issue of free and informed consent. The principles of autonomy, of benefiting the patient and not causing any harm to her should guide the strategy chosen, also respecting the opinion of a child if she is in a position to understand what is occurring (Shenfield *et al*, 2004).A multidisciplinary approach is essential, with an integrated action of physicians and psychologists in order to permit conscious decision making since the vulnerability of, and enormous pressure suffered by, everybody when a diagnosis of cancer is made directly interfere with their ability to understand and accept.

Questions related to the period of storage of frozen tissues in banks, as well as their posthumous use and donation to recipients or for research continue to be ethical dilemmas. Despite efforts to regulate this new field of medicine (Shenfield *et al*, 2002; Shenfield *et al*, 2004; Pennings *et al*, 2006; Pennings *et al*, 2007), only its evolution will permit us to obtain replies.

References

[1] Arnon, J; Meirow, D; Lewis-Roness H; Ornoy, A. (2001). Genetic and teratogenic effects of cancer treatments on gametes and embryos. *Hum. Reprod. Update,* 7, 394-403.

[2] Ataya, KM; Palmer, KC; Blacker, CM; Moghissi, KS; Mohammad, SH. (1988). Inhibition of rat ovarian [3H]thymidine uptake by luteinizing hormone-releasing hormone agonists: a possible mechanism for preventing damage by cytotoxic agents. *Cancer Res*, 48, 7252-7256.

[3] Ataya, K and Moghissi, K. (1989). Chemotherapy-induced premature ovarian failure: mechanisms and prevention. *Steroids,* 54, 607-626.

[4] Azim, A and Oktay, K. (2007). Letrozole for ovulation induction and fertility preservation by embryo cryopreservation in young women with endometrial carcinoma. *Fertil Steril*, 88, 657-664.

[5] Bines, J; Oleske, DM; Cobleigh, MA. (1996). Ovarian function in premenopausal women treated with adjuvant chemotherapy for breast cancer. *J. Clin. Oncol,* 14, 1718-1729.

[6] Blatt J. (1999). Pregnancy outcome in long-term survivors of childhood cancer. *Med. Pediatr. Oncol,* 33, 29–33.

[7] Blumenfeld, Z; Avivi, I; Linn, S; Epelbaum, R; Ben-Shahar, M; Haim, N. (1996). Prevention of irreversible chemotherapy-induced ovarian damage in young women with lymphoma by a gonadotropin-releasing hormone agonist in parallel to chemotherapy. *Human. Reprod*, 11, 1620-1626.

[8] Blumenfeld Z; Avivi I; Ritter M; Rowe JM. (1999). Preservation of fertility and ovarian function and minimizing chemotherapy-induced gonadotoxicity in young women. *J. Soc. Gynecol. Investig*, 6, 229-39.

[9] Blumenfeld Z, Shapiro D, Shteinberg M, Avivi I, Nahir M. (2000). Preservation of fertility and ovarian function and minimizing gonadotoxicity in young women with systemic lupus erythematosus treated by chemotherapy. *Lupus;* 9(6):401-5.

[10] Blumenfeld Z; Avivi I; Eckman A; Epelbaum R; Rowe JM; Dann EJ. (2007). Gonadotropin-releasing hormone agonist decreases chemotherapy-induced gonadotoxicity and premature ovarian failure in young female patients with Hodgkin lymphoma. *Fertil. Steri.*, [Epub ahead of print].

[11] Borini A, Bonu MA, Coticchio G, Bianchi V, Cattoli M, Flamigni C. (2004). Pregnancies and births after oocyte cryopreservation. *Fertil. Steril.* 82(3):601-5.

[12] Buckett WM; Chian RC, Dean NL; Sylvestre C; Holzer HE; Tan SL. (2007). Pregnancy loss in pregnancies conceived after in vitro oocyte maturation, conventional in vitro fertilization, and intracytoplasmic sperm injection. *Fertil. Steril*, [Epub ahead of print].

[13] Chapman RM; Sutcliffe SB; Malpas JS. (1979). Cytotoxic-induced ovarian failure in women with Hodgkin's disease. I. Hormonal function. *JAMA*, 242, 1877-81.

[14] Chen C. (1986). Pregnancy after human oocyte cryopreservation. *Lancet*, 1, 884-6.

[15] Clayton RN; Eccleston L; Gossard F; Thalbard JC; Morel G. (1992). Rat granulosa cells express the gonadotropin-releasing hormone gene: evidence from in-situ hybridization histochemistry. *J. Mol. Endocrinol*, 9, 189-95.

[16] Clough KB; Goffinet F; Labib A; Renolleau C; Campana F; de la Rochefordiere A; Durand JC. (1996). Laparoscopic unilateral ovarian transposition prior to irradiation: prospective study of 20 cases. *Cancer*, 77, 2638-45.

[17] Cobo A; Kuwayama M; Pérez S; Ruiz A; Pellicer A; Remohí J. (2007). Comparison of concomitant outcome achieved with fresh and cryopreserved donor oocytes vitrified by the Cryotop method. *Fertil. Steril*, [Epub ahead of print].

[18] Deanesly R. Egg survival in immature rat ovaries grafted after freezing and thawing. (1957). *Proc. R. Soc. Lond. B. Biol. Sci,* 147, 412-21.

[19] Donnez J; Dalmans MM; Demylle D; Jadoul P; Pirard C; Squifflet J; Martinez-Madrid B; van Langendonckt A. (2004). Livebirth after orthotopic transplantation of cryopreserved ovarian tissue. *Lancet*, 364, 1405-10.

[20] Dudzinski DM. (2004). Ethical issues in fertility preservation for adolescent cancer survivors: oocyte and ovarian tissue cryopreservation. *J. Pediatr. Adolesc. Gynecol*, 17, 97-102.

[21] Edgar DH; Bourne H; Speirs AL; McBain JC. (2000). A quantitative analysis of the impact of cryopreservation on the implantation potential of human early cleavage stage embryos. *Hum. Reprod*, 15, 175-9.

[22] Fabbri R; Porcu E; Marsella T; Rocchetta G; Venturoli S; Flamigni C. (2001). Human oocyte cryopreservation: new perspectives regarding oocyte survival. *Hum. Reprod*, 16, 411-6.

[23] Familiari G; Caggiati A; Nottola SA; Ermini M; Di Benedetto MR; Motta PM. (1993). Ultrastructure of human ovarian primordial follicles after combination chemotherapy for Hodgkin`s disease. *Hum. Reprod*, 8, 2080-7.

[24] Fauser BC and van Heusden AM. (1997). Manipulation of human ovarian function: Physiological concepts and clinical consequences. *Endocr. Rev*, 18, 71-106.

[25] Gelbaya TA; Nardo LG; Hunter HR; Fitzgerald CT; Horne G; Pease EEH; Brison DR; Lieberman BA. (2006). Cryopreserved-thawed embryo transfer in natural or down-regulated hormonally controlled cycles: a retrospective study. *Fertil. Steril*, 85, 603-9.

[26] Gradishar WJ and Schilsky RL. (1989).Ovarian function following radiation and chemotherapy for cancer. *Semin. Oncol,* 16(5):425-36.

[27] Holm K; Nysom K; Brocks V; Hertz H; Jacobsen N; Müller J. (1999). Ultrasound B-mode changes in the uterus and ovaries and Doppler changes in the uterus after total

body irradiation and allogeneic bone marrow transplantation in childhood. *Bone Marrow Transplant,* 23, 259-63.

[28] Hotamisligil S; Toner M; Powers RD. (1996). Changes in membrane integrity, cytoskeletal structure, and developmental potential of murine oocytes after vitrification in ethylene glycol. *Biol. Reprod*, 55, 161–8.

[29] Hovatta O. (2003). Cryobiology of ovarian and testicular tissue. *Best. Pract. Res. Clin. Obstet. Gynaecol*, 17, 331-42.

[30] Hovatta O. (2004). Cryopreservation and culture of human ovarian cortical tissue containing early follicles. *Eur. J. Obstet. Gynecol. Reprod. Biol*, 113 Suppl 1, S50-4.

[31] Isachenko E; Isachenko V; Rahimi G; Nawroth F. (2003). Cryopreservation of human ovarian tissue by direct plunging into liquid nitrogen. *Eur. J. Obstet. Gynecol. Reprod. Biol*, 108, 186-93.

[32] Jarrell JF; McMahon A; Barr RD; YoungLai EV. (1991). The agonist (d-leu-6, des-gly-10) - LHRH - ethylamide does not protect the fecundity of rats exposed to high dose unilateral ovarian irradiation. *Reprod. Toxicol*, 5, 385-8.

[33] Jemal A; Murray T; Ward E; Samuels A; Tiwari RC; Ghafoor A; Feuer EJ; Thun MJ. (2005). Cancer Statistics, 2005. *CA Cancer J. Clin.*, 55, 10-30.

[34] Johnson, M.H.; Pickering, S.J.; George, M.A. (1988). The influence of cooling on the properties of the zona pellucida of the mouse oocyte. *Hum. Reprod, 3*, 383-7.

[35] Juretzka, M.M.; O'Hanlan, K.A.; Katz, S.L.; El-Danasouri, I.; Westphal, L.M. (2005). Embryo cryopreservation after diagnosis of stage IIB endometrial cancer and subsequent pregnancy in a gestational carrier. *Fertil. Steril, 83*, 1041.

[36] Killick, S.R.; Eyong, E.; Elstein, M. (1987). Ovarian follicular development in oral contraceptive cycles. *Fertil. Steril, 48*, 409-13.

[37] Kim, S.S.; Battaglia, D.E.; Soules, M.R. (2001a). The future of human ovarian cryopreservation and transplantation: fertility and beyond. *Fertil. Steril, 75*, 1049.

[38] Kim, S.S.; Radford J.; Harris M.; Varley J.; Rutherford A.J.; Lieberman B.; Shalet S.; Gosden R. (2001b). Ovarian tissue harvested from lymphoma patients to preserve fertility may be safe for autotransplantation. *Hum Reprod, 16*, 2056-60.

[39] Kwon J.S. and Case A.M. (2004). Preserving reproductive function in women with cancer. *Sexuality, Reproduction and Menopause, 2*, 222-29.

[40] Lee S.J.; Schover L.R.; Partridge A.H.; Patrizio P.; Wallace W.H.; Hagerty K.; Beck L.N.; Brennan L.V.; Oktay K. (2006). American Society of Clinical Oncology Recommendations on Fertility Preservation in Cancer Patients. *J. Clin. Oncol, 24*, 1-15.

[41] Leung P.C.K.; Cheng C.K.; Zhu X. (2003). Multi-factorial role of GnRH-I and GnRH-II in the human ovary. *Mol. Cell Endocrinol, 202*, 145-53.

[42] Levi Setti PE, Albani E, Novara PV, Cesana A, Bianchi S, Negri L. (2005) Normal birth after transfer of cryopreserved human embryos generated by microinjection of cryopreserved testicular spermatozoa into cryopreserved human oocytes. *Fertil. Steril.* 83(4):1041.

[43] Longhi A.; Pignotti E.; Versari M.; Asta S.; Bacci G. (2003). Effect of oral contraceptive on ovarian function in young females undergoing neoadjuvant chemotherapy treatment for osteosarcoma. *Oncol. Rep, 10*, 151-5.

[44] Mandelbaum J.; Junca A.M.; Tibi C.; Plachot M.; Alnot M.O.; Rim H.; Salat-Baroux J.; Cohen J. (1988). Cryopreservation of immature and mature hamster and human oocytes. *Ann. N. Y. Acad. Sci, 541*, 550-61

[45] Mathur R.; Evbuomwan I.; Jenkins J. (2005). Prevention and management of ovarian hyperstimulation syndrome. *Curr. Obstet. and Gynaecol, 15*, 132–8.

[46] Mazur P. (1963). Kinetics of water loss from cells at subzero temperatures and the likelihood of intracellular freezing. *J. Gen. Physiol, 47*, 347-69.

[47] Michelmann H.W.; Nayudu P. (2006). Cryopreservation of human embryos. *Cell Tissue Bank, 7*, 135-41.

[48] Modan B.; Ron E.; Lerner-Geva L.; Blumstein T.; Menczer J.; Rabinovici J.; Oelsner G.; Freedman L.; Mashiach S.; Lunenfeld B. (1998). Cancer incidence in a cohort of infertile women. *Am. J. Epidemiol, 147*, 1038-42.

[49] Newton H.; Aubard Y.; Rutherford A.; Sharma V.; Gosden R. (1996). Low temperature storage and grafting of human ovarian tissue. *Hum. Reprod, 11*, 487-91.

[50] Oda K.; Gibbons W.E.; Leibo S.P. (1992). Osmotic shock of fertilized mouse ova. *J. Reprod. Fertil, 95*, 737–47.

[51] Oehninger S. (2005). Strategies for fertility preservation in female and male cancer survivors. *J. Soc. Gynecol. Investig, 12*, 222-31.

[52] Oktay K.; Nugent D.; Newton H.; Salha O.; Gosden R.G. (1997). Isolation and characterization of primordial follicles from fresh and cryopreserved human ovarian tissue. *Fertil. Steril, 67*, 481–6.

[53] Oktay K., Newton H., Aubard Y., Gosden R.G. (1998). Cryopreservation of human oocytes and ovarian tissue: an emerging technology? *Fertil. Steril, 69*, 1–7.

[54] Oktay, K. and Gosden, R.G. (1999). Cryopreservation of human oocytes and ovarian tissue. In: Brinsden, P.R. (Ed.), *A Textbook of in vitro fertilization and assisted reproduction* (3rd Edition., pp. 303-10). Lancaster, UK: Parthenon Inc.

[55] Oktay, K. and Karlikaya, G. (2000). Ovarian function after transplantation of frozen, banked autologous ovarian tissue. *N. Engl. J. Med, 342*, 1919.

[56] Oktay, K.; Buyuk, E.; Rosenwaks, Z. (2003a). Novel use of an aromatase inhibitor for fertility preservation via embryo cryopreservation in endometrial cancer: a case report. *Fertil. Steril, 80*, 144.

[57] Oktay, K.; Buyuk, E.; Davis, O.; Yermakova, I.; Veeck, L.; Rosenwaks, Z. (2003b). Fertility preservation in breast cancer patients: IVF and embryo cryopreservation after ovarian stimulation with tamoxifen. *Hum. Reprod, 18*, 90-5.

[58] Oktay, K.; Sonmezer, M. (2004). Ovarian tissue banking for cancer patients. Fertility preservation, not only ovarian preservation. *Hum. Rep, 19*, 477-80.

[59] Oktay, K. (2005). Further evidence on the safety and success of ovarian stimulation with letrozole and tamoxifen in breast cancer patients undergoing in vitro fertilization to cryopreserve their embryos for fertility preservation. *J. Clin. Oncol, 23*, 3858-9.

[60] Oktay, K.; Cil, A.P.; Bang, H. (2006). Efficiency of oocyte cryopreservation: a meta-analysis. *Fertil. Steril, 86*, 70-80.

[61] Ortin, T.T.; Shoshlak, C.A.; Donaldson, S.S. (1990). Gonadal status and reproductive function following treatment for Hodgkin's disease in childhood: the Stanford experience. *Int. J. Radiol. Oncol. Biol. Phys, 19*, 873-80.

[62] Pegg, D.E.; Diaper, M.P. (1988). On the mechanism of injury to slowly frozen erythrocytes. *Biophys. J, 54*, 471-88.

[63] Peng, C.; Fan, N.C.; Ligier, M.; Vännänen, J.; Leung, P.C.K. (1994). Expression and regulation of gonadotropin-releasing hormone (GnRH) and GnRH receptor messenger ribonucleic acids in human granulosa-luteal cells. *Endocrinology, 135*, 1740-6.

[64] Pennings, G.; de Wert, G.; Shenfield, F.; Cohen, J.; Tarlatzis, B.; Devroey P. (2006). ESHRE Taskforce on Ethics and Law 11: posthumous assisted reproduction. *Hum. Reprod, 21*, 3050-3.

[65] Pennings, G.; de Wert, G.; Shenfield, F.; Cohen, J.; Tarlatzis, B.; Devroey P. (2007). ESHRE Taskforce on Ethics and Law 12: oocyte donation for non-reproductive purposes. *Hum. Reprod, 22*, 1210-3.

[66] Poirot, C.J.; Vacher-Lavenu, M.C.; Helardot, P.; Guibert, J.; Brugières, L.; Jouannet, P. (2002). Human ovarian tissue cryopreservation: indications and feasibility. *Hum. Reprod, 17*, 1447-52.

[67] Porcu, E.; Fabbri, R.; Seracchioli, R.; Ciotti, P.M.; Magrini, O.; Flamigni, C. (1997). Birth of a healthy female after intracytoplasmic sperm injection of cryopreserved human oocytes. *Fertil. Steril, 68*, 724-6.

[68] Recchia, F.; Sica, G.; De Filippis, S.; Saggio, G.; Rosselli, M.; Rea, S. (2002). Goserelin as ovarian protection in the adjuvant treatment of premenopausal breast cancer: a phase II pilot study. *Anticancer Drugs, 13*, 417-24.

[69] Revel, A.; Davis, V.J.; Casper, R.F. (2000). Ovarian cortex cryopreservation in pediatric and adolescent medicine. *J. Pediatr. Adolesc. Gynecol, 13*, 95.

[70] Ries, L.A.G.; Smith, M.A.; Gurney, J.G.; Linet, M.; Tamra, T.; Young, J.L.; Bunin G.R. (Eds) (1999). *Cancer Incidence and Survival among Children and Adolescents: United States SEER Program 1975-1995*, National Cancer Institute, SEER Program. NIH Pub. No. 99-4649. Bethesda, MD.

[71] Ries, L.A.G.; Melbert, D.; Krapcho, M.; Mariotto A.; Miller, B.A.; Feuer, E.J.; Clegg, L.; Horner, M.J.; Howlader, N.; Eisner, M.P.; Reichman, M.; Edwards, B.K. (Eds). *SEER Cancer Statistics Review, 1975-2004*, National Cancer Institute, Bethesda, MD [online]. Dec 4th 2007. Available from: URL: http://seer.cancer.gov/csr/1975_2004/.

[72] Roberts, J.E. and Oktay, K. (2005). Fertility preservation: A comprehensive approach to the young woman with cancer. *J. Natl. Cancer Inst. Monogr*, 57-9.

[73] Rosa e Silva, A.C.J.S. (2006). Fertility Preservation. *Rev. Bras. Ginecol. Obstet, 28*, 365-72.

[74] Rosa e Silva, A.C.J.S.; Rosa e Silva, J.C.; Reis, R.M.; Tone, L.G.; Sá, M.F.S.; Ferriani, R.A. (2007). Gonadal function in adolescent patients submitted to chemotherapy during childhood or during the pubertal period. *J. Pediatr. Adolesc. Gynecol, 20*, 89-91.

[75] Shamberger RC, Sherins RJ, Ziegler JL, Glatstein E, Rosenberg SA. (1981). Effects of postoperative adjuvant chemotherapy and radiotherapy on ovarian function in women undergoing treatment for soft tissue sarcoma. *J. Natl. Cancer Inst.,* 67(6): 1213-8.

[76] Shenfield, F.; Pennings, G.; Sureau, C.; Cohen, J.; Devroey, P.; Tarlatzis, B. (2002). ESHRE Taskforce on Ethics and Law III: gamete and embryo donation. *Hum. Reprod, 17*, 1407-8.

[77] Shenfield, F.; Pennings, G.; Cohen, J.; Devroey, P.; Sureau, C.; Tarlatzis, B. (2004). ESHRE Taskforce on Ethics and Law 7: Ethical considerations for the cryopreservation of gametes and reproductive tissues for self use. *Hum. Reprod, 19*, 460-2.

[78] Shüffner, A.G.; Piazza, M.J.; Costa, S.L.; Centa, L.J.R. (2003). Criopreservação de tecido ovariano. Revisão Histórica. *Femina, 31*, 63-6.

[79] Shushan, A.; Paltiel, O.; Iscovich, J.; Elchalal, U.; Peretz, T.; Schenker, J.G. (1996). Human menopausal gonadotropin and the risk of epithelial ovarian cancer. *Fertil. Steril, 65*, 13-8.

[80] Trounson, A.O. and Mohr, L. (1983). Human pregnancy following cryopreservation, thawing and transfer of an eight-cell embryo. *Nature, 305*, 707-9.

[81] Tucker, M.J.; Wright, G.; Morton, P.C.; Massey, J.B. (1998). Birth after cryopreservation of immature oocytes with subsequent in vitro maturation. *Fertil. Steril, 70*, 578-9.

[82] Vincent, C. and Johnson, M.H. (1992). Cooling, cryoprotectants, and the cytoskeleton of the mammalian oocyte. *Oxf. Rev. Reprod. Biol, 14*, 73–100.

[83] White, J.; Serafini, P.; De Martin, H.; Peterle, M. (1998). Criopreservação de tecido ovariano humano: uma nova perspectiva em fertilização assistida. *Femina, 26*, 831-32.

[84] Whitelaw, P.F.; Eidne, K.A.; Sellar, R.; Smyth, C.D.; Hillier, S.G. (1995). Gonadotropin-releasing hormone receptor ribonucleic acid expression in rat ovary. *Endocrinology, 136*, 172-9.

[85] Williams RS, Littell RD, Mendenhall NP. (1999). Laparoscopic oophoropexy and ovarian function in the treatment of Hodgkin disease. *Cancer.* 86(10):2138-42.

[86] Woods, E.J.; Benson, J.D.; Agca, Y.; Critser, J.K. (2004). Fundamental cryobiology of reproductive cells and tissues. *Cryobiology, 48*, 146-56.

In: Cancer in Female Adolescents
Editor: Margarite T. Moorland
ISBN: 978-1-60456-421-1

Chapter V

Solid-Pseudopapillary Tumor of the Pancreas: Characteristic Clinicopathological Features and Implications for Surgical Management

Masanao Kurata,[1] Terumi Kamisawa,[2] Shin-ichiro Horiguchi[3] and Atsutake Okamoto[1]
[1] Departments of Surgery, [2] Internal Medicine, and [3] Pathology
Tokyo Metropolitan Komagome Hospital, Tokyo, Japan

Abstract

Solid-pseudopapillary tumor (SPT) of the pancreas is an uncommon malignant tumor that predominantly affects young females. In this study, the clinical and histological features of pancreatic SPT are reviewed.

Over 19 years, 5 patients with SPT were seen in our practice. They were all females, ranging in age from 21 - 66 years. Three tumors were located in the head of the pancreas, and two were located in the body and tail of the pancreas. Clinically, pancreatic SPT patients usually have vague abdominal symptoms, including discomfort, abdominal pain, increased abdominal girth, and the presence of a palpable mass. Three patients had pancreaticoduodenectomy, and two patients had distal pancreatectomy. No patients had metastasis to other sites. All patients are currently alive without recurrent disease. The histological findings were similar in all patients, and included: fairly uniform, round or oval eosinophilic cells concomitant with numerous thin-walled blood vessels in the solid component; red blood cells in the spaces between the pseudopapillary structures; and rare mitoses. The following immunohistochemical findings were confirmed: no reaction was evident with anti-chromogranin A, amylase, lipase or pancreatic polypeptide antibodies. The most useful markers for making a conclusive diagnosis were alpha-1-antitrypsin, neuron-specific enolase (NSE), and vimentin. Alpha-1-antitrypsin- and NSE-positive cells were present in all cases. All tumor cells were progesterone receptor-positive and estrogen receptor-negative. These findings show a close relationship between the tumor and sex hormones.

Pancreatic SPT occurs most frequently in young females and has low-grade malignant potential; it is associated with distinctive pathological and immunohistochemical features. Surgical resection should be considered even if metastases or local invasion is present, since it offers the patients an excellent prognosis.

Introduction

Solid-pseudopapillary tumor (SPT) of the pancreas is an uncommon malignant tumor that predominantly affects young females. Although the tumor has been studied closely, and its clinical characteristic features have been gradually identified, its pathogenesis and the optimal therapeutic approach remain unclear. The pathogenic features of pancreatic SPT include the presence of a relatively benign-looking solid lesion with a cystic component, which is associated with an area of limited degeneration and occasional neurosecretory granules. Most examples of SPT can be readily diagnosed on routine histological examination; additional immunohistochemical studies are frequently used to make a conclusive diagnosis. Despite the presence of malignant morphological features, SPT usually has a low-grade malignant potential, and the development of tumor metastasis to other sites is exceptional. Surgical excision is the treatment of choice, and patient prognosis is good. In the present study, 5 cases of SPT are described and the literature is reviewed to identify the characteristic features of pancreatic SPT and the surgical outcomes.

Case 1

A 32-year-old woman presented with continuous dull pain in the upper abdomen that had been present for six years. She was also aware of the same pain during menstruation. A fist-sized abdominal mass was detected, but all laboratory data, including tumor marker levels, were within normal range. Ultrasonography (US) revealed a large, round, well-circumscribed mass (74×59×72 mm in diameter) located in the pancreatic tail, with multicystic lesions that contained a solid component. Computed tomography (CT) scan showed a round, encapsulated mass with a non-homogeneous density and a fibrotic capsule. Celiac and superior mesenteric angiography was done to exclude major vascular tumor invasion. The main feeding artery of the tumor was the great pancreatic artery; it and the transverse pancreatic artery were stretched in an arc. However, these arteries were not encased by the tumor, and tumor staining was not detected. Pancreatic tail SPT was suspected prior to surgery. Operative findings included: a large and well-defined mass located in the pancreatic tail; no distant metastases; and no involvement of the adjacent organs. Radical tumor removal involving a distal pancreatectomy combined with splenectomy was performed (figure 1A). On histology, the characteristic findings of SPT were identified. The tumor was globular and consisted of solid and cystic components surrounded by a fibrous pseudocapsule. The cystic lesion was filled with old blood clots and fibrin. Some areas, where the tumor tissue broke the pseudocapsule and penetrated to peripancreatic soft tissue, had no capsule. Microscopically, the tumor tissue exhibited a solid monomorphic pattern with variable sclerosis; a pseudopapillary pattern was present in the more central portion. These components gradually merged into each other. In the papillary part, the thick fibrovascular core showed prominent mucinous change. The tumor cells had eosinophilic or clear vacuolar cytoplasm with centrally located nuclei. Glycogen and mucin could not be found (figure 2). No mitotic activity was visible. No vascular invasion or lymph node metastasis was detected. The results of immunostaining are summarized in table 2. The tumor cells were reactive for vimentin, alpha-1-antitrypsin (figure 3A), NSE (figure 3B), and progesterone receptor (figure 3C), but not for chromogranin A, synaptophysin, amylase, or estrogen receptor. The patient's postoperative course was uneventful. At 7-year follow-up, the patient is alive and disease-free.

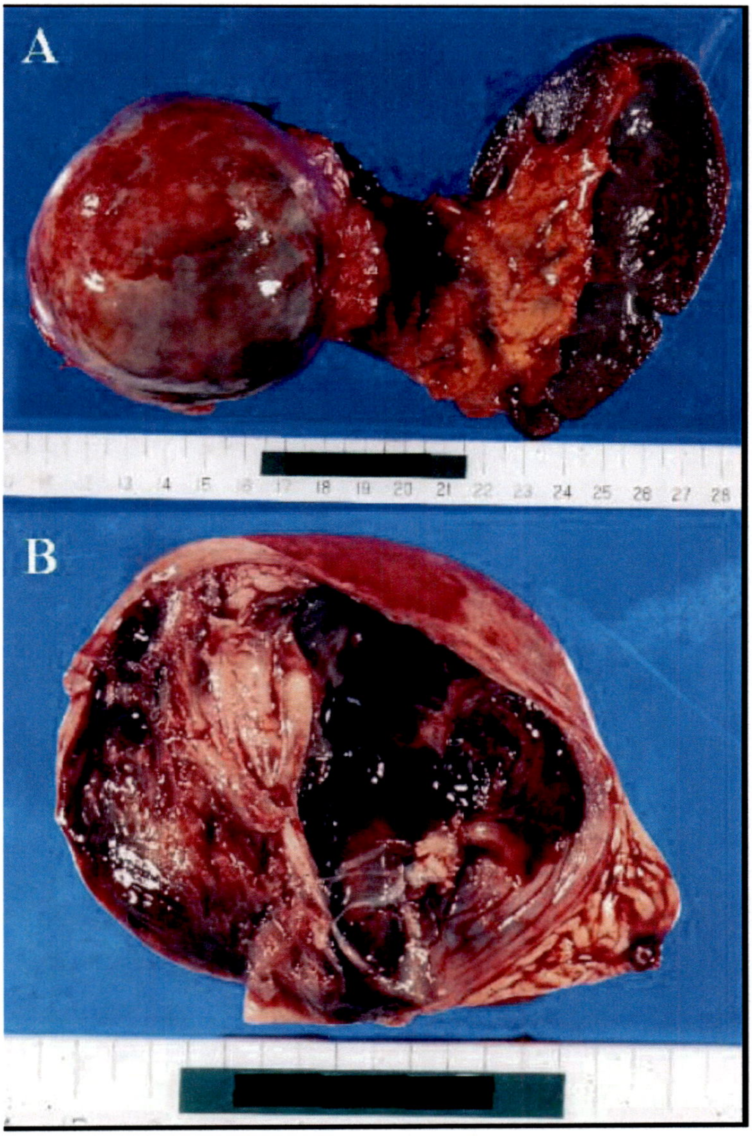

Figure 1. Gross appearance of resected specimens of case 1. A heterogeneous mass consisting of solid, cystic, and hemorrhagic components is seen.

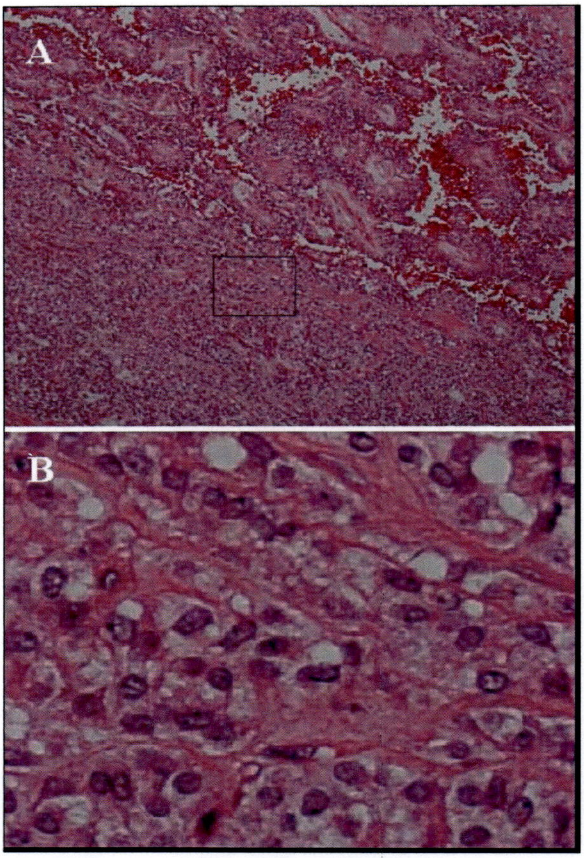

Figure 2. Histology of the tumor shows a solid monomorphous pattern and a pseudopapillary pattern (A). Higher magnification of the tumor reveals solid sheets of uniform cells containing eosinophilic cytoplasm (*arrows*). Some of the cells are vacuolated (B). (Hematoxylin and eosin stain).

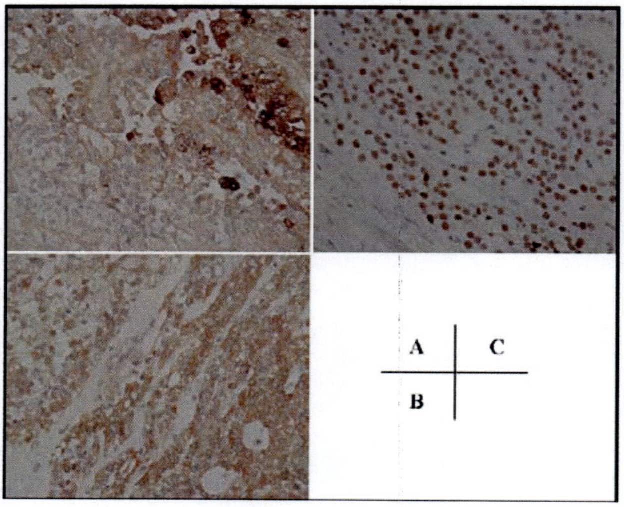

Figure 3. Immunohistochemical staining is diffusely positive for alpha-1-antitrypsin (A), positive for NSE in the cytoplasm of the tumor cells (B), and positive for progesterone receptor in the nuclei of the tumor cells (C).

Table 1. Clinical data with Solid-pseudopapillary Tumor of the Pancreas

Case No.	Age/ Sex	Symptoms	Location	Tumor Size (mm)	Metastasis	Operation
1	32/F	Abdominal pain	body	60x53x45	No	DP+S
2	66/F	No symptoms	tail	17x16x13	No	DP+S
3	31/F	Fatigue, jaundice	head	70x65x60	No	PD
4	21/F	Nausea	head	50x40x35	No	PD
5	-/F		head	150x110x100	No	PD

DP: distal pancreatectomy; S: slenectomy; PD: pancreaticoduodenectomy

Table 2. Immunostaining study of Solid-pseudopapillary Tumor of the Pancreas

Case	Vim	AAT	NSE	S-100	Synp	Chro	Amy	Lipase	ER	PR
1	+	+	+		–	–	–	–	–	+
2	+	+	+	–	+		–	–	–	+
3		+	+		+	–	–	–		
4		+	+			–	–	–		
5		+	+			–	–			

Vim: vimentin; ATT: alpha-1-antitrypsin; NSE: neuron specific enolase; Synp: synaptophysin; Chro: chromoglanin A; Amy: amylase; ER: estrogen receptor; PR: progesterone receptor.

Case 2

A 66-year-old woman was referred to our hospital for the evaluation of hyperglycemia (HbA_{1C} 8.4%) and the treatment of a pancreatic mass. She had no complaints or any past history of pancreatic disorders. Laboratory data showed normal serum amylase, lipase, carcinoembryonic antigen (CEA), and CA 19-9 levels. On endoscopic ultrasonography (EUS), a well-defined, non-homogeneous, hypo-echoic mass (14×15 mm in diameter) with a fibrotic capsule and a central septum was found in the pancreatic tail. A CT scan demonstrated a slightly enhanced mass in the tail of the pancreas without dilatation of the main pancreatic duct. There was no evidence of metastasis to lymph nodes and other organs (figure 4A). On magnetic resonance imaging (MRI), the lesion had low signal intensity on the T1-weighted image and high signal intensity on the T2-weighted image (figure 4B). A preoperative diagnosis of mucinous cystic neoplasm (MCN) was made. To remove the tumor, the patient had a distal pancreatectomy with regional lymphadenectomy. Neither extrapancreatic invasion nor metastases to lymph nodes were observed during the operation. Macroscopic examination of the resected pancreatic specimens showed a solid, yellow mass that had cystic components and was hemorrhagic. The tumor was 17×16×13 mm in size. The fibrous capsule of the tumor was exposed to the surface of the normal pancreas (figure 5). On histology, the tumor tissue was composed of a solid monomorphous pattern with a thick fibrovascular network; a pseudopapillary pattern was found in very focal areas. Tumor cells were dyscohesive, with uniform, small, round to oval, grooved, centrally located nuclei and eosinophilic cytoplasm. Some areas were characterized by a variable zone of hyalinization and myxomatous change. Mitotic activity or tumor vascular invasion was not found. The cut end of the residual pancreas was free of tumor cells, but nuclear atypia, pyknotic nuclei, and moderately large nucleoli were seen in the branched pancreatic ducts.

On immunohistochemistry, vimentin, alpha-1-antitrypsin, NSE, synaptophysin, and progesterone receptor stained positive. No reactivity was observed with estrogen receptor, S-100 protein, amylase, or lipase (table 2). The patient's postoperative course was uneventful. At 4-year follow-up, the patient is alive and disease-free. The patient's preoperative hyperglycemia was not related to SPT; her diabetes mellitus has been treated separately.

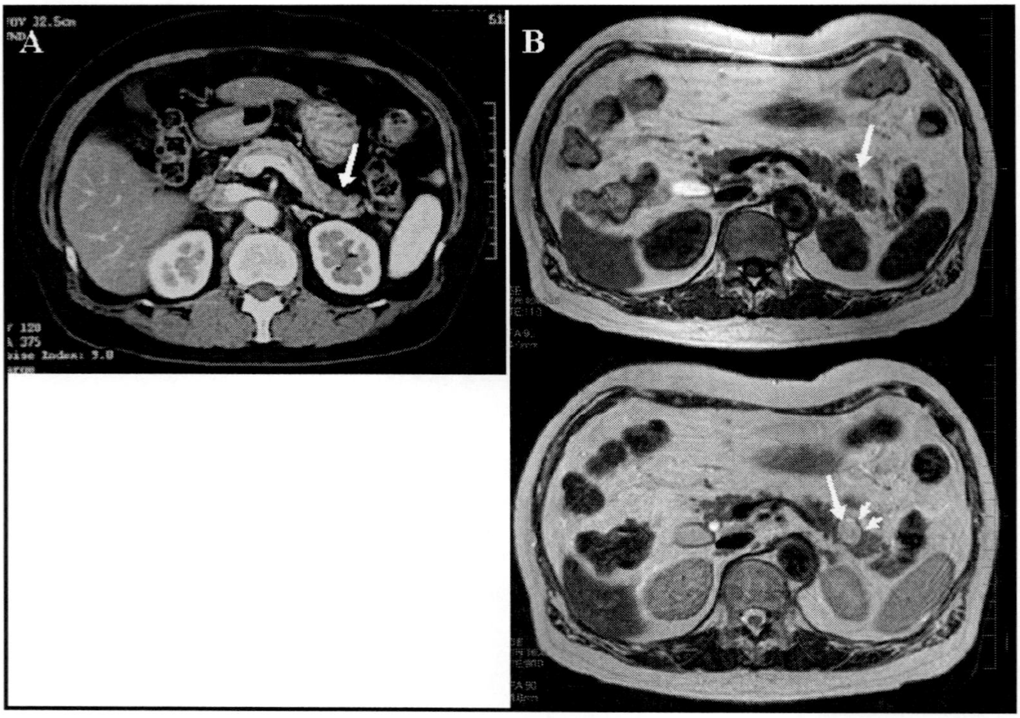

Figure 4. The CT of case 2 shows a round, 15 × 14 mm mass located in the pancreatic tail without lymph node metastasis (A). T1-weighted MRI image (upper column) shows a mass with low signal intensity (*arrows*), and the T2-weighted image (lower column) shows heterogeneous high intensity (*long arrows*) (B). Note the presence of the hypo-intense capsule (*short arrows*).

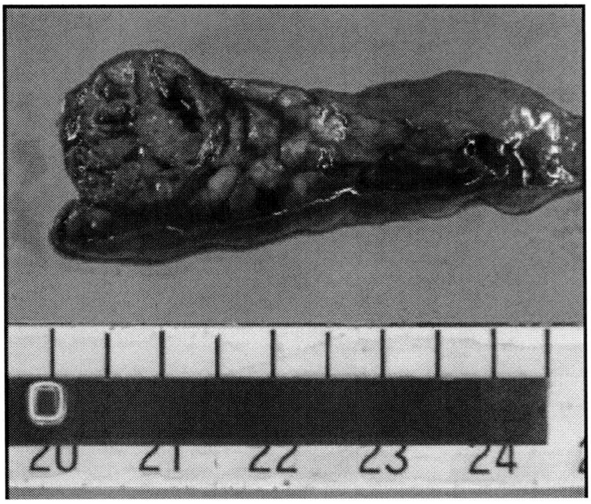

Figure 5. Gross appearance of resected specimens of case 2. The cut surface of the tumor shows a uniloculated cystic appearance.

Case 3

A 31-year-old woman was admitted to our hospital because of general fatigue and mild jaundice. Six years before admission, a mass had been detected in the head of the pancreas on US and diagnosed as SPT. However, she refused surgery at that time. Laboratory data showed elevated serum aspartate aminotransferase (AST) (275 IU/L), alanine aminotransferase (ALT) (476 IU/L), total bilirubin (1.7 mg/dL), amylase (223 IU/L), alkaline phosphatase (ALP) (846 IU/L), and CA19-9 (48.3 U/mL) levels. The serum CEA level was normal. On US, a large hypo-echoic mass was present in the upper abdomen. CT scan showed a solid round mass in the head of the pancreas measuring 70 mm in diameter that was slightly enhanced and associated with dilatation of the main pancreatic duct (MPD). There was no evidence of metastases to lymph nodes and other organs (figure 6A). On MRI, a well-defined lesion was found; it had a heterogeneously high or low signal intensity on T1-weighted images and heterogeneously high signal intensity on T2-weighted images (figure 6B). The tumor was contiguous to the common bile duct (CBD), and the intrahepatic bile duct was slightly dilated. On angiography, the feeding arteries were the gastroduodenal, superior pancreaticoduodenal, and inferior pancreaticoduodenal arteries, all of which were stretched by the tumor (figure 6C). Furthermore, these arteries were encased by the tumor to a marked degree, and the circumference of the tumor was highly stained. Endoscopic retrograde cholangiopancreatography demonstrated compression and flexion but no interruption of the CBD and the MPD in the distal pancreas. With a preoperative diagnosis of SPT, the tumor was removed. The encapsulated tumor was localized in the pancreatic head without tumor invasion to adjacent organs but with invasion to the middle colic vein and artery. The splenic and superior mesenteric veins adhered tightly to the tumor due to concomitant inflammation. A pancreaticoduodenectomy with partial resection of the transverse colon was successfully performed. No lymph node metastases were observed. The resected specimen was elastic, soft, and 70×65×60 mm in size; it had a small lobular pattern and a slit. The tumor was confirmed to be an SPT on microscopic examination and immunostaining. At 7-year follow-up, the patient is alive and disease-free.

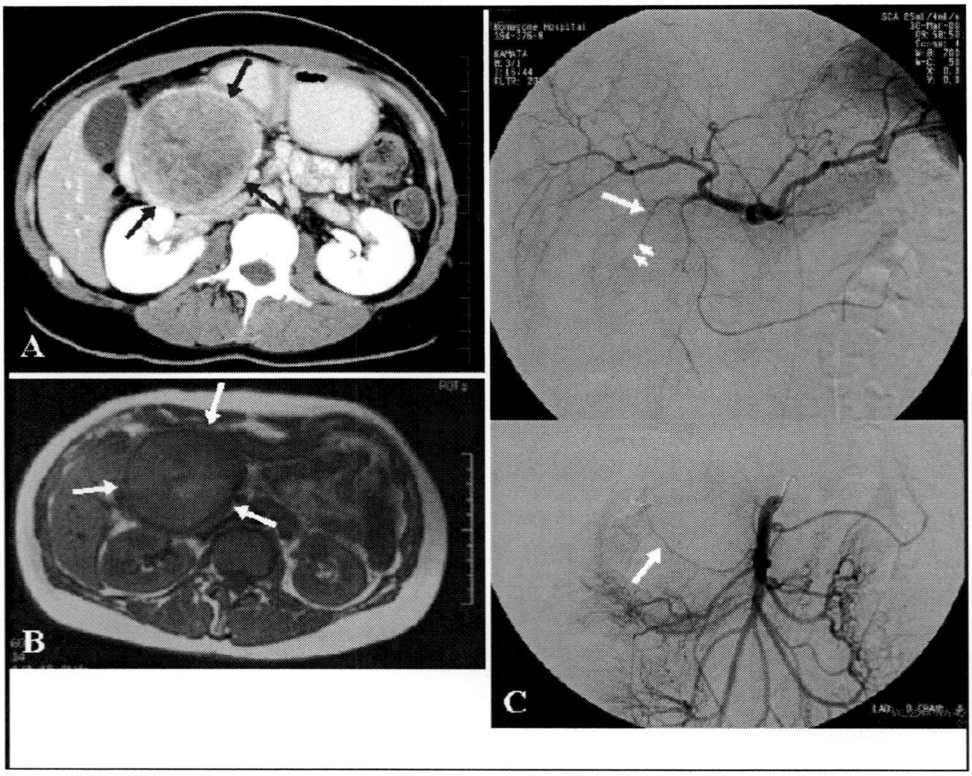

Figure 6. The CT of case 3 shows a huge complex mass surrounded by a well-defined capsule that includes a disrupted area (A). A T1-weighted MRI image shows a well-defined, heterogeneous, high intensity mass (*arrows*) located in the pancreatic head (B). Celiac angiography (upper column) shows stretching (*arrow*) and encasement (*short arrows*) of the gastroduodenal and superior pancreaticoduodenal arteries; superior mesenteric angiography (lower column) shows a stretched inferior pancreaticoduodenal artery (*arrow*) (C).

Case 4

A 21-year-old woman was admitted to our hospital due to nausea. She had no abdominal pain, tenderness, or weight loss. On CT and US, a cystic mass was found in the pancreatic head. The mass was not palpable, and the patient's laboratory findings were not contributory. The imaging findings of this tumor were similar to those described in the other patients, and included: a 6-cm mass that showed a focal high echo-pattern on US; a low density area with local irregular borders on CT; and stretched arterial branches of the pancreatic head arcade and compression of the superior mesenteric vein by the tumor on angiography. The liver and lymph nodes were free of metastases. A pancreaticoduodenectomy was performed, which resulted in successful removal of the tumor.

Case 5

The histological findings of this patient's tumor were similar to those described above, and included: prominent solid and cystic patterns; a dark red mass surrounded by a fibrous pseudocapsule; and a central component filled with a large amount of old blood, whereas the peripheral area had calcification. Tumor tissues were exposed through the pseudocapsule into the peripancreatic soft tissue. In the solid areas, there were sheets and cords of polygonal cells with eosinophilic cytoplasm and fine chromatin structure. The tumor cells tended to surround thin-walled blood vessels. Pseudopapillary structures were formed by the disintegration of tumor cells. Mitotic activity or vascular invasion was not found. On immunohistochemistry, alpha-1-antitrypsin and NSE were strongly positive. No reactivity was observed to chromogranin A, pancreatic polypeptide, amylase, or insulin.

Discussion

Pancreatic SPT is a rare exocrine tumor that accounts for about 2% of all pancreatic tumors [1]. Frantz first described SPT in 1959 [2], and the distinctive characteristics of the tumor have been gradually identified. In the last decade, the incidence of this disease has increased, and many case reports of SPT have appeared, since the pathological features of this entity have become widely known. In 1981, Kloppel et al. clearly described the evidence for the acinar origin of SPT and suggested the name "solid and cystic acinar cell tumor" [3]. Recently, the World Health Organization, in its classification of exocrine pancreatic tumors, referred to these tumors as "solid pseudopapillary tumors" of the pancreas [4].

Papavramidis reported that 91% of patients were females with a mean age of 21.97 years [5]. Up to 1999, approximately 90 children (≤18 years) with SPT had been reported [6]. Pancreatic SPT tends to be diagnosed in young females. However, the age of our five patients ranged from 21 to 66 years old, which suggests that the tumor may develop not only in young but also in older patients.

The most common clinical signs are vague gastrointestinal symptoms, such as upper abdominal discomfort or pain, followed by gradual enlargement of a palpable abdominal mass. Due to slow tumor growth, about 9% of patients remain completely asymptomatic until the tumor has enlarged considerably [7]. Therefore, the tumor is sometimes detected incidentally on imaging studies done as part of a routine physical examination. In our experience, one of the five patients presented no symptoms, and the tumor was detected on US imaging done as part of a routine physical checkup. Jaundice is an uncommon symptom that is documented in 1% patients who are hospitalized for the treatment of SPT [5]. Tumor size does not predict tumor resectability, since even very large tumors do not invade adjacent organs and do not occlude the CBD. Indeed, the tumor that was removed in case 3 had tight adhesions to contiguous structures due to concomitant inflammation but no tumor invasion.

The body and tail of the pancreas are more frequently affected (64%) than the head [8]. Interestingly, tumor growth into extrapancreatic sites has also been reported [3].

Laboratory examination results, such as serum amylase, blood sugar, and pancreatic cancer markers, are frequently normal, though case 3 had abnormal liver function and an elevated serum CA19-9 level.

On US, CT, MRI, and angiography, the characteristic imaging findings of SPT typically include the presence of a large, round, well-circumscribed tumor that consists of solid and cystic components. Occasionally, some cases have calcifications or internal septations in the tumor[9]. On US, the tumor is well encapsulated, homogeneous or heterogeneous, and consists of echogenic solid and hypoechogenic cystic components. On CT, a well-encapsulated and circumscribed tumor with various solid and cystic components caused by hemorrhagic degeneration is seen. Usually, the cystic spaces are located centrally, and the enhanced solid components are located peripherally [10].

MRI is better for diagnosing SPT than CT, since it allows certain tissue characteristics, such as hemorrhagic or cystic degeneration and the presence of a capsule, to be visualized. Typical findings on MRI include a well-defined heterogeneous lesion with high or low signal intensity on T1-weighted images and heterogeneous high signal intensity on T2-weighted images [11, 12].

On angiography, the tumor is usually found to be avascular, though it is sometimes hypovascular or mildly hypervascular. Angiography and MRI may be helpful to delineate the mass from adjacent structures and other structures that could be involved.

The differential diagnoses of SPT include other solid or cystic pancreatic tumors, such as microcystic adenoma, MCN, islet cell tumor, cystadenocarcinoma, acinar cell carcinoma, inflammatory pseudocyst, and pancreatoblastoma. The first four tumors seldom develop in patients younger than 30 years of age and have no particular gender preponderance. Microcystic adenoma is composed of innumerable tiny cysts that display a honeycomb appearance. MCN consists of large, unilocular or multilocular cysts. Pancreatoblastoma is usually found in younger individuals of either gender and has more aggressive tumor behavior than SPT. Islet cell tumors have radiological findings that are similar to those of SPT, though SPT is generally hypovascular on angiography, and it is less enhanced on the CT contrast study than an islet cell tumor [6].

Many reports recommend US-guided fine needle aspiration (FNA) or pancreatic duct brush cytology for preoperative diagnosis. However, SPT can be diagnosed easily due to the recent increasing incidence and the well-known findings of the tumor on various imaging studies. Thus, FNA or pancreatic duct brush cytology might not be necessary for preoperative diagnosis. FNA may be unacceptable because it has a risk of spreading tumor cells.

On gross appearance, the resected tumors are soft, yellow-red in color and consist of solid and cystic areas. The variegated appearance reflects the variable combination of hemorrhage, cystic degeneration, and cyst wall irregularity [8, 13]. Microscopically, there are solid areas composed of sheets and cords of polygonal or low columnar cells whose cytoplasm is eosinophilic and contains clear vacuoles, and whose nuclei are ovoid with fine chromatin structures. The tumor cells tend to surround blood vessels. Pseudopapillary structures are the result of tumor cell disintegration and the creation of fibrovascular stalks or pseudorosettes. Neither cellular atypia nor mitotic activity is usually observed [3]. The presence of necrosis, vascular or perineural invasion, high nuclear grade, and prominent necrobiotic nests suggest greater malignant potential [14]. However, in the absence of the various criteria mentioned above, aggressive tumor behavior cannot be excluded. While most SPTs can be regarded as being relatively indolent tumors, further studies, such as gene mutation, are needed to determine their malignant potential.

Immunohistochemical studies are frequently done to confirm the diagnosis. Most tumor cells are diffusely positive for vimentin, NSE, alpha-1-anitrypsin, and progesterone receptors, and they are sometimes reactive for S-100 protein. Markers of acinar differentiation, including trypsin and chymotrypsin, were consistently negative (data not shown). The neuroendocrine marker synaptophysin is sometimes positive, but chromogranin A is always negative. The positive NSE and synaptophysin results suggest that SPT has an endocrine cell origin [15]. The strong tendency for the tumor to be found in young females and the fact that it usually expresses progesterone receptors suggest that during early embryogenesis, the close relationship between the left genital ridge and the pancreas could conduct tumor precursor cells into pancreatic tissue [16].

Surgical removal of the tumor should be the treatment of choice for SPT, as it provides patients with a good prognosis. It is important to make a correct diagnosis of SPT prior to surgery, since SPT is a low-grade malignant tumor that appears to be curable by surgical excision. Pathologic factors, including the mitotic rate and vascular invasion, are not related to the prognosis [17]. Since the tumor has a mild biological character and is usually localized and well encapsulated, tissue-preserving tumor removal is feasible. Under such circumstances, tumor enucleation may be possible. A spleen-preserving distal pancreatectomy is also feasible for tumors located in the body or tail, and a pylorus-preserving pancreaticoduodenectomy is suitable for tumors located in the head. Limited surgery seems to be currently in vogue; a laparoscopic approach could be used in patients for whom enucleation or distal pancreatectomy is considered [18]. Extensive lymph node clearance or more radical approaches are not always necessary since, in approximately 85% of patients, the SPT is limited to the pancreas. However, in about 10% to 15% of patients, metastases to extra-pancreatic tissues have already developed at the time of clinical presentation. The most common sites of metastasis are the liver, regional lymph nodes, mesentery, omentum, and peritoneum [19, 20]. Although there is no one particular approach to the treatment of lymph node, liver, and other organ metastases, many surgeons agree that surgical debulking, such as hepatic resection or tumor enucleation, is required. Papavramidis reported an overall 2-year survival rate of 97% and a 5-year survival rate of about 95% [5]. In our experience, all tumors were removed surgically along with lymph node clearance near the tumor, and all patients have achieved long-term survival without recurrent disease. Thus, tumor removal along with lymph node clearance is our basic treatment policy for SPT. In addition, persistent patient follow-up is important, since recurrent lesions may develop in 2-6% of elderly patients 7 to 8 years after tumor removal [21, 22].

Several interesting cases have been reported in which the tumors had been treated by neo-adjuvant chemotherapy and radiotherapy, since the tumors were unresectable due to their locally advanced condition. After reducing tumor size with chemotherapy employing cis-platinum and 5-fluorouracil [23], or gemcitabine [24], the tumors were removed successfully. Thus, even a patient with a large SPT that appears unresectable may be cured.

In conclusion, pancreatic SPT is a rare and low-grade malignant tumor of unknown etiology that typically occurs in young females. It is diagnosed according to its characteristic imaging and pathological features, which include a large well-encapsulated mass with solid and cystic components caused by hemorrhage. Since surgical removal of the primary tumor and metastatic lesions improves patient survival, surgeons, radiologists, and pathologists should be aware of this entity, as they play an important role in ensuring that patients with SPT receive appropriate treatment.

References

[1] MorohashiT, Held G, Kloppel G. Exocrine pancreatic tumors and their histological classification: a study based on 167 autopsy and 97 surgical cases. *Histopathology.* 1983; 7: 645-661.

[2] Frantz VK. Papillary tumors of the pancreas: Benign or malignant? Tumors of the pancreas. Atlas of the tumor Pathology, 1st Series, Fascicles 27 and 28. Frantz VK (ed). Washinton. DC, *Armed Forces Institute of Pathology,* 1951:32-33.

[3] Kloppel G, Morohashi T, John HD, Oehmichen W, Opitz K, Angelkort A, Lietz H, Rückert K. Solid and cystic acinar cell tumour of the pancreas. A tumour in young women with favourable prognosis. *Virchows Arch. A Pathol. Anat. Histol.* 1981;392:171-183.

[4] Kloppel G, Solcia E, Longnecker DS, Capella C, Sobin LH. World Health Organization, Institutional histological classification of the Tumors. Histological Typing of Tumors of the Exocrine Pancreas, 2nd ed. Springer-Verlag, Berlin, 1996.

[5] Papavramidis T, Papavramidis S. Solid pseudopapillary tumors of the pancreas: review of 718 patients reported in English literature. *J. Am. Cioll. Surg.* 2005; 200: 965-972.

[6] Huang HL, Shih SC, Chang WH, Wang TE, Chen MJ, Chan J. Solid-pseudopapillary tumor of the pancreas: Clinical experience and literature review. *World J. Gastroenterol.* 2005; 11: 1403-1409.

[7] Crawford BE 2nd. Solid and papillary epithelial neoplasm of the pancreas, diagnosis by cytology. *South. Med. J.* 1998; 91: 973-977.

[8] Rebhandl W, Felberbauer FX, Puig S, Paya K, Hochschorner S, Barlan M, Horcher E. Soid-Pseudopapillary Tumor of the Pancreas (Frantz tumor) in Children: Report of Four Cases and Reviw of the Literature. *J. Surg. Oncol.* 2001; 76: 289-296.

[9] Friedman AC, Lichtenstein JE, Fishman EK, Oertel JE, Dachman AH, Siegelman SS. Solid and papillary epithelial neoplasm of the pancreas. *Radiology.* 1985; 154: 333-337.

[10] Choi BI, Kim KW, Han MC, Kim YI, Kim CW. Solid and Papillary Epithelial Neoplasms of the Pancreas: CT FIndinfs. *Radiology.* 1988; 166: 413-416.

[11] Dong PR, Lu DS, Degregario F, Fell SC, Au A, Kadell BM. Solid and papillary neoplasm of the pancreas: radiological - pathological study of five cases and review of the literature. *Clin. Radiol.* 1996; 51: 702-705.

[12] Cantisani V, Mortele KJ, Levy A, Glickman JN, Ricci P, Passariello R, Ros PR, Silverman SG. MR imaging features of solid pseudopapillary tumor of the pancreas in adult and pediatric patients. *Am. J. Roentgenol.* 2003; 181: 395-401.

[13] Pettinato G, Manivel JC, Ravetto C, Terracciano LM, Gould EW, di Tuoro A, Jaszcz W, Albores-Saavedra J. Papillary cystic tumor of the pancreas. A clinicopathologic study of 20 cases with cytologic, immunohistochemical, ultrastructural, and flow cytometric observations, and a review of the literature. *Am. J. Clin. Pathol.* 1992; 98: 478-488.

[14] Nishihara K, Nagoshi M, Tsuneyoshi M, Yamaguchi K, Hayashi I. Papillary cystic tumors of the pancreas. Assessment of their malignant potential. *Cancer.* 1993;71:82-92.

[15] Martin RC, Klimstra DS, Brennan MF, Conlon KC. Solid-pseudopapillary umor of the pancreas: a surgical enigma? *Ann. Surg. Oncol.* 2002; 9: 35-40.

[16] Kusmahl M, Seada LS, Janig U, Harms D, Kloppel G. Solid-pseudopapillary tumor of the pancreas: its origin revisited. *Virchows Arch.* 2000;436: 473-480.

[17] Adair CF, Wenig BM, Haffess CS. Solid and papillary cystic carcinoma of the pancreas: a tumor of low malignant potential. *Int. J. Surg. Pathol.* 1995;2:326.

[18] Carricaburu E, Enezian G, Bonnard A, Berrebi D, Belarbi N, Hout O, et al. Laparoscopic distal pancreatectomy for Frantz's tumor in a child. *Surg. Endosc.* 2003;17:2028-2031.

[19] Mao C, Guvendi M, Donenico DR, Kim K, Thomford NR, Howard JM. Papillary cystic and solid tumors of the pancreas: a pancreatic embryonic tumor? Studies of three cases and cumulative review of the world's literature. *Surgery.* 1995; 188: 821-828.

[20] Andronikou S, Moon A, Ussher R. Peritoneal metastatic disease in a child after excision of a solid pseudopapillary tumour of the pancreas: a unique case. *Pediatr. Radiol.* 2003; 33: 269-271.

[21] Matsunou H, Konishi F. Papillary-cystic neoplasm of the pancreas. A clinicopathologic study concerning the tumor aging and malignancy of nine cases. *Cancer.* 1990; 65: 283-291.

[22] Avdiner F, Erinanç H, Savaş B, Erden E, Karayalçin K. Solid pseudopapillary tumor of the pancreas: emphasis on differential diagnosis from aggressive tumors of the pancreas. *Turk. J. Gastroenterol.* 2006; 17: 219-222.

[23] Strauss JF, Hirsch VJ, Rubey CN, Pollock M. Resection of a Solid and Papillary Epithelial Neoplasm of the Pancreas Following Treatment With Cis-Platinum and 5-Fluorouracl: A Case Report. *Medical and Pediatric Oncology.* 1993; 21:365-367.

[24] Maffuz A, Bustamante F, Silva A, Vargas ST. Preoperative gemcitabine for unresectable, solid psudopapillary tumour of the pancreas. *Lancet Oncol.* 2005; 6: 185-186.

In: Cancer in Female Adolescents
Editor: Margarite T. Moorland

ISBN: 978-1-60456-421-1

Chapter VI

Early Puberty Onset and Female Cancers—Is There a Link?

Christian L. Roth[1*] and Claudio Mastronardi[2*]
[1]Division of Endocrinology, Seattle Children's Hospital Research Institute, WA, USA
[2]Department of Psychiatry, University of Miami, FL, USA

Introduction

Breast cancer etiology researchers and those examining puberty regulation may think they have little in common, yet the conclusion that, "...breast feeding and late age at menarche protect against both ER^+PR^+ and ER^-PR^- breast cancer" (estrogen/progesterone receptor status) from the 2006 publication of Ma et al. a meta-analysis of reproductive factors and breast cancer risk [1] would argue otherwise. In a number of studies, early menarche has been identified as an important risk factor for breast cancer which has been explained by increased hormonal exposure. But among monozygotic twins, this risk becomes much stronger, implicating genetic factors as well [2]. The focus of recent female cancer epidemiological study designs has shifted from adult cohort studies to the ontogeny of female reproductive organs [2–5], presenting potential causal data either leading to or resulting from precocious puberty, late versus early breast development, parity and age at first birth.

In a recent microarray gene expression study we found a group of related genes known to regulate the cell cycle and suppression of tumor growth (termed tumor related genes or TRGs) to be one of the most prominent groups of genes to increase hypothalamic expression throughout female puberty [6]. When the above factors are considered within the context of the newly unveiled hypothalamic polygenic TRG network, compelling research questions

* Address all correspondence and requests for reprints to: Christian L. Roth, MD; Division of Endocrinology; Seattle Children's Hospital Research Institute; 1900 Ninth Avenue, Seattle, WA 98101; E-mail: christian.roth@seattlechildrens.org; Tel: +1 (206) 9875428; Fax: +1 (206) 9877661

* Claudio Mastronardi, PhD; Department of Psychiatry, University of Miami, Miami, Florida 33101; E-mail: CMastronardi@med.miami.edu

demanding multi-dimensional approaches emerge to investigate possible links. They also cast new hope for understanding and managing cancer predispositions as we expand the dimensions and details regarding this genetic network operating within the neuroendocrine brain.

Physiological Regulation of Puberty

Physiologically, gonadotropin secretion is elevated during neonatal development and early childhood, presumably as a consequence of enhanced pulsatile release of gonadotropin releasing hormone (GnRH), also known as luteinizing hormone-releasing hormone (LHRH). This phase of increased activity is followed by a rather protracted pause during childhood, which ends with the reactivation of the pulse generator at the beginning of the second decade of postnatal life. Such a change in pulsatile gonadotropin secretion is necessary for normal gonadal development and function. GnRH secretion is regulated by both transsynaptic and glial inputs. The search for the neuronal networks most critically involved in controlling GnRH release during sexual development includes systems that utilize excitatory/inhibitory amino acids, and the recently identified neuropeptide metastin/kisspeptin [6-8] for neurotransmission. Cell-cell signaling molecules which are produced in astroglial cells have now been identified and in silico analyses of genomes are being employed to define the physiological contribution of these molecules to the pubertal process.

Female Cancers in Industrialized Nations

The specter of female cancers in industrialized nations is alarming: breast cancer causes the highest female mortality due to cancer in developed countries, it is the most common non-skin cancer among women in the United States [4] and in the 40 years between 1960 and 2000, its incidence doubled in most areas as mortality continued to increase despite herculean efforts to combat this disease [9]. Coupled with these data is the fact that primary carcinoma of the ovary is the fourth most common cancer among women in the United Kingdom [5]. An intriguing Belgian study published this year surveyed birth to puberty (mean age 13 y) parental and lifestyle data of 1146 girls [3]. Their basal study platform was that earlier menarche in the Western hemisphere is associated with earlier onset of hyperinsulinemia, with numerous case-control studies reporting fasting hyperinsulinemia as a marker of increased breast cancer risk [10] and they wanted to investigate the sequence of endocrine events in early life. An increased body-mass index (BMI), whether familially predispositioned (implied by higher weight of mother at beginning of pregnancy) or life-style induced (correlating with sugar-sweetened drinks known to be associated with obesity in children [11]), was significantly related with both early breast development and menarche. Early menarche, as well as increased height and weight, are all recognized as important determinants for breast cancer [12,13]. This seems to be BMI-specific as tall girls at birth, girls with tall parents, and girls engaging in physical activity all had a trend toward delayed age at menarche. As insulin is one of the key factors in human breast development, it follows that inappropriate secretion of insulin might induce lesions in breast cells which could lead to breast cancer later in life [14]. In addition to classical risk factors for breast cancer, the metabolic syndrome, obesity, type 2 diabetes, hyperinsulinemia, overstimulation of the breast epithelium by estrogens and testosterone, plus direct and indirect effects of altered adipocytokine production on mammary tissue are discussed as additional breast cancer risk factors [15]. Aromatase activity in adipose tissue converts androstenedione secreted by the adrenal gland into estrone by aromatase in adipose tissue stroma, leading to increased estrogen levels, especially in obese postmenopausal women. But younger obese women are also vulnerable to increased estrogen levels. At certain risk are premenopausal African American women who have lower sex-hormone binding globulin levels (SHBG) compared to caucasian women and tend to have upper body obesity, both of which are factors that increase levels of circulating biologically active estrogen [16]. Insulin might promote breast cancer by causing a reduction in SHBG production or inducing aromatase activity, leading to estrogen production and stimulation of breast cancer cell growth by endocrine, paracrine or autocrine mechanisms [17,18].

Newly Discovered Genes in the Regulation of Puberty

In an attempt to unlock some of these mysteries related to genes that are involved in the onset of puberty, we employed new systems biology technology and developed a hierarchically arranged gene network underlying female puberty in the monkey [6]. Moreover, our examination of changes in gene expression in the rodent hypothalamus at the time of female puberty resulted in similar findings. Selected genes from the microarray experiments were validated by real-time PCR and localization of the sites of brain expression of these genes was performed by *in situ* hybridization. Using "guilt-by-association" and "retrospective" approaches and bioinformatics, a hierarchically arranged gene set containing five major hubs was revealed (CDP/CUTL1, MAF, p53, YYi, and USF2) controlling the hypothalamic TRG network at the transcriptional level, hubs which in turn are heavily connected to non-TRGs involved in the pubertal process. The guilt-by-association approach led us to the examination of p53 which is one of the most prominent suppressor genes in cancers and central to maintaining cellular differentiation by regulating expression of hundreds of downstream genes [7,19]. We found that p53 increased specifically in the hypothalamus but not in the cerebral cortex [6].

Tumor Related Genes and Genes Associated with Female Cancers Expressed in the Hypothalamus

When the gene expression profiles were performed we uncovered eleven genes associated to the TRG network that were also involved in the regulation of female puberty. Six of these eleven genes were identified as tumor suppressor genes (TSGs) and the remaining five were identified as oncogenes [6]. The recent overwhelming evidence that one of the major stimulatory inputs triggering the onset of puberty is exerted by one of these TSGs, kisspeptin, a metastasis suppressor peptide whose biological roles were mainly studied until recently in the context of tumor suppression upon binding to its G-coupled protein receptor 54 (GPR54), constituted the first landmark that related a TSG with the onset of puberty [20–23]. This foundation stone for our emerging concept of the TRG network regulating female puberty was concomitantly laid by two research teams in 2003 when they reported that inactivating mutations in GPR54 were associated with hypogonadotropic hypogonadism in humans [24,25]. Moreover, subsequent studies carried-out in the rhesus monkey model have shown that GPR54 and KiSS-1 are expressed in the mediobasal hypothalamus (MBH) and their expression within the MBH increases at the time of the pubertal increase of GnRH release [23].

Of the eleven TRGs showing a hypothalamic-specific pubertal increase in expression, two TSGs (SASH1 and CUTL1) and two oncogenes (CCND1 and AF1Q) have been identified to be altered in breast and/or ovarian carcinoma [26-30]. SASH1 (containing SAM And SH3 domains-1) encodes a protein that participates in signal transduction to maintain differentiated functions and has been shown to be down-regulated in a majority of breast cancer cases [26]. Like other proteins containing SH3 and SAM domains (including Eph receptors and ETS transcription factors), SASH1 appears to maintain differentiated functions via protein-protein interactions related to signal transduction [26,27]. CUTL1 (CDP/cux), an evolutionary conserved homeobox gene, has been shown to function as a transcriptional repressor in several systems [28] and has been identified as a TSG in occurrences of breast cancer. Interestingly, CUTL1-null mutant has also been shown to exhibit a severe reduction in male fertility [29], suggesting that this gene encodes a protein that exerts stimulatory input during the onset of puberty. In addition, CUTL1-null mutant has also been shown to display defects in skin and lung development [29,30].

CCND1 (cyclin D1), shown to be a positive regulator of the start checkpoint in the cell cycle [31], has been found to be overexpressed in both breast [32,33] and ovarian cancer [34,35]. The idea that CCND1 plays non-pathogenic roles in neuroendocrinological events is supported by the fact that even though deregulation of cyclin D1 has been shown to result in unchecked cell growth and division, expression of cyclin D1 appears to be associated with growth factor-dependent neuronal differentiation in the mature brain [36,37]. The overexpression of the fourth TRG network gene associated with female cancers, AF1Q (ALL1-fused gene from chromosome 1q), has been implicated in the progression of human breast cancer through a mechanism that involves, at least in part, the regulation of the expression of integrin alpha3, transcription factor ETS1 and matrix metalloproteinase MMP-2 [37-39].

The TSGs identified by retrospective examination of the literature and the guilt-by-association approach were examined to test the possibility that changes in the expression of the four TRG discussed in the previous section—given their non-pathogenic involvement in the regulation of female puberty as well as their pathological expression in female cancers—could reflect a larger cluster of functionally connected TRGs in the neuroendocrine brain. These three genes were the previously mentioned p53 whose expression has been shown to be altered in several types of malignancies, including ovarian [34] and breast cancers [19];

SynCam, a TSG which has been shown to play a major role in the onset of puberty in mutant mice displaying an aberrant erbB4-directed signaling in astrocytes and whose expression has been shown to be downregulated in breast cancer [40] and possibly also in ovarian cancer [41]; and DNMT1, which encodes the most important enzyme in cytosine methylation-dependent TSG silencing [42] and has also been associated with ovarian [43] and breast cancers [44].

Role of the TRG Network in Cell Cycle and Hypothalamic Activity

Basically, the proteins encoded by tumor suppressor genes (TSGs) protect the cells from undergoing malignant transformation by exerting repressive effects on the regulation of the cell cycle, causing cell arrest and/or promoting programmed cell death. A major action of TSGs is to protect the organism by impeding the division of cells that have undergone mutagenic events. If this molecular damage is reparable, the cell cycle continues. If the genetic damage cannot be repaired, the cell initiates programmed cell death to remove the perceived threat it poses to the organism. Generally, it is believed that TSGs acquire loss of function by inactivating mutations or deletions that block their biological activity to protect and/or rescue the cell from genetic deleterious events. Alternatively, TSGs may undergo aberrant promoter methylation, producing "gene silencing" which leads to a similar inactivating effect.

Evidence to date suggests that in normal individuals, the TRG network exerts an overall inhibitory action on the onset of puberty that is partly counterbalanced by the action of some of the components of this network that trigger an opposite, stimulatory, effect (see also our model Fig. 1). However, the possibility also exists that as genes with tumor-promoting activity become activated at puberty in the presence of hormonal influences (e.g. estrogen) favoring the initiation of malignant growth, there is a concomitant upregulation of TSG expression to maintain the developmental process focused on differentiated functions, rather than on proliferative activity.

The physiological importance of this tightly regulated balance among stimulatory and inhibitory inputs is probably associated with the central morphological changes that occur within the mediobasal hypothalamus during sexual development. It is also likely that growth factors such as neuregulins (NRGs) which induce cell growth and differentiation [45] and insulin-like growth factor I [46] which have been shown to play important central stimulatory roles within the mediobasal hypothalamus during sexual maturation orchestrate, at least in part, some of the changes occurring in these tumor related genes (TRGs). Interestingly, but at this point not so surprisingly, these growth factors have also been shown to increase tumorigenesis in different types of cancers, including ovarian and breast carcinoma [47–50].

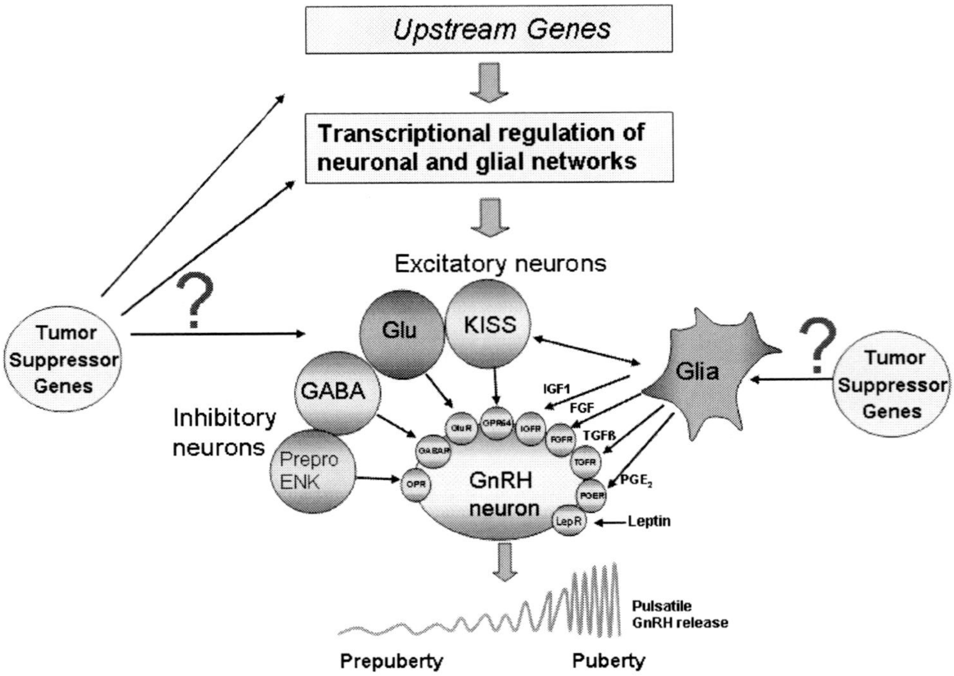

Figure 1. Schematic overview on the transcriptional control of the GnRH neuronal network at puberty by "upper-echelon" genes. Changes in the secretory activity of GnRH neurons are specified by neuronal and glial inputs. Physiological modification of these inputs requires a host of subordinate genes that, differentially expressed in neurons and glia, are necessary for the integration of neuron-to neuron, glia-neuron, and glia-to-glia communication. In turn, upper-echelon genes control expression of these subordinate genes at the transcriptional level. It is envisioned that tumor suppressor genes might interact on different levels of this hierarchical arrangement. GABA: GABAergic neurons, GLU: glutamatergic neurons, PreproENK: opiatergic neurons, KISS: KISS neurons (see references 6, 7, 13).

Conclusion

It has now been discovered that about 10% of hypothalamic genes that increase their expression at the time of puberty are genes previously implicated in tumorigenesis or tumor suppression. The mechanism needs to be further elucidated as these genes appear to have non-pathogenic functions beyond their tumor regulation roles, playing a part in the normal regulatory GnRH regulating network. This network is specifically activated around puberty, coordinating expression and transcription of downstream components. Given the massive cell building that occurs at the onset of and throughout puberty and again during pregnancy, their activation could also be to modulate the effects of sex steroids leading to maturation of the hypothalamic network. Although there are some limitations, as gene profiling using mRNA depends on changes in patterns of gene expression, the bioinformatics high-throughput approach that uncovered the TRG hypothalamic network is a powerful tool, and the identification of genes involved in both tumor regulation as well as female puberty begs the question of a cancer presupposition in cases of pubescent morbidities occurring in this complex neuroendocrine regulatory network [13], especially given the extreme vulnerability of the human juvenile breast for toxins such as radiation, unbalanced hormones, and nutrition [14]. Associations between early menarche and breast cancer may occur as a result of different genotypes in the TRG network. It would be intriguing to explore in large field studies whether abnormal early onset of puberty might be an indicator for a genetically-determined higher risk of cancer, even though some of the responsible genes are not yet known.

All of this and more weighs heavily toward the hypothetical conclusion that major components of the TRG network constitute an "endogenous physiological brake" system to ensure that stimulatory input triggering the onset of puberty exerted by growth factors occurs without eliciting an undesirable exacerbated cell proliferation. In view of the emerging stage of the TRG brain network, clearly more studies will be necessary to establish if indeed, and if so to what extent, a functional relationship between early puberty and the development of breast and ovarian cancers exists. What is clear is that these new research directions and unveilings cast fresh hope for understanding and managing of potential cancer predispositions as we expand the dimensions and details regarding this genetic network operating within the neuroendocrine brain that could also result in a predictive treatment model for patients.

References

[1] Ma H, Bernstein L, Pike MC, Ursin G 2006 Reproductive factors and breast cancer risk according to joint estrogen and progesterone receptor status: a meta-analysis of epidemiological studies. *Breast Cancer Res.* 8:R39

[2] Hamilton AS, Mack TM 2003 Puberty and genetic susceptibility to breast cancer in a case-control study in twins. *N. Engl. J. Med.* 348:2313-2322

[3] Vandeloo M, Bruckers LM, Janssens JP 2007 Effects of lifestyle on the onset of puberty as determinant for breast cancer. *Eur. J. Cancer Prev.* 16:17–25

[4] Fenton SE 2006 Endocrine-Disrupting Compounds and Mammary Gland Development: Early Exposure and Later Life Consequences. *Endocrinology.* 147 (Supplement):S18–S24

[5] Elmasry K, Gayther SA 2006 Ovarian cancer aetiology: facts and fiction. *J. Fam. Plann. Reprod. Health Care.* 32:82–86

[6] Roth CL, Mastronardi C, Lomniczi A, Wright H, Cabrera R, Mungenast AE, Heger S, Jung H, Dubay C, Ojeda SR 2007 Expression of a tumor-related gene network increases in the mammalian hypothalamus at the time of female puberty. *Endocrinology.* 148:5147-5161

[7] Ojeda SR, Roth C, Mungenast A, Heger S, Mastronardi C, Parent AS, Lomniczi A, Jung H 2006 Neuroendocrine mechanisms controlling female puberty: new approaches, new concepts. *Int. J. Androl.* 29:256-263

[8] Seminara SB 2005 Metastin and its G protein-coupled receptor, GPR54: critical pathway modulating GnRH secretion. *Front. Neuroendocrinol.* 26:131-138

[9] Coebergh JW 2003 Early breast cancer in Europe: progress and pitfalls in detection and management at the start of the new century *Eur. J. Cancer.* 39:1645-1647

[10] Fairfield KM, Hankinson SE, Rosner BA, Hunter DJ, Colditz GA, Wilett WC 2001 Risk of ovarian carcinoma and comsumption of vitamins A, C, and E and specific carotenoids: a prospective analysis. *Cancer.* 92:2318–2326

[11] Bray GA 2002 The underlying basis for obesity: relationship to cancer. *J. Nutr.* 2002 132:3451S-3455S

[12] Risch HA, Howe GR 1995 Pelvic inflammatory disease and the risk of epithelial ovarian cancer. *Cancer Epidemiol. Biomarkers Prev.* 4:447–451

[13] Ojeda SR, Lomniczi A, Mastronardi C, Heger S, Roth CL, Parent AS, Matagne V, Mungenast AE 2005 Minireview: The neuroendocrine regulation of puberty: Is the time ripe for a systems biology approach? *Endocrinology.* 147:1166–1174

[14] Baanders AN, de Waard F 1992 Breast cancer in Europe. The importance of factors operating at an early age. *Eur. J. Cancer Prev.* 1:285–291

[15] Rose DP, Haffner SM,. Baillargeon 2007 Adiposity, the Metabolic Syndrome, and Breast Cancer in African-American and White American Women. *Endocrine Reviews.* 28: 763-777

[16] Berman DM, Rodrigues LM, Nicklas BJ, Ryan AS, Dennis KE, Goldberg AP 2001 Racial disparities in metabolism, central obesity, and sex hormone-binding globulin in postmenopausal women. *J. Clin. Endocrinol. Metab.* 86:97–103

[17] Plymate SR, Matej LA, Jones RE, Friedl KE 1988 Inhibition of sex hormone-binding globulin production in the human hepatoma (Hep G2) cell line by insulin and prolactin. *J. Clin. Endocrinol. Metab.* 67:460–464

[18] Ternan PG, Anwar A, Eggo MC, Barnett AH, Stewart PM, Kumar S 2000 Gender differences in the regulation of P450 aromatase expression and activity in human adipose tissue. *Int. J. Obes. Relat. Metab. Disord.* 24:875–881

[19] Vogelstein B, Lane D, Levine AJ 2000 Surfing the p53 network. *Nautre.* 408:307–310

[20] Gottsch ML, Cunningham MJ, Smith JT, Popa SM, Acohido BV, Crowley WF, Seminara S, Clifton DK, Steiner RA. 2004 A role for kisspeptins in the regulation of gonadotropin secretion in the mouse. *Endocrinology.* 145:4073–4077

[21] Irwig MS, Fraley G S, et al. 2004 Kisspeptin activation of gonadotropin releasing hormone neurons and regulation of KiSS-1 mRNA in the male rat. *Neuroendocrinology.* 80:264–272

[22] Navarro VM, Fernández-Fernández R, Castellano JM, Roa J, Mayen A, Barreiro ML,Gaytan F, Aguilar E, Pinilla L, Dieguez C, Tena-Sempere M 2004 Advanced vaginal opening and precocious activation of the reproductive axis by KiSS-1 peptide, the endogenous ligand of GPR54. *J. Physiol.* 561:379-386.

[23] Shahab M, Matronardi C, Seminara SB, Crowley WF, Ojeda SR, Plant TM 2005 Increased hypothalamic GPR54 signaling: a potential mechanism for initiation of puberty in primates. *Prc. Natl. Acad. Sci. USA.* 102:2129–2134

[24] de Roux N, Genin E, Carel J-C, Matsuda F, Chaussain J-L, Milgrom E 2003 Hypogonadotropic hypogonadism due to loss of function of the KiSS1-derived peptide receptor GPR54. *Proc. Natl. Acad. Sci. USA.* 100:10972–10976

[25] Seminara SB, Messager S, Chatzidaki EE, Thresher RR, Aciemo Jr JS, Shagoury JK, Bo-Abbas Y, Kuohung W, Schwinof KM, Hendrick AG, Zahn D, Dixon J, Haiser UB, Slaugenhaupt SA, Gusella JF, O'Rahilly S, Carlton MB, Crowley Jr WF, Aparicio SA, Colledge WH 2003 The GPR54 gene as a regulatory of puberty. *N. Engl. J. Med.* 349:1614–1627

[26] Zeller C, Hinzmann B, Seitz S, Prokoph H, Burkhard-Goettges E, Fischer J, Jandrig B, Schwarz L-E, Rosenthal A, Scherneck S 2003 SASH1: a candidate tumor suppressor gene on chromosome 6q24.3 is downregulated in breast cancer. *Oncogene.* 22:2972–2983

[27] Claudio JO, Zhu YX, Benn SJ, Skukla AH, McGlade CJ, Falcioni N, Stewart AK 2001 HACS1 encodes a novel SH3-SAM adaptor protein differentially expressed in normal and malignant hematopoietic cells. *Oncogene.* 20:5373–5377

[28] Nepveu A 2001 Role of the multifunctional CDP/Cut/Cux homeodomain transcription factor in regulating differentiation, cell growth and development. *Gene.* 270:1–15

[29] Luong MX, van der Meijden CM, Xing DX, Hesselton R, Monuki ES, Jones SN, Lian JB, Stein JL, Stein GS, Neufeld EJ, van Wijnen AJ 2002 Genetic ablation of the CDP/Cux protein C terminus results in hair cycle defects and reduced male fertility. *Mol. Cell Biol.* 22:1424–1437

[30] Ellis T, Gambardella L, Horcher M, Tschanz S, Capol J, Bertram P, Jochum W, Barrandon Y, Busslinger M 2001 The Transcriptional repressor CDP (Cutl1) is essential for epithelial cell differentiation of the lung and the hair follicle. *Genes Dev.* 15:2307–2319

[31] Hunter T, Pines J 1994 Cyclins and cancer. II. Cyclin D and CDK inhibitors come of age. *Cell.* 79:573–582

[32] Chodosh LA 2002 The reciprocal dance between cancer and development. *N. Engl. J. Med.* 347:134–136

[33] Roy PG, Thompson AM 2006 Cyclin D1 and breast cancer. *Breast.* 15:718–727

[34] Shigemasa K, Tanimoto H, Parham GP, Parmley TH, Ohama K, O'Brien TJ 1999 Cyclin D1 overexpression and p53 mutation status in epithelial ovarian cancer. *J. Soc. Gynecol. Investig.* 6:102–108

[35] Barbieri F, Lorenzi P, Ragni N, Schettini G, Bruzzo C, Pedullà F, Alama A 2004 Overexpression of cyclin D1 is associated with poor survival in epithelial ovarian cancer. *Oncology.* 66:310–315

[36] Yan G Z, Ziff EB 1995 NGF regulates the PC12 cell cycle machinery through specific inhibition of the Cdk kinases and induction of cyclin D1. *J. Neurosci.* 15:6200–6212

[37] Xiong W, Pestell R, Rosner MR 1997 Role of cyclins in neuronal differentiation of immortalized hippocampal cells. *Mol. Cell Biol.* 17:6585–6597

[38] Li D-Q, Hou Y-F, Wu J, Chen Y, Lu J-S , Di G-H , Ou Z-L , Shen Z-Z , Ding J, Shao Z-M 2006 Gene expression profile analysis of an isogenic tumour metastasis model reveals a functional role for oncogene AF1Q in breast cancer metastasis. *Eur. J. Cancer.* 42:3274–3286

[39] Chang, XZ, Li DQ, Hou YF, Wu J, Lu JS, Di GH, Jin W, Ou ZL, Shen ZZ, Shao ZM 2007 Identification of the functional role of AF1Q in the progression of breast cancer. *Breast Cancer Res. Treat.* [Epub ahead of print]

[40] Heller G, Geradts J, Ziegler B, Newsham I, Filipits M, Markis-Ritzinger EM, Kandioler D, Berger W, Stiglbauer W, Depisch D, Pirker R, Zielinski CC,Zöchbauer-Müller S 2007 Downregulation of TSLC1 and DAL-1 expression occurs frequently in breast cancer. *Breast Cancer Res. Treat.* 103:283–291

[41] Fukami T, Fukuhara H, Kuramochi M, Maruyama T, Isogai K, Sakamoto M, Takamoto S, Murakami Y 2003 Promoter methylation of the TSLC1 gene in advanced lung tumors and various cancer cell lines. *Int. J. Cancer.* 107:53-59

[42] Robert MF, Morin S, Beaulieu N, Gauthier F, Chute IC, Barsalou A, MacLeod AR 2003 DNMT1 is required to maintain CpG methylation and aberrant gene silencing in human cancer cells. *Nat. Genet.* 33(1):61-65

[43] Chen CL, Yan X, Gao YN, Liao QP 2005 Expression of DNA methyltransferase 1, 3A and 3B mRNA in the epithelial ovarian carcinoma. *Zhonghua Fu. Chan. Ke Za Zhi.* 40:770–774

[44] Agoston AT, Argani P, Yegnasubramanian S, De Marzo AM, Ansari-Lari MA, Hicks JL, Davidson NE, Nelson WG 2005 Increased protein stability causes DNA methyltransferase 1 dysregulation in breast cancer. *J. Biol. Chem.* 280:18302–18310

[45] Ojeda SR, Prevot V, Heger S, Lomniczi A, Dziedzic B, Mungenast A 2003 Glia-to-neuron signaling and the neuroendocrine control of female puberty. *Ann. Med.* 35:244–255

[46] Hiney JK, Srivastava V, Nyberg CL, Ojeda SR, Dees WL 1996 Insulin-like growth factor I of peripheral origin acts centrally to accelerate the initiation of female puberty. *Endocrinology.* 137:3717–3728

[47] Karasik A, Menczer J, Pariente C, Kanety H 1994 Insulin-like growth factor-I (IGF-I) and IGF-binding protein-2 are increased in cyst fluids of epithelial ovarian cancer. *J. Clin. Endocrinol. Metab.* 78:271–276

[48] Hankinson SE, Willett WC, Colditz GA, Hunter DJ, Michaud DS, Deroo B, Rosner B, Speizer FE, Pollak M 1998 Circulating concentrations of insulin-like growth factor-I and risk of breast cancer. *Lancet.* 351:1393–1396

[49] Li Q, Ahmed S, Loeb JA 2004 Development of an autocrine neuregulin signaling loop with malignant transformation of human breast epithelial cells. *Cancer Res.* 64:7078–7085

[50] Renehan AG., Zwahlen M, Minder C, O'Dwyer ST, Shalet SM, Egger M 2004 Insulin-like growth factor (IGF)-I, IGF binding protein-3, and cancer risk: systematic review and meta-regression analysis. *Lancet.* 363:1346–1353

In: Cancer in Female Adolescents
Editor: Margarite T. Moorland

ISBN: 978-1-60456-421-1

Chapter VII

Ovarian Malignancies in Adolescents – A Pathologic Perspective

***Atif Ali Ahmed**[*1] **and Debra S. Heller**[2]*

Departments of Pathology,

[1] Children's National Medical Center, Washington, DC and

[2] University of Medicine and Dentistry, Newark, New Jersey

Abstract

Ovarian masses in children and adolescents are a heterogeneous group of lesions that are predominantly neoplastic. Ovarian malignancies are uncommon, accounting for 1% of all malignant pediatric neoplasms. The pathology of ovarian neoplasms differs significantly from those occurring in adults. The majority of ovarian neoplasms in the pediatric and adolescent age group are of germ cell origin, as opposed to the predominance of surface epithelial-derived neoplasms in adults. Metastatic tumors to the ovary such as rhabdomyosarcoma are rare and are often bilateral.

Ovarian tumors usually present as abdominal or pelvic masses and may secrete hormones and other tumor markers that help in preoperative diagnosis and monitoring. However, preoperative evaluation alone is insufficient in the evaluation of these neoplasms. Pathology of the resected ovarian tissue remains an important tool for accurate diagnosis and staging. Histology with the aid of immunohistochemistry, as well as chromosomal karyotyping in some cases is an important tool in making accurate diagnosis and predicting patient's prognosis.

[*] Corresponding Address: Atif Ali Ahmed, MD; Anatomic Pathology; 111 Michigan Avenue, NW; Washington, DC 20010; T: 202-476-2051; F: 202-476-4030; E-mail: aahmed@cnmc.org

Introduction

Ovarian masses in children and adolescents are heterogenous group of lesions and are mostly neoplastic. The majority of these neoplasms are benign and only 10-30% are malignant. Ovarian cancer is one of the most common causes of cancer deaths in adults. In children, malignant ovarian neoplasms constitute only 1% of all pediatric malignancies [1,2]. However this percentage may not be entirely accurate as the distinction between benign and malignant tumors is frequently blurred. Malignant tumor foci can frequently develop in otherwise benign tumors. Similarly other tumors may have spectrum of behavioral patterns depending on their degree of differentiation and rate of proliferation. The incidence of ovarian neoplasia is higher in western countries compared to African or Asian countries. Ovarian tumors in children and adolescents are more frequently seen in non-white population than whites.

Few types of ovarian neoplasia have familial or genetic association. Examples include patients with gonadal dysgenesis (chromosomal karyotypes 46,XY and mosaic 45,X/46,XY) who are more likely to develop gonadoblastoma. Increased incidence of benign ovarian tumors such as Sertoli cell tumor and fibroma occurs in patients with Peutz-Jeghers syndrome and nevoid basal cell carcinoma syndrome respectively. BRCA1 and BRCA2 gene mutations do not play a major role in the pathogenesis of ovarian malignancies in children, as these are mostly of germ cell origin. Similarly, environmental factors that are known to influence the development of ovarian neoplasia in adults [3] have much less role to play in children, simply because of limited exposure duration time. However, obesity was mentioned a possible contributing factor to the causation of ovarian cancers in adolescents [4].

Most patients with ovarian neoplasia present as stage I disease with abdominal or adnexal mass. Patients may also have abdominal pain simulating the pain of acute appendicitis. The presence of ascites, vaginal bleeding or urinary symptoms correlates with locally spreading disease. The development of virilization and/or precocious puberty indicates the presence of hormonally active tumors, particularly sex cord stromal tumors, and necessitate complete endocrinologic evaluation. Serum markers such as CA125, carcinoembryonic antigen, alpha-fetoprotein (AFP) and human chorionic gonadotrophin (β-hCG) may be elevated and may prove useful in initial diagnostic suspicion. These markers, however, proved to be more important in post-surgical fellow-up and monitoring of tumor recurrence. Imaging studies are frequently performed in the preoperative evaluation process. Ultrasound examination, transabdominal or transvaginal, is a safe noninvasive technique that is also useful in differentiating benign from malignant and cystic versus solid lesions [5,6]. In some cases, preoperative evaluation can not distinguish benign from malignant tumors and accurate diagnosis and tumor staging depend largely on pathologic evaluation of the resected specimen.

In this chapter, we review the major malignant pathologic entities in adolescent ovaries in comparison to adults and shed light on the importance of histology in making the diagnosis and judging the prognosis. This review is intended for scientists and researchers aiming at basic understanding of different morphologic types of ovarian tumors in attempt to bridge the gap between molecules, neoplastic cell types and patient's outcome.

Pathogenesis

Ovarian tumors arise from the celomic epithelium, germ cells or stromal cells. Germ cell tumors constitute the majority (>60%) of ovarian cancers in children. Unlike adults, epithelial surface tumors occur in approximately 20% of cases while sex-cord stromal tumors are seen in 15% [1,6]. Most of ovarian tumors in adolescents are benign and only about 4.2 % are malignant.

Tumors can spread to the other ovary and through the lymphatics to the regional lymph nodes. Peritoneal dissemination is a common type of extraovarian spread and results in peritoneal or omental implants that may be invasive and change the prognosis of the patient. Treatment depends largely on accurate staging which also depends on pathologic classification and clinical and histologic extension of the tumor. Detailed staging of ovarian cancer can be found in the American Cancer Society website at: http://www.cancer.org/docroot/CRI/content/CRI_2_4_3X_How_is_ovarian_cancer_staged_33.asp?sitearea=CRI.

Morphology

Germ Cell Tumors

Germ cell tumors account for more than 60% of ovarian tumors in the pediatric population and approximately one-third of these are malignant. Germ cell tumors represent a heterogenous group of neoplasms arising from stem cells that show different levels and different lines of differentiation. The primitive germ cell gives rise to dysgerminoma. Teratoid and endodermal differentiation can result in yolk sac tumor or embryonal carcinoma. Foci of neuroectodermal and trophoblastic differentiation can occur in many germ cell tumors as well. More than 90% of ovarian germ cell tumors are benign and composed of mature teratomatous tissue [7]. Mixed germ cell tumor is the term used when 2 or more germ cell tumors are present. Isochromosome 12p, i(12p) is a cytogenetic structural rearrangement, occasionally found in germ cell tumors, particularly dysgerminomas and malignant germ cell tumors with a yolk sac component. Isochromosome (12p) is, however, more prevalent in testicular rather than ovarian germ cell tumors [7].

Dysgerminoma

Dysgerminoma is the most common malignant tumor of the ovary in children and adolescents [7,8]. The tumor is unilateral in most cases and appears well-encapsulated with fibrous tissue septa. This germ cell tumor has a seminoma-like morphology that is characterized by monomorphic proliferation of germ cells associated with varying amount of infiltrating lymphocytes and macrophages (Figure 1A). Areas of hemorrhage, necrosis, cystic change or calcifications may be present [9]. The tumor cells are characteristically positive for placental alkaline phosphatase (PLAP), CD117 (Figure 1B) and OCT3/4.

Approximately 65% of dysgerminomas present as stage I disease and can be primarily treated with surgery. Advanced stages may require chemotherapy and/or radiotherapy. 10-15% of cases have bilateral tumor in initial diagnosis. In other cases, bilateral disease may later develop in the contralateral ovary after surgical resection of the diseased ovary.

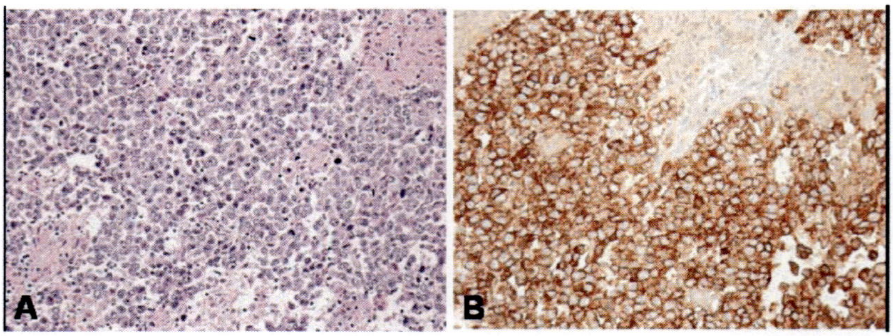

Figure 1. Dysgerminoma forms diffuse sheets of monomorphic cells (figure A, H&E x20) that are frequently infiltrated by lymphocytes. The tumor cells are highlighted with CD117 immunostain (figure B).

Immature Teratoma

Teratoma is the most common neoplasm in the ovary [10]. Most teratomas in the ovaries are mature and contain various endodermal, mesodermal and ectodermal elements. The presence of neuroectodermal elements, in the form of rosettes and tubules, leads to the designation of immature teratoma. The number of microscopic foci with immature elements forms the basis of a grading system that correlates with the prognosis and is often used to guide patient's management (Figure 2). [11]. Immature teratoma is not synonymous with malignant teratoma. The clinical behavior of these tumors will additionally depend on the clinical stage and the concomitant presence of yolk sac components [12,13]. Grade I stage I immature teratoma is expected to have 100% survival and the survival decreases with higher grade and advanced stage.

Malignancy can arise in otherwise mature cystic teratoma. Such malignant transformation is very rare in children but has been well-documented [14]. Carcinomas and glial tumors have been reported to arise within mature cystic teratoma.

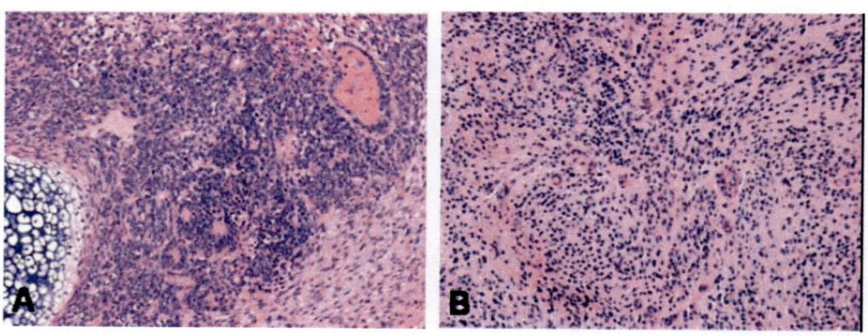

Figure 2. The presence of immature neuroepithelium is the hallmark of immature teratoma, as seen in this patient who presented with ovarian mass and ascites (A, H&Ex20). Peritoneal implants were also present composed of immature glial tissue (B, H&Ex20).

Yolk Sac Tumor

Yolk sac tumor has a heterogenous histologic morphology [15] with multiple lines of differentiation and characteristically expresses AFP. A characteristic histologic reticular pattern is identified by labyrinthine microcystic arrangement of tumor cells in loose myxoid stroma. Numerous and less common histologic variants also exist, including polyvesicular vitelline, solid, intestinal (glandular) and hepatoid variants. Schillar-Duval bodies are characteristic but are less frequently identified. The tumor cells show varying degrees of nuclear atypia and hyperchromatism, and may have eosinophilic hyaline globules in the cytoplasm (Figure 3).

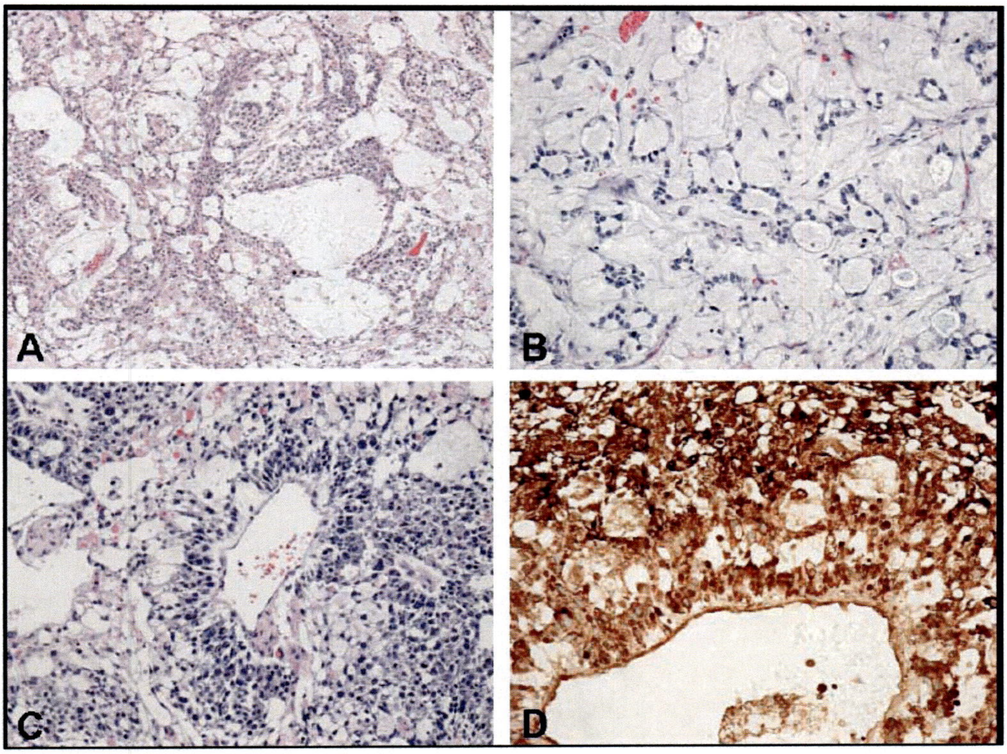

Figure 3. Yolk sac tumor shows variety of histologic pattern, including most commonly polyvesicular (A, H&Ex10) and reticular patterns (B,H&E x20). Tumor cells tend to form concentric layers around blood vessels (C, H&E x20). Alpha-fetoprotein (D) diffusely stains tumor cells.

The prognosis of Yolk sac tumor depends primarily on the clinical stage. Stage I tumors have more favorable prognosis [16]. Following removal of the tumor, serum levels of AFP should fall dramatically. Subsequent rising levels of AFP are of value in detecting early recurrence and metastasis.

Embryonal Carcinoma

Embryonal carcinoma is a highly malignant tumor with aggressive local spread and early metastasis. It is composed of epithelial cells resembling the primitive stages of embryonic differentiation. This rare tumor occurs commonly as a component of mixed germ cell tumor and is characteristically positive for CD30 and AFP by immunohistochemistry. The tumor cells are large polygonal or ovoid with ample amount of pale cytoplasm and show prominent mitotic activity (Figure 4). The nuclei are large irregular vesicular or hyperchromatic and have more than one nucleolus. The cells may grow in solid patterns or may form papillae. Very rarely the tumor exhibits prominent differentiation towards embryoid structures resembling presomite embryos and is hence called polyembryoma.

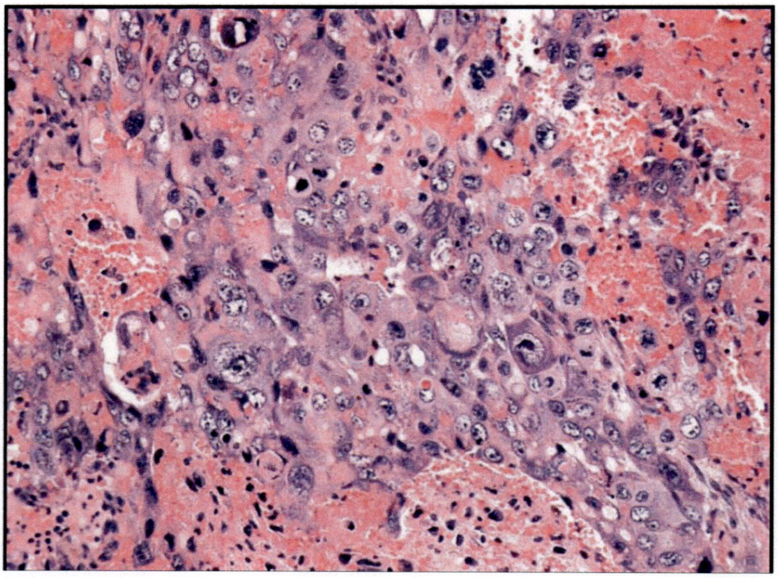

Figure 4. Embryonal carcinoma cells are large pleomorphic polygonal cells and frequently undergo necrosis and hemorrhage (H&Ex20).

Mixed Germ Cell Tumor

Mixed germ cell tumors are composed of more than one neoplastic germ cell element. The presence of malignant components within a tumor, depending on their relative amount, is usually associated with more aggressive behavior. Examples include yolk sac tumor components that are frequently found in teratomas. Choriocarcinoma is rarely present alone, and is commonly seen as a component of mixed germ cell tumor. In these situations choriocarcinoma renders a less favorable prognosis. Elevated AFP or β-hCG serum levels in a patient with an immature teratoma should raise suspicion of the concomitant presence of yolk sac tumor or choriocarcinoma respectively and should prompt extensive sampling of the tumor.

Gonadoblastoma

Gonadoblastoma is a very rare bilateral tumor occurring exclusively in patients with gonadal dysgenesis or pseudohermaphroditism [17]. Patients are usually phenotypically females who have amenorrhea and signs of virilization. In more than 90% of patients a Y chromosome is present and the karyotype is commonly 46,XY. Some patients have associated Turner syndrome. The typical karyotype of Turner syndrome is (45,XO). Up to 6% of patients, however, have mosaic patterns including Y chromosome or fragments of Y chromosome and hence become at risk for developing a dysgerminoma [18].

Gonadoblastoma is characterized by dual proliferation of germ cells and sex cord derivatives resembling immature sex cord derivatives. The tumor is arranged in nests surrounded by connective tissue stroma (Figure 5). Inside the nests, small round spaces containing eosinophilic hyaline material are identified. Calcification is very frequent in these hyaline spaces and may progress to involve the whole lesion. Dysgerminoma or another malignant germ cell tumor may arise from gonadoblastoma in a large percentage of cases. Gonadoblastoma is a small lesion confined to the gonad and can be treated with surgical excision alone. The concomitant presence of dysgerminoma or another malignant germ cell tumor increases the risk for spread. In these situations, surgical staging and postoperative combination chemotherapy may be required.

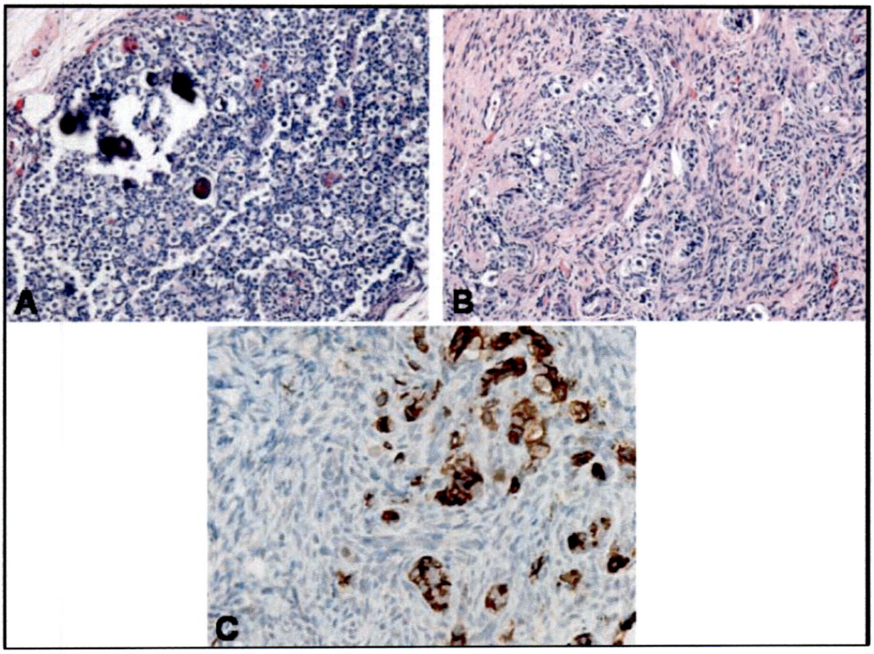

Figure 5. Nests of gonadoblastoma tumor cells with calcification (H&E,x20) were identified in a young patient with mixed gonadal dysgenesis. An invasive tumor component was also seen infiltrating the ovarian stroma (B,H&Ex20), highlighted by staining with CD117 (C).

Surface Epithelial Tumors

Surface epithelial tumors of the ovary compromise less than 20% of all ovarian neoplasms in adolescents and may occasionally be bilateral. They are characterized by a spectrum of biologic behavior from benign, low malignant potential (borderline tumors), to frankly malignant tumors [19]. The latter two non-benign groups compromise less than 50% of all ovarian epithelial tumors. Patients with malignant surface epithelial tumors have a poor prognosis. Borderline tumors have increased incidence during adolescent period. Tumors are classified, according to the morphology of the epithelial component as serous, mucinous, endometrioid, transitional or undifferentiated.

Serous Tumors

Serous epithelial tumors are characterized by epithelium resembling that of the Fallopian tube. Increased familial risk is attributed to BRCA1 and BRCA2 gene mutations. Patients with hereditary nonpolyposis colon cancer syndrome have slightly increased risk for development of ovarian carcinoma. Tumor cells are positive for cytokeratin 7, epithelial membrane antigen and CAM5.2 and are negative for cytokeratin 20. Serous adenocarcinoma is an invasive tumor (Figure 6) with a 5-year survival rate of 40%. Histology shows various architectural organizational patterns including glandular, papillary, cystic and solid components. Lack of frank stromal invasion in the presence of atypia and epithelial hyperplasia classifies the tumor as "borderline tumor". Borderline tumors have better prognosis than serous adenocarcinoma and the 5-year survival rate of localized tumors approaches 100%. Serous borderline tumors may be associated with tumor on the surface of the ovary, non-invasive peritoneal implants, or lymph node involvement without significant change in the prognosis. Invasive omental implants correlate with poor prognosis [19].

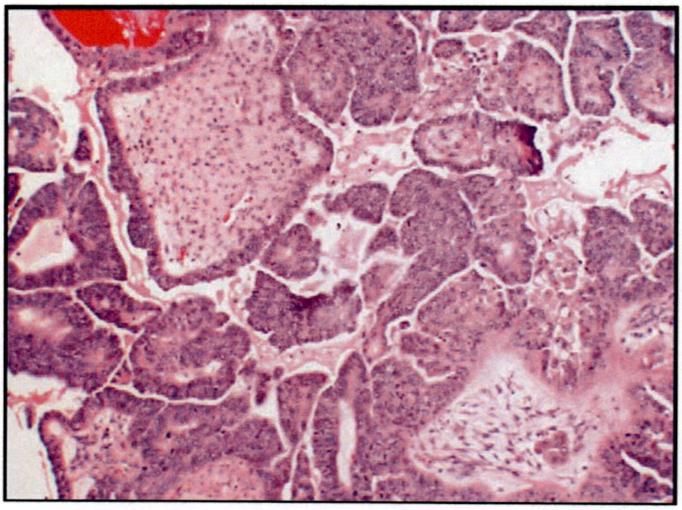

Figure 6. Serous carcinoma of the ovary commonly has papillary architecture (H&E, x20).

Mucinous Tumors

Mucinous tumors are derived from epithelial cells containing intracytoplasmic mucin and thus may resemble the epithelium of endocervix, gastric pylorus or intestine. Mucinous tumors have increased frequency of KRAS mutations. These tumors are usually multilocular or unilocular large cystic masses that contain watery or viscid mucoid material.

Other Types of Carcinoma

Endometrioid carcinoma is extremely rare in adolescents and children [20]. More frequent is the presence of endometrioid-like areas in yolk sac tumors [21]. Small cell carcinoma of the ovary has also been rarely reported [22,23]. Malignant Brenner's tumor and transitional cell carcinoma are exceptionally rare in adolescents and pediatric patients

Sex Cord Stromal Tumors

These tumors are composed of granulosa cells, theca cells, Sertoli cells, Leydig cells and fibroblast stromal cells in various combinations [24]. Immunoreactivity for inhibin is characteristic and correlates with the presence of hormone secreting cells [25]. Inhibin immunostaining is currently used effectively as a diagnostic marker for sex cord stromal cells, particularly granulosa cell tumors [26].

Granulosa Cell Tumor

Granulosa cell tumor (GCT) in adolescence is almost always of the juvenile type and is associated with precocious puberty in 80% of cases due to production of pituitary gonadotrophins. Adult type GCT and tumors with androgen production leading to virilization have been reported in rare cases [27,28]. These tumors may also be associated with Maffucci syndrome and Ollier's disease [29,30].

Histologically, the neoplastic granulosa cells show nodular or diffuse proliferation with focal follicle formation (Figure 7). Unlike the adult variant, the cells lack nuclear grooves and may have more eosinophilic (luteinized) cytoplasm. Cytomegaly and multi-nucleation may occasionally be present. No Call-Exner bodies are present. In addition to inhibin the tumor cells may react to vimentin, cytokeratin and calretinin.

Granulosa cell tumor is commonly unilateral and confined to the ovary and thus presents as stage I. There is however potential for aggressive behavior including recurrence and nodal metastasis [31]. Factors related to poor prognosis include advanced stage [32], bilaterality [33], atypia and high mitotic rate [34] Aggressive JGC tumors apparently lose expression of FOXL2, a marker of normal folliculogenesis [35].

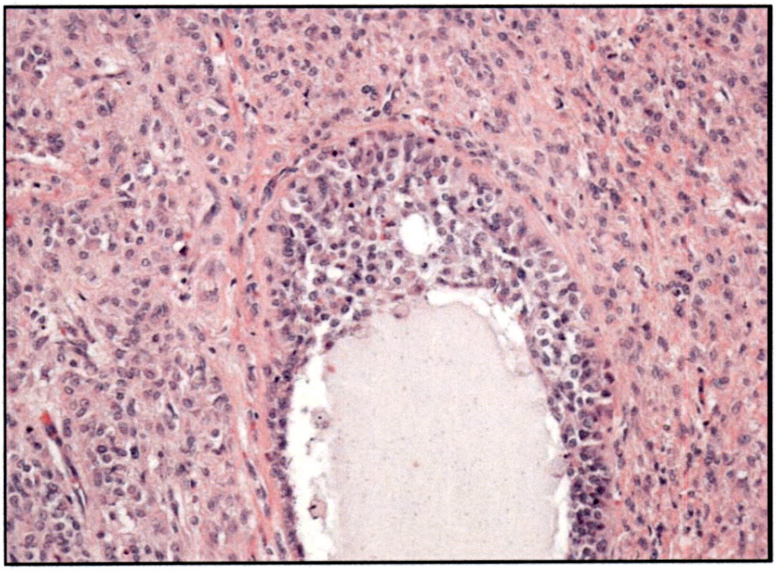

Figure 7. Solid sheets of juvenile granulosa cells are frequently interspersed by follicles of varying sizes.

Sertoli-Leydig Stromal Cell Tumors

This group of tumors is rare and contains various combinations of Sertoli cells, stromal cells and Leydig cells in various degrees of differentiation. Most of these tumors are unilateral and benign and are otherwise well-known for their endocrine manifestations which appear in up to 50% of cases [24]. Unlike granulosa cell tumors androgens are more commonly produced than estrogens. Prognosis of patients is closely related to stage and histologic degree of differentiation. Clinically malignant tumors are most likely to be poorly differentiated or have a retiform component (Figure 8). The presence of mesenchymal heterologous elements carries a bad prognosis as well. Intermediately differentiated tumors with calcifications and tubular patters are seen in patients with Peutz-Jeghers syndrome and some of these cases may have a malignant course [36,37,38].

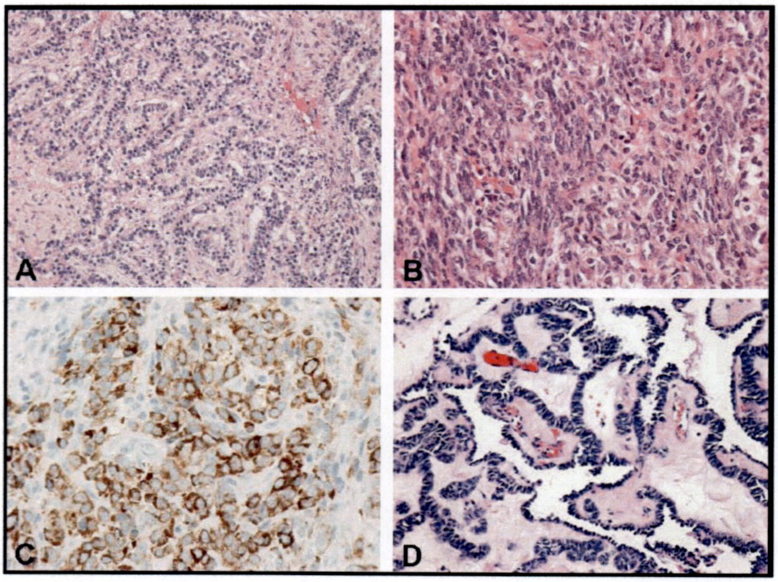

Figure 8. Moderately (A,H&Ex20) and poorly differentiated (B,H&Ex40) areas were present in this Seroli-Leydig cell ovarian tumor of a 14-year old girl. Tumor cells were diffusely positive with inhibin immunostain ©. Aggressive clinical course is seen in tumors with retiform elements, present either focally or diffusely throughout the tumor (D, H&E,x20).

Metastatic Ovarian Tumors

Tumors metastatic to the ovary in adults are mostly carcinomas. In adolescents and pediatric patients, neuroblastoma is the most common malignancy metastasizing to the ovary, followed by rhabdomyosarcoma, Ewing's family tumors and other small round cell tumors. Clinical features and frequent bilaterality of ovarian metastatic tumors are helpful diagnostic features in many cases [39].

Conclusion

Ovarian malignancies in adolescents have variable clinicopathologic and histologic patterns which may differ from those seen in adults. Clinical and endocrine features, serologic data, surgical resection and pathologic examination are often needed to reach an accurate diagnosis. The prognosis of patients should be determined using a multidisciplinary approach that includes surgical staging, and histologic sub-typing. The behavior of these tumors is frequently unpredictable and close oncologic follow-up is needed.

References

[1] Fotiou SK. Ovarian malignancies in adolescence. Ann. N. Y. Acad. Sci. 1997; 17;816:338-46

[2] de Silva KS, Kanumakala S, Grover SR, Chow CW, Warne GL. Ovarian lesions in children and adolescents--an 11-year review. *J. Pediatr. Endocrinol. Metab.* 2004 Jul;17(7):951-7.

[3] Chiaffarino F, Parazzini F, Bosetti C, Franceschi S, Talamini R, Canzonieri V, Montella M, Ramazzotti V, Franceschi S, La Vecchia C. Risk factors for ovarian cancer histotypes. *Eur. J. Cancer.* 2007 May;43(7):1208-13. Epub 2007 Mar 21.

[4] Olsen CM, Green AC, Whiteman DC, Sadeghi S, Kolahdooz F, Webb PM. Obesity and the risk of epithelial ovarian cancer: a systematic review and meta-analysis. *Eur. J. Cancer.* 2007 Mar;43(4):690-709.

[5] Stankovic ZB, Djukic MK, Savic D, Lukac BJ, Djuricic S, Sedlecki K, Zdravkovic D.Pre-operative differentiation of pediatric ovarian tumors: morphological scoring system and tumor markers. *J. Pediatr. Endocrinol. Metab.* 2006 Oct;19(10):1231-8

[6] Deligeoroglou E, Eleftheriades M, Shiadoes V, Botsis D, Hasiakos D, Kontoravdis A, Creatsas G.Ovarian masses during adolescence: clinical, ultrasonographic and pathologic findings, serum tumor markers and endocrinological profile. *Gynecol. Endocrinol.* 2004 Jul;19(1):1-8.

[7] Thomas M Ulbright. Germ cell tumors of the gonads: a selective review emphasizing problems in differential diagnosis, newly appreciated, and controversial issues. *Modern Pathology.* (2005) 18, S61–S79;

[8] Marshall Stepanian, David E. Cohn. Gynecologic malignancies in adolescents. *Adolesc. Med.* 15 (2004) 549–568

[9] Song ES, Lee JP, Han JH, Kim HY, Mun SH, Ryu HS, Chang KH. Dysgerminoma of the ovary with precocious puberty: a case report. *Gynecol. Endocrinol.* 2007 Jan; 23(1):34-7.

[10] de Silva KS, Kanumakala S, Grover SR, Chow CW, Warne GL. Ovarian lesions in children and adolescents--an 11-year review. *J. Pediatr. Endocrinol. Metab.* 2004 Jul;17(7):951-7

[11] O'Connor DM, Norris HJ. The influence of grade on the outcome of stage I ovarian immature (malignant) teratomas and the reproducibility of grading. *Int. J. Gynecol. Pathol.* 1994 Oct;13(4):283-9

[12] J.I. Einarsson, C.L. Edwards, and R.K. Zurawin. Immature ovarian teratoma in an adolescent: A case report and review of the literature. *J. Pediatr. Adolesc. Gynecol.* (2004) 17:187–189;

[13] Harms D, Zahn S, Göbel U, Schneider DT. Pathology and molecular biology of teratomas in childhood and adolescence. *Klin. Padiatr.* 2006 Nov-Dec;218(6):296-302.

[14] Biskup W, Calaminus G, Schneider DT, Leuschner I, Göbel U. Teratoma with malignant transformation: experiences of the cooperative GPOH protocols MAKEI 83/86/89/96. *Klin. Padiatr.* 2006 Nov-Dec;218(6):303-8

[15] Dällenbach P, Bonnefoi H, Pelte MF, Vlastos G. Yolk sac tumours of the ovary: an update. *Eur. J. Surg. Oncol.* 2006 Dec;32(10):1063-75. Epub 2006 Sep 22

[16] Nawa A, Obata N, Kikkawa F, Kawai M, Nagasaka T, Goto S, Nishimori K, Nakashima N. Prognostic factors of patients with yolk sac tumors of the ovary. *Am. J. Obstet. Gynecol.* 2001 May;184(6):1182-8

[17] Looijenga LH, Hersmus R, Oosterhuis JW, Cools M, Drop SL, Wolffenbuttel KP. Tumor risk in disorders of sex development (DSD). *Best Pract. Res. Clin. Endocrinol. Metab.* 2007 Sep;21(3):480-95

[18] Maggio MC, Liotta A, De Grazia E, Cimador M, Di Pace R, Corsello G. Polycystic ovary and gonadoblastoma in Turner's syndrome. *Minerva Pediatr.* 2007 Aug;59(4):397-401

[19] Marshall Stepanian, David E. Cohn. Gynecologic malignancies in adolescents. *Adolesc. Med.* 15 (2004) 549–568

[20] Fink D, Plaxe SC, Brown JF, Baergen RN. Endometrioid ovarian carcinoma in a premenarchal girl: report of a case. *Gynecol. Oncol.* 1997 Nov;67(2):222-5.

[21] Clement PB, Young RH, Scully RE. Endometrioid-like variant of ovarian yolk sac tumor. A clinicopathological analysis of eight cases. *Am. J. Surg. Pathol.* 1987 Oct;11(10):767-78

[22] Ferrera PC, Whitman MC. Ovarian small cell carcinoma: a rare neoplasm in a 15-year-old female. *Pediatr. Emerg. Care.* 2000 Jun;16(3):170-2.

[23] Sholler GL, Luks F, Mangray S, Meech SJ. Advanced small cell carcinoma of the ovary in a pediatric patient with long-term survival and review of the literature. *J. Pediatr. Hematol. Oncol.* 2005 Mar;27(3):169-72

[24] Pathology and genetics. Tumours of the breast and female genital organs 2002

[25] Kommoss F, Oliva E, Bhan AK, Young RH, Scully RE. Inhibin expression in ovarian tumors and tumor-like lesions: an immunohistochemical study. *Mod. Pathol.* 1998 Jul;11(7):656-64.

[26] Rishi M, Howard LN, Bratthauer GL, Tavassoli FA. Use of monoclonal antibody against human inhibin as a marker for sex cord-stromal tumors of the ovary. *Am. J. Surg. Pathol.* 1997 May;21(5):583-9.

[27] Nomelini RS, Micheletti AM, Adad SJ, Murta EF. Androgenic juvenile granulosa cell tumor of the ovary with cystic presentation: a case report. *Eur. J. Gynaecol. Oncol.* 2007;28(3):236-8.

[28] Kabaca C, Karateke A, Gurbuz A, Cesur S. Androgenic adult granulosa cell tumor in a teenager: a case report and review of the literature. *Int. J. Gynecol. Cancer.* 2006 Jan-Feb;16 Suppl 1:368-74

[29] Vaz RM, Turner C. Ollier disease (enchondromatosis) associated with ovarian juvenile granulosa cell tumor and precocious pseudopuberty . *J. Pediatr.* 1986 Jun;108(6):945-7.;

[30] Tanaka Y, Sasaki Y, Nishihira H, Izawa T, Nishi T. Ovarian juvenile granulosa cell tumor associated with Maffucci's syndrome. *Am. J. Clin. Pathol.* 1992 Apr;97(4):523-7.

[31] Abu-Rustum NR, Restivo A, Ivy J, Soslow R, Sabbatini P, Sonoda Y, Barakat RR, Chi DS.Retroperitoneal nodal metastasis in primary and recurrent granulosa cell tumors of the ovary. *Gynecol. Oncol.* 2006 Oct;103(1):31-4. Epub 2006 Mar 13.

[32] Powell JL, Connor GP, Henderson GS. Management of recurrent juvenile granulosa cell tumor of the ovary. *Gynecol. Oncol.* 2001 Apr;81(1):113-6.

[33] Lancaster EJ, Muthuphei MN.Bilateral juvenile granulosa--cell tumour with multiple metastases. A case report. *Cent. Afr. J. Med.* 1998 Jun;44(6):158-60.

[34] Schneider DT, Calaminus G, Harms D, Göbel U.Ovarian sex cord-stromal tumors in children and adolescents. *J. Reprod. Med.* 2005 Jun;50(6):439-46

[35] Kalfa N, Philibert P, Patte C, Ecochard A, Duvillard P, Baldet P, Jaubert F, Fellous M, Sultan C.Extinction of FOXL2 expression in aggressive ovarian granulosa cell tumors in children. *Fertil. Steril.* 2007 Apr;87(4):896-901.

[36] Lantzsch T, Stoerer S, Lawrenz K, Buchmann J, Strauss HG, Koelbl H. Sertoli-Leydig cell tumor. *Arch. Gynecol. Obstet.* 2001 Jan;264(4):206-8.

[37] Borer JG, Tan PE, Diamond DA. The spectrum of Sertoli cell tumors in children. *Urol. Clin. North Am.* 2000 Aug;27(3):529-41

[38] Robert H. Young, Robert Scully. Sex cord-stromal, steroid cell, and other ovarian tumors with endocrine, paraendocrine, and paraneoplastic manifestations. In Blaustein's *Pathology of the female genital tract*, 5th edition, Springer-Verlag New York, 2002, pp 905-966

[39] Young RH, Kozakewich HP, Scully RE. Metastatic ovarian tumors in children: a report of 14 cases and review of the literature. *Int. J. Gynecol. Pathol.* 1993 Jan;12(1):8-19

Index

A

B

C

D

H

I

J

K

L

M

N

O

P

Q

R

S

T

U

V

W

X

Y